STUDIES OF RHEUMATOID DISEASE

The Conference was held under the auspices of
The Canadian Rheumatism Association
and
The Canadian Arthritis and Rheumatism Society

Studies of Rheumatoid Disease

PROCEEDINGS OF THE
THIRD CANADIAN CONFERENCE
ON RESEARCH IN THE
RHEUMATIC DISEASES
TORONTO, FEBRUARY 25–27
1965

University of Toronto Press

Copyright, Canada, 1966 by
University of Toronto Press
Reprinted 2017
ISBN 978-1-4875-9817-4 (paper)

Preface

RESEARCH in rheumatoid arthritis is now quite properly dominated by intensive efforts to determine the pathogenesis of this disease. Sufficient circumstantial evidence implicating a distorted and excessive activity of immune mechanisms has accumulated to allow a strong indictment to be drawn: a formal written statement charging the immunologically competent cells with the crime of auto-aggression. In this symposium, the opening address for the prosecution is delivered by Professor Mellors, who describes with rigorous clarity the alleged chain of events, detailing the extensive evidence that has accumulated at each key point. The bulk of the symposium is given to a detailed examination of various aspects of this charge. At the outset, it must be admitted that the initiating factor remains unknown, and an exogenous agent may play a primary role. The important accessory role of lysosomes is also indicated, these agents being charged with the actual work of destruction.

The line that the defence may take is more subtle. The activity of the immunologic system, it is argued, is protective, not aggressive. The complexes formed by the union of rheumatoid factor with gamma globulin are apparently well tolerated by the host, and may exist in the circulation of patients or recipients of transfused rheumatoid plasma without visible ill-effect, and certainly without the glomerulitis or widespread anaphylactic responses characteristic of the reaction to soluble antigen–antibody complexes.

It is argued that the initial event in the chain (or cycle) of events is a stimulation of immunogenic mechanisms. The nature of this stimulus is not clear, but one assumes that the stimulating factor is an antigen, either exogenous or endogenous, although other driving forces could be imagined. If the cells are stimulated to proliferate and function by one specific antigen, then it is odd that such a variety of antibodies should be produced in patients with rheumatoid disease. Should it be argued that the primary response to a single antigen is obscured by secondary non-specific responses to products of tissue damage, then a whole series of weaknesses in the line of argument appear. All the morphological and serological evidence of immunologic activity then could be attributed to these responses, which have been dismissed as secondary, and in fact no evidence of a primary antigenic challenge and immunologic response exists at all.

For most of us, the original attractiveness of the auto-immune theory arose from the discovery of rheumatoid factor, which behaved as an auto-antibody and was characteristic of this disease. But Dr. Ziff has suggested that we all have a little rheumatoid factor and that production of this protein is a predictable and unsurprising response to the alterations in gamma globulin associated with its union with antigen. Thus it is far from clear that this perhaps non-specific and well-tolerated factor is the single agent by which a (possibly) subverted immunologic system attacks cartilage, synovial cells, fibrous connected tissues, or the microcirculation. The rheumatoid factor could have about the same specificity and fundamental importance as the Wasserman reagent in syphilis, in which disease the evidence of immunologic activity and response is strikingly similar to that in rheumatoid arthritis.

It is apparent that an exclusive commitment to the auto-immune hypothesis cannot be made at this time. After hearing the arguments, a jury could only return the old Scottish verdict of "not proved." Thus a broadly based enquiry into the structure and function of connective tissues is continuing, in order to open many avenues of exploration from which the long-sought advances in the knowledge of fundamental mechanisms may derive.

Meanwhile, patients with rheumatoid arthritis continue to appear, and methods of improving their treatment must be explored, using the disciplined empirical approach, which is so difficult to apply in clinical situations. Those of our colleagues who work with model systems in laboratories must appreciate the extreme difficulties of clinical science. When even the simplest of clinical trials is planned, the factors of sample size and time loom very large, and the supply of trained personnel and facilities so inadequate. The populations cannot with certainty be defined and the methods of measurement are extremely crude and difficult to apply, so that adequately controlled trials are always difficult and often impossible. However, these difficulties must be faced squarely by clinicians, and the necessary tasks of organization and discipline attacked with the concentration and serious effort required by the magnitude of the problem.

This publication is derived from the proceedings of the Third Canadian Conference on Research in the Rheumatic Diseases, sponsored jointly by the Canadian Rheumatism Association (the professional organization) and The Canadian Arthritis and Rheumatism Society (the voluntary association). Like the previous conferences on Research in Rheumatic Diseases held in 1955 and 1960, this gathering served as a meeting ground for the exchange of information and the re-examination of the correlations suggested by the observations gathered and arranged by investigators using differing tools and hypothetical models. As in previous conferences, the discussions were enlivened and enriched by the forceful presence of two visitors invited as Devil's Advocates. This role was admirably fulfilled and the participants were much indebted to Professor R. C. Mellors, of Cornell University Medical College, and to Dr. Morris Ziff, of Dallas, Texas. Some of the most spirited discussion was sacrificed in the interests of brevity in the course of converting the transcript into book form. These decisions were made with regret, and the readers should know that grey words on paper could not hope to convey the pleasure and interest of the gathering, or the personality of the participants.

THE SPONSORS

Contents

PART I

Morphological Studies and Experimental Arthritis
Chairman: Dr. H. A. Smythe, Toronto

Morphologic Methods in the Investigation of Rheumatic Diseases: The Pathogenesis of Rheumatoid Arthritis*

ROBERT C. MELLORS, M.D., PH.D.†

DURING THE LAST FEW YEARS I have examined some 10,000 pathological specimens in the field of rheumato-orthopaedic diseases. More than 2000 were examples of common rheumatic diseases and, of these, 250 were manifestations of rheumatoid arthritis mainly affecting adults and involving large and small joints of the upper and the lower extremities. These studies have made it clear, confirming others (5), that in so far as the articular disease is concerned rheumatoid arthritis begins as a proliferative and exudative inflammatory lesion of the synovial membrane which thereafter by adhesion and infiltration gradually destroys the articular cartilage, invades subchondral bone, and contributes to the weakening of the fibrous capsule, the tendon sheaths, and the tendons themselves. The studies show that the dramatis personae in this theatre of action are proliferating synoviocytes, immunologically competent cells (lymphocytes and plasma cells), and inflammatory cells (macrophages and polymorphonuclear leucocytes).

Recent studies in several laboratories (3, 9, 10, 13, 14, 16, 20, 21, 26, 27, 31) and observations to be presented by participants in this conference can now be brought to focus in a working concept of the pathogenesis of common typical rheumatoid arthritis. The sequence of events, beginning in the synovial membrane, may be somewhat as follows: unknown initiating mechanism leading to immunogenic stimulation by exogenous or endogenous antigens; formation, in turn, of antibodies, rheumatoid factors, and rheumatoid factor–antibody (γ_M–γ_G) complexes; phagocytosis and intracellular lysosomal

*This work was supported in part by research grants from the National Institute of Arthritis and Metabolic Diseases, United States Public Health Service.

†The Hospital for Special Surgery, P. D. Wilson Research Foundation, Affiliated with the New York Hospital–Cornell University Medical College and the Department of Pathology, Cornell University Medical College, New York, New York.

enzymatic degradation of the macromolecular complexes; extracellular liberation of lysosomal enzymes which degrade the organic matrix of articular cartilage; perpetuation of these immunological and enzymatic reactions; continuing and progressive destruction of the joint cartilage.

Let us now examine the evidence for this 1965 pathogenic model of North America's number one crippling disease.

1/ Immunogenic stimulation in active rheumatoid arthritis is indicated morphologically by the abundance of plasma cells (5, 22) and occasional germinal centres (1, 5) in the synovial membrane and by the hyperplasia of regional and distant lymph nodes containing numerous germinal centres and plasma cells (Figs. 1–8). For it is now well recognized that plasma cells are the main source of antibodies (8), and germinal centres are sites of proliferation of immunologically competent cells as they are transformed into antibody-forming cells (24).

2/ Immunoglobulins of all classes, $\gamma_G(7S)$, $\gamma_M(19S)$, γ_A, are formed by plasma cells and germinal centres in the synovial membranes and lymph nodes in active rheumatoid arthritis, as shown by immunofluorescence (21–23); see Figs. 11 and 12. This "polyclonal" microscopic picture is correlated with electrophoretically diffuse or broad-banded hypergammaglobulinaemia.

3/ Rheumatoid factors demonstrable by their *in vitro* reactivity with aggregated human γ_G-globulins (4, 7) and rabbit (γ_G-globulin) immune complexes (7) are formed by plasma cells and germinal centres in the synovial membranes and lymph nodes in active rheumatoid arthritis, again as shown by immunofluorescence (21, 22); see Figs. 13–15. This cellular formation correlates with the presence of circulating rheumatoid factors but occurs also in early or seronegative cases (Table I).

TABLE I

PATIENTS WITH RHEUMATOID ARTHRITIS AND CELLULAR RHEUMATOID FACTORS:* STAGES OF JOINT INVOLVEMENT AND RESULTS OF SERUM LATEX TESTS

Stage†	No. of patients	Serum latex globulin test		
		Strongly pos. (3+ to 4+)	Weakly pos. (1+ to 2+)	Neg.
I	5	2	1	2
II	1	1		
III	7	2	3	1
IV	4	2	2	
?	3		1	2
I–IV	20	7	7	5

*Published (21, 22) and unpublished work; tissues positive with fluorescent aggregated human γ-globulin and/or fluorescent rabbit immune complex.

†Evaluated by Dr. Alice Garrett according to A.R.A. criteria: I, no destruction of articular cartilage; II, slight destruction of articular cartilage; III, destruction of joint with deformity; IV, marked destruction of joint with ankylosis.

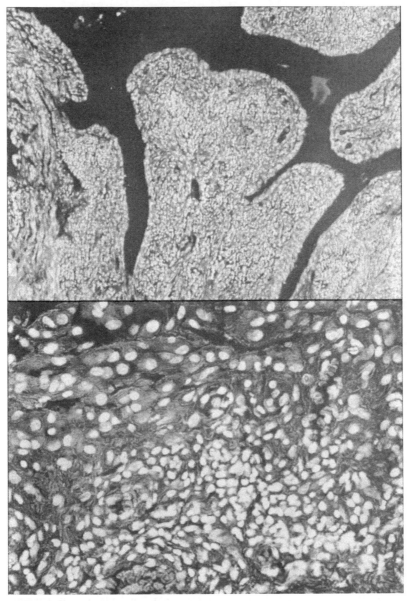

FIG. 1 (*top*). Chronic proliferative and exudative rheumatoid synovitis of wrist joint. Haematoxylin-eosin. 90×.

FIG. 2 (*bottom*). Surface stratification of proliferated synoviocytes, underlain mainly by lymphocytes. Haematoxylin-eosin. 365×.

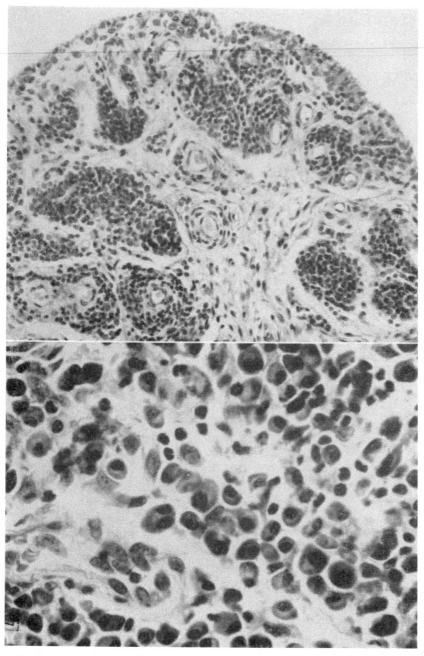

Fig. 3 (*top*). Plasma cells in great number, cuffing and presumably emerging from small blood vessels in rheumatoid synovitis of knee joint. Haematoxylin-eosin. 240×.

Fig. 4 (*bottom*). Higher-power view showing the characteristic morphology—eccentric nucleus, basophilic cytoplasm—of mature plasma cells in rheumatoid synovitis, with some polymorphonuclear leucocytes near by. Needle biopsy of knee joint. Haematoxylin-eosin. 420×.

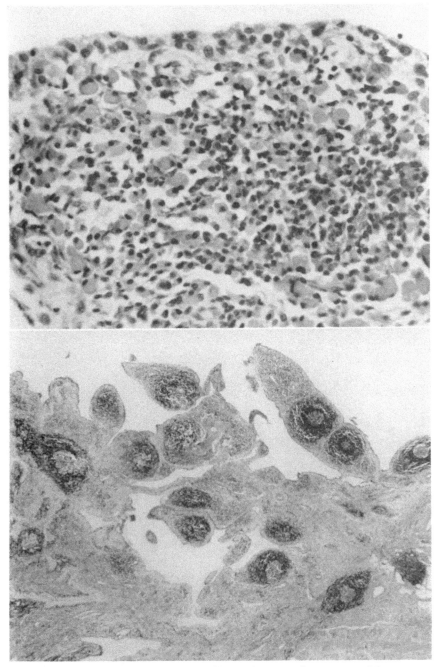

Fig. 5 (*top*). Russell-body plasma cells in rheumatoid synovitis of knee joint.
Haematoxylin-eosin. 384×.

Fig. 6 (*bottom*). The lymphoid nodules in rheumatoid synovitis occasionally
contain active germinal centres, as shown here in rheumatoid synovitis of knee
joint. Haematoxylin-eosin. 24×.

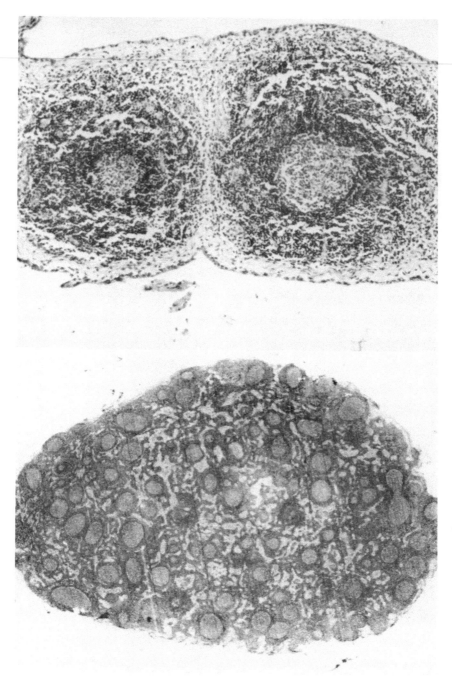

FIG. 7 (*top*). High-power view of large synovial villus containing two germinal centres. Haematoxylin-eosin. 120×.

FIG. 8 (*bottom*). Hyperplastic lymph nodes in rheumatoid arthritis may contain, in addition to numerous plasma cells, many germinal centres as shown here. Haematoxylin-eosin. 11×.

4. Rheumatoid factor-γ_G[22S] as well as intermediate complexes are demonstrable in rheumatoid serum by ultracentrifugal analysis (10, 16). Localized depositions of rheumatoid factors (21) and immunoglobulins (15, 29, 30) resolved into γ_M- and γ_G-globulins are present in extracellular tissue spaces in rheumatoid synovitis (Fig. 16) and in rheumatoid granulomas (Figs. 9, 18, and 19).

5. γ_M-Globulins, presumably rheumatoid factors, associated with γ_G globulins are phagocytized by polymorphonuclear leucocytes, thus forming the so-called R.A. or inclusion-body cells as demonstrated in rheumatoid *synovial fluids* by Hollander and his associates (13, 14, 27) and also by Astorga and Bollet (2). Rheumatoid factors are also present in cytoplasmic vacuoles and granules of macrophages and polymorphonuclear leucocytes in the rheumatoid synovial membrane (Fig. 17).

6. Phagocytic vacuoles (11, 25) and leucocyte granules (12) of this sort correspond to various forms of lysosomes.

7. Studies of the fine structure of the synovial membrane by Barland and his associates (3) have shown that rheumatoid synoviocytes also contain large numbers of cytoplasmic granules, rich in acid phosphatase, one of the histochemically demonstrable lysosomal enzymes (Figs. 20 and 21) and corresponding to altered lysosomes.

8. Lysosomal enzymes have been shown by Fell and Dingle (9) to be capable of degrading the organic matrix (the protein-polysaccharide complex) of cartilage *in vitro*. An increase in lysosomal enzyme activity, as compared with the normal, has been demonstrated by Carol Smith and Hamerman (28) in synovial fluid and by Mollie Luscombe (18) in synovial tissue of patients with rheumatoid arthritis.

9. A characteristic microscopic feature of rheumatoid arthritis is the aggressive destruction of articular cartilage at sites of attachment of synovial inflammatory granulation tissue (i.e., pannus); see Fig. 10. The destruction of cartilage is presumably a consequence of impaired nutrition of cells and chemical degradation of matrix by lysosomal enzymes liberated locally and in synovial fluid.

10. Immunological responses are perpetuated by the persistence of antigen. The most lasting of antigens are self-components in auto-immunity (19); examples in the connective-tissue and allied diseases include γ_G-globulin, deoxyribonucleoprotein, thyroglobulin, and red blood cells. It should also be added that immunological reactions of the auto-immune and delayed hypersensitivity types can be mediated by sensitized lymphocytes in the absence of plasma cells and demonstrable circulating antibodies (17).

Needless to say, much more work has yet to be done on the nature of rheumatoid arthritis. Also, the search for a satisfactory experimental model continues. Two studies of recent date are especially relevant to initiating and perpetuating mechanisms in experimental arthritis. Weissmann and his associates (31), basing their experiments on the lysosomal concept, have

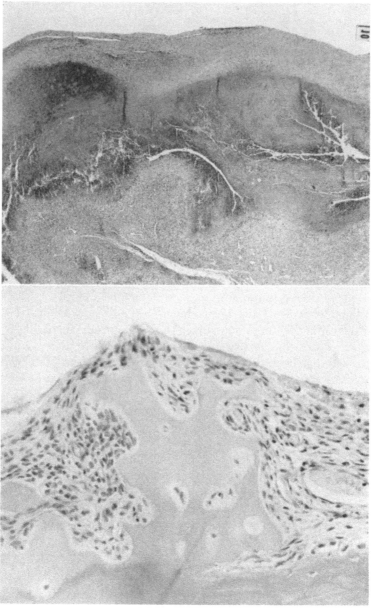

FIG. 9 (*top*). Confluent rheumatoid granulomas in dense fibrous extensor tendon of the hand. Haematoxylin-eosin. 27×.

FIG. 10 (*bottom*). Destruction of articular cartilage in rheumatoid arthritis at site of adhesion and infiltration of synovial inflammatory granulation tissue (pannus). Haematoxylin-eosin. 240×.

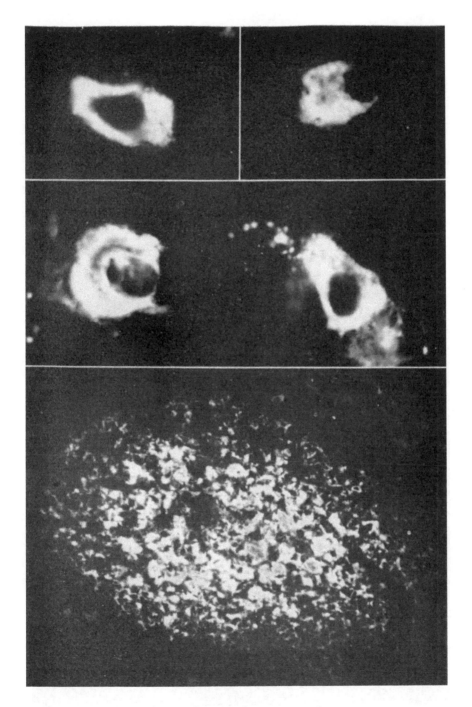

Fig. 11 (*top*). Plasma cells in rheumatoid synovitis conform to immature, mature, and Russell-body types and form immunoglobulins of all classes, here γ_M-globulins. Immunofluorescence. 1500×.

Fig. 12 (*bottom*). The germinal centres of hyperplastic lymph nodes form immunoglobulins of all classes, such as γ_G-globulin as shown here. Immunofluorescence. 244×.

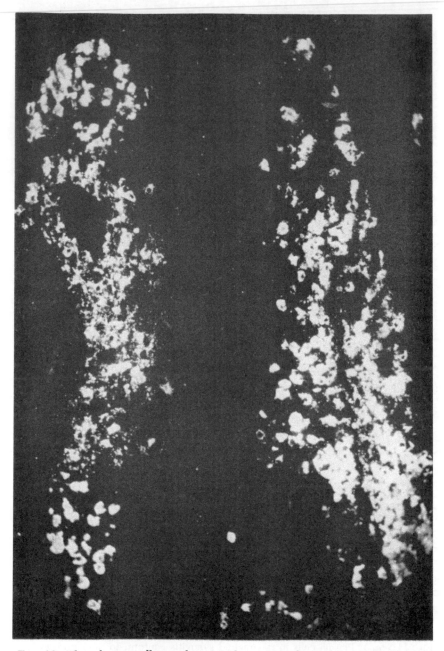

FIG. 13. The plasma cells in rheumatoid synovitis form rheumatoid factor, as shown here in the stalks of two vertically oriented hypertrophic villi (21). Fluorescent aggregated human γ_G-globulins. 245×.

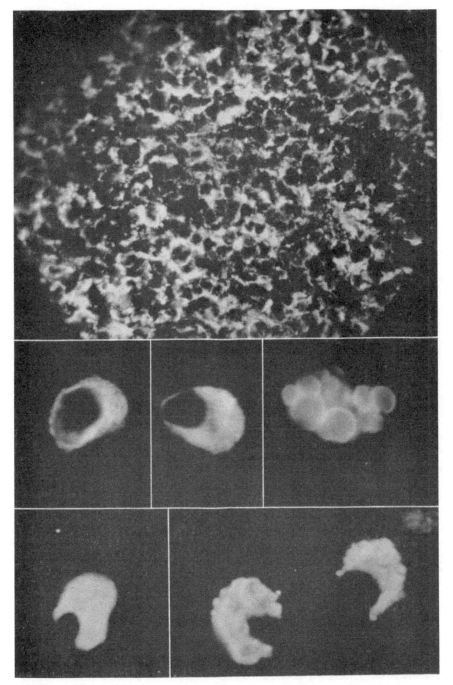

Fig. 14 (*top*). The germinal centres of the hyperplastic lymph nodes, an example of which is shown here, as well as the rare centres in rheumatoid synovitis, form rheumatoid factor. Fluorescent rabbit (γ_G-globulin) immune complexes. 400×.

Fig. 15 (*bottom*). The plasma cells, as well as germinal centres, show remarkable specificity, some forming rheumatoid factors reacting either with fluorescent rabbit (γ_G-globulin) immune complexes (top) or with fluorescent aggregated γ_G-globulins (bottom) and a few (not shown) forming both types of rheumatoid factors (22). 1500×.

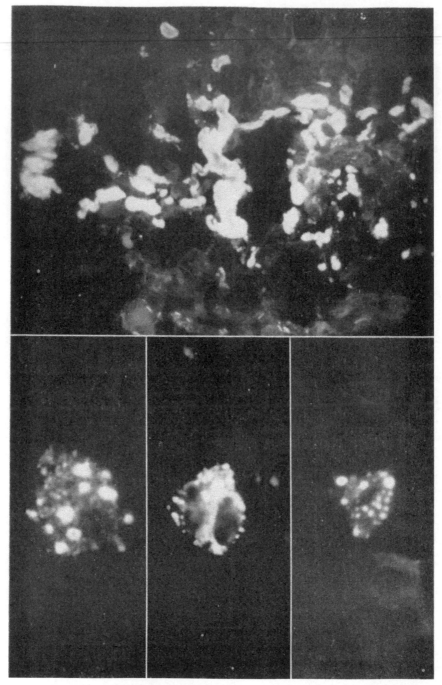

Fig. 16 (*top*). Extracellular deposits of γ_M-globulins in rheumatoid synovial membrane. Immunofluorescence. 1000×.

Fig. 17 (*bottom*). Polymorphonuclear leucocytes as well as a macrophage (left) in rheumatoid synovial membrane with cytoplasmic particulates containing rheumatoid factor. Fluorescent aggregated human γ_G-globulins. 1500×.

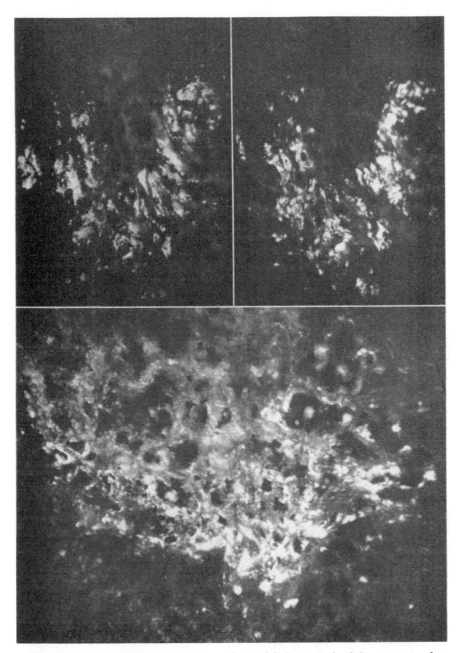

FIG. 18 (*top*). Localized depositions of γ_M-globulins, on the left, occur in close association with γ_G-globulins, shown in a similar field on the right, in rheumatoid granuloma. Immunofluorescence. 170×.

FIG. 19 (*bottom*). The γ_M-globulins deposited in rheumatoid granuloma are demonstrable as rheumatoid factors after γ_G-globulins are eluted by exposure of section to acid buffer. Fluorescent aggregated human γ_G-globulins. 280×.

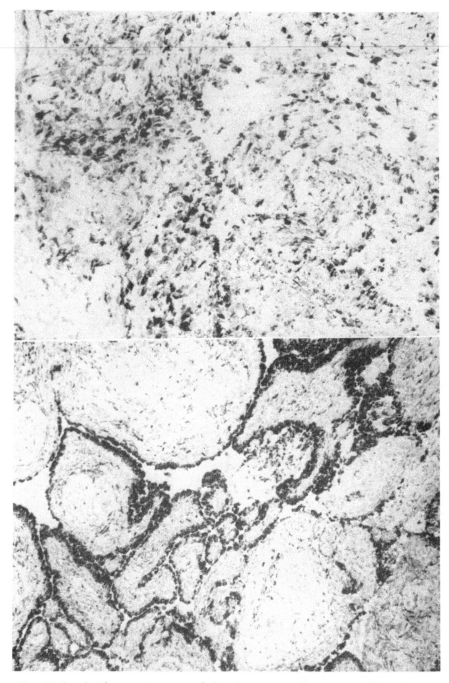

Fig. 20 (*top*). The synoviocytes and the phagocytic inflammatory cells in rheumatoid synovitis contain cytoplasmic granules rich in acid phosphatase. Gomori method, Novikoff modification; β-glycerophosphate substrate. 144×.

Fig. 21 (*bottom*). Proliferative synovitis in gouty arthritis. Here too synoviocytes and phagocytic inflammatory cells show intense activity of acid phosphatase enzymes. Gomori method. Novikoff modification. 120×.

produced chronic arthritis in rabbits by repeated intra-articular injections of a non-antigenic material capable of disrupting lysosomes in synovial lining cells. The ensuing joint-lesions resembled human rheumatoid disease in several respects: proliferation of synoviocytes, exudation of plasma cells, formation of lymphoid nodules in the synovial membrane, and erosion of articular cartilage by inflammatory granulation tissue. A surprising finding was the appearance of antibodies directed *not* against the injected material but against constituents of the animal's own tissues, that is, auto-antibodies to subcellular constituents which presumably had been denatured or otherwise rendered auto-antigenic by the action of lysosomal enzymes.

Dumonde and Glynn (6) have produced chronic arthritis in rabbits by inducing auto-immunity to fibrin, which is in reality denatured or partially degraded fibrinogen, followed by a single intra-articular injection of fibrin. In this work, the degraded and denatured products of inflammation, including fibrinous inflammation, were *themselves* thought to provide continuing auto-antigenic stimulation and in turn to contribute to chronicity of the articular disease. As is known, fibrinous exudation is a feature of the human connective-tissue diseases, and sometimes a prominent one in rheumatoid arthritis.

If these experimental results have bearing on the human disease, then the initiating mechanism in rheumatoid arthritis could be connective-tissue injury produced by a variety of biological, chemical, or physical agents; and the perpetuating mechanism could be auto-immunity. The further deliberations of this conference will almost certainly bring one or the other, or even a newer, aspect of this problem into clearer focus. While I am loathe to use an unduly optimistic expression, somehow I believe that a "breakthrough" in the understanding of this and other mysterious articular diseases is occurring, hopefully with ultimate benefit to those who suffer from them. In the meantime I am sure that you and I will be reasonably satisfied provided that steady progress continues to be made by many small steps if not by a giant one!

REFERENCES

1. Allison, N., and Ghormley, R. K. Diagnosis in Joint Disease (Wm. Broad and Co., New York, 1931).
2. Astorga, G., and Bollet, A. J. Diagnostic specificity and possible pathogenetic significance of inclusion-body cells in synovial fluid (Abstract). Arth. & Rheum. 7: 288 (1964).
3. Barland, P., Novikoff, A. B., and Hamerman, D. Fine structure and cytochemistry of the rheumatoid synovial membrane, with special reference to lysosomes. Am. J. Path. 44: 853 (1964).
4. Christian, C. L. Characterization of the "reactant" (gamma globulin factor) in the FII precipitin reaction and the FII tanned sheep cell agglutination test. J. Exper. Med. 108: 139 (1958).
5. Collins, D. H. The Pathology of Articular and Spinal Diseases (Edward Arnold & Co., London, 1949).
6. Dumonde, D. C., and Glynn, L. E. The production of arthritis in rabbits by an immunological reaction to fibrin. Brit. J. Exper. Path. 43: 373 (1962).
7. Edelman, G. M., Kunkel, H. G., and Franklin, E. C. Interaction of the rheumatoid factor with antigen-antibody complexes and aggregated gamma globulin. J. Exper. Med. 108: 105 (1958).

8. FAGRAEUS, A. Antibody production in relation to the development of plasma cells. In vivo and in vitro experiments. Acta med. scandinav. *130*: suppl. 204, 3 (1948).

9. FELL, H. B., and DINGLE, J. T. Studies on the mode of action of excess of vitamin A. 6. Lysosomal protease and the degradation of cartilage matrix. Biochem. J. *87*: 403 (1963).

10. FRANKLIN, E. C., HOLMAN, H. R., MÜLLER-EBERHARD, H. J., and KUNKEL, H. G. An unusual protein component of high molecular weight in the serum of certain patients with rheumatoid arthritis. J. Exper. Med. *105*: 425 (1957).

11. GOLDFISCHER, S., ESSNER, E., and NOVIKOFF, A. The localization of phosphatase activities at the level of ultrastructure. J. Histochem. *12*: 72 (1964).

12. HIRSCH, J. G., BERNHEIMER, A. W., and WEISSMANN, G. Motion picture study of the toxic action of streptolysins on leucocytes. J. Exper. Med. *118*: 223 (1963).

13. HOLLANDER, J. L., RAWSON, A. J., RESTIFO, R. A., and LUSSIER, A. J. Studies on the pathogenesis of rheumatoid joint inflammation (Abstract). Arth. & Rheum. 7: 314 (1964).

14. HOLLANDER, J. L., McCARTY, D. J., ASTORGA, G., and CASTRO-MURILLO, E. Studies on the pathogenesis of rheumatoid joint inflammation. I. The "R.A. cell" and a working hypothesis. Ann. Int. Med. *62*: 271 (1965).

15. KAPLAN, M. H. *In* Immunologic Aspects of Rheumatoid Arthritis and Systemic Lupus Erythematosus (Grune and Stratton, Inc., New York, 1963), p. 475.

16. KUNKEL, H. G., MÜLLER-EBERHARD, H. J., FUDENBERG, H. H., and TOMASI, T. B. Gamma globulin complexes in rheumatroid arthritis and certain other conditions. J. Clin. Invest. *40*: 117 (1961).

17. LAWRENCE, H. S. (ed.). Cellular and Humoral Aspects of the Hypersensitive States (Hoeber and Harper, Medical Book Department, New York, 1959).

18. LUSCOMBE, MOLLIE. Acid phosphatase and catheptic activity in rheumatoid synovial tissue. Nature, *197*: 1010 (1963).

19. MACKAY, I. R., and BURNET, F. M. Autoimmune Diseases: Pathogenesis, Chemistry and Therapy (Charles C. Thomas, Springfield, Ill., 1963).

20. McCARTY, D. J. Phagocytosis of urate crystals in gouty synovial fluid. Am. J. Med. Sci. *243*: 288 (1962).

21. MELLORS, R. C., HEIMER, R., CORCOS, J., and KORNGOLD, L. Cellular origin of rheumatoid factor. J. Exper. Med. *110*: 875 (1959).

22. MELLORS, R. C., NOWOSLAWSKI, A., and KORNGOLD, L. Rheumatoid arthritis and the cellular origin of rheumatoid factors. Am. J. Path. *39*: 533 (1961).

23. MELLORS, R. C., and KORNGOLD, L. The cellular origin of human immunoglobulins (γ_2, γ_{1M}, γ_{1A}). J. Exper. Med. *118*: 387 (1963).

24. NOSSAL, G. J. V. Genetic control of lymphopoiesis, plasma cell formation, and antibody production. Internat. Rev. Exper. Path. *1*: 1 (1962).

25. NOVIKOFF, A. B., and ESSNER, E. The liver cell, some new approaches to its study. Am. J. Med. *29*: 102 (1960).

26. PARKER, R. L., and SCHMID, F. R. Phagocytosis of particulate complexes of gamma globulin and rheumatoid factor. J. Immunol. *88*: 519 (1962).

27. RAWSON, A. J., ABELSON, N. M., and HOLLANDER, J. L. Studies on the pathogenesis of rheumatoid joint inflammation. II. Intracytoplasmic particulate complexes in rheumatoid synovial fluids. Ann. Int. Med. *62*: 281 (1965).

28. SMITH, CAROL, and HAMERMAN, D. Acid phosphatase in human synovial fluid. Arth. & Rheum. 5: 411 (1962).

29. TAYLOR, H. E., and SHEPHERD, W. E. The immunohistochemical interaction of autologous rheumatoid serum with subcutaneous rheumatoid nodules. Lab. Invest. 9: 603 (1960).

30. VAZQUEZ, J. J., and DIXON, F. J. Immunohistochemical study of lesions in rheumatic fever, systemic lupus erythematosus, and rheumatoid arthritis. Lab. Invest. 6: 205 (1957).

31. WEISSMANN, G., BECHER, B., WIEDERMANN, G., and BERNHEIMER, A. W. Studies on lysosomes. VII. Acute and chronic arthritis produced by intra-articular injections of streptolysin S in rabbits. Am. J. Path. *46*: 129 (1965).

Electron Microscopic Studies of
Normal Guinea-Pig Synovium*

M. DARIA HAUST, M.D.,
JOHN C. WYLLIE, M.D., and
ROBERT H. MORE, M.D.

IN THE COURSE of our studies on rheumatoid arthritis (1) it became essential to establish a baseline of normality of the synovial lining. Since it appeared from the literature that there is no significant morphological difference in the synovium from one species to another (2–6), the guinea pig was utilized in the study of normal synovium.

Strips of synovium excised from the knee joints of five healthy albino guinea pigs were fixed in 1 per cent osmium tetroxide and processed for electron microscopy as described in detail elsewhere (7). Thin sections were examined in an RCA EM-3D electron microscope.

The synovial membrane is composed of loose, vascularized connective tissues lined towards the joint cavity by a layer of synovial cells two to three cells thick (Fig. 1). These cells are arranged loosely, in a ground substance containing only sparse collagen fibrils. The synovial cell layer is not separated from the underlying supporting tissue by a basement membrane, and there is a close and intimate relation between these cells and the vessels (Fig. 1). There are two distinct types of synovial cells: one has an abundant rough-surfaced endoplasmic reticulum (Fig. 1), whereas a prominent Golgi apparatus characterizes the other (Fig. 2). However, cells intermediate between the two types were most common (Figs. 1 and 3). Cellular processes of all sizes overlap and interdigitate with those of neighbouring cells. The most superficial cells often extend slender cell processes (filopodia) into the joint cavity (Fig. 1). Each synovial cell is surrounded by an incomplete cellular basement membrane, which is moderately electron dense, structureless, and measures approximately 200 Å in thickness. While it is usually separated

*From the Department of Pathology, Kingston General Hospital and Queen's University, Kingston, Ontario.

Supported by grant-in-aid of research from the Canadian Arthritis and Rheumatism Society, Toronto, Ontario.

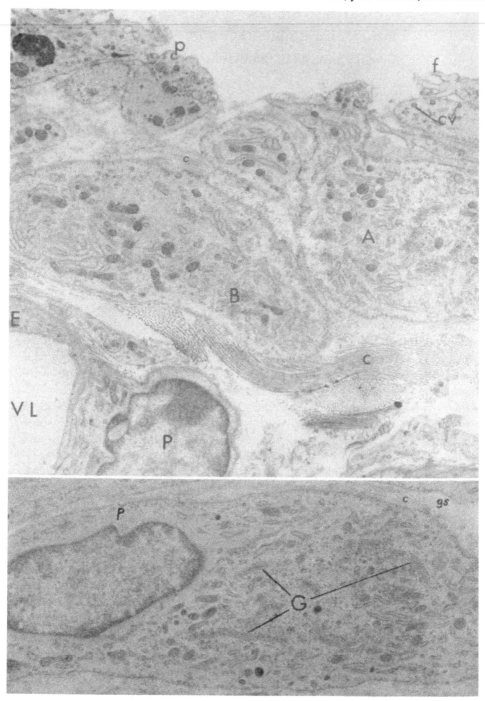

from the cytoplasmic membrane by an electron-lucent zone 300 Å thick, it is at times in direct contact with the cell membrane (Figs. 3 and 4). The nucleus of the synovial cells is large, ovoid to round, and occasionally undulation or indentation is seen (Figs. 2 and 3). The nucleoplasm is finely granular and it condenses in triangular or oval-shaped areas along the nuclear membrane (Figs, 2 and 3). Occasionally, a centrosome consisting of a pair of centrioles is present and rarely cilia are found (Fig. 4).

Rough-surfaced endoplasmic reticulum is present in all cells but in one cell type it is particularly abundant (Fig. 1).

The Golgi zone is present in almost all cells, and in many it is prominent and occupies a large part of the cytoplasm (Figs. 2 and 3). This organelle is composed of groups of parallel, elongated flattened lamellae, many small sacs, and vesicles. They are all limited by a smooth membrane. Finely granular material of slightly intenser electron density than that of the surrounding hyaloplasm is present in the lamallae and in small saccules on their surface. These saccules have a diameter of approximately 400 Å and resemble pinocytotic vesicles (Fig. 3). Cells with prominent Golgi complex have more mitochondria than other cells. In the vicinity of the Golgi zone two types of microbodies are usually observed. One is small, measuring 450 to 650 Å in diameter, does not have a sharply delineated limiting membrane, and is composed of electron-dense, finely granular material (Fig. 3). The other microbody measures 1200 to 2000 Å in diameter and is bounded by a membrane (Fig. 3). It contains a core of electron-dense material surrounded by a less dense zone. Round to oval membrane-limited bodies slightly larger than mitochondria are occasionally seen in the cytoplasm. They contain granules which vary in size and electron density (Fig. 5).

Two types of vesicles are observed in addition, in synovial cells. The smaller, more numerous ones are pinocytotic vesicles. They are found along the cell membranes and measure 600 to 900 Å in diameter (Figs. 1-5). They are often fused with the cellular membrane and occasionally contain basement membrane material in continuation with it (Figs. 1-5). The second vesicle is larger, measuring 1200 to 1500 Å. It is usually slightly elongated, and has an electron-dense wall of 70 Å which is covered by perpendicular spines measuring 150 to 200 Å in length. This vesicle also contains electron-dense,

FIG. 1 (*top*). The joint cavity (top) is lined by a layer two to three cells thick, arranged loosely in ground substance. Sparse collagen (c) fibrils are present within the synovial cell layer, but thick collagen bundles are seen in the subsynovial connective tissue layer. A small blood vessel lies in close proximity to synovial cells. A = cell type A; B = cell type B; C = collagen; P = pericyte; VL = lumen of small vessel; E = endothelium; f = filopodium; p = "pit"; cv = "coated" vesicle. Magnification, 9600×.

FIG. 2 (*bottom*). Synovial cell with a prominent Golgi complex (G) (cell type A). Numerous pinocytotic vesicles and occasional "pits" (p) are seen along the cellular membrane. The nucleus is elongated and slightly indented. The intercellular space contains ground substance (gs) and collagen fibrils (c). Magnification, 9600×.

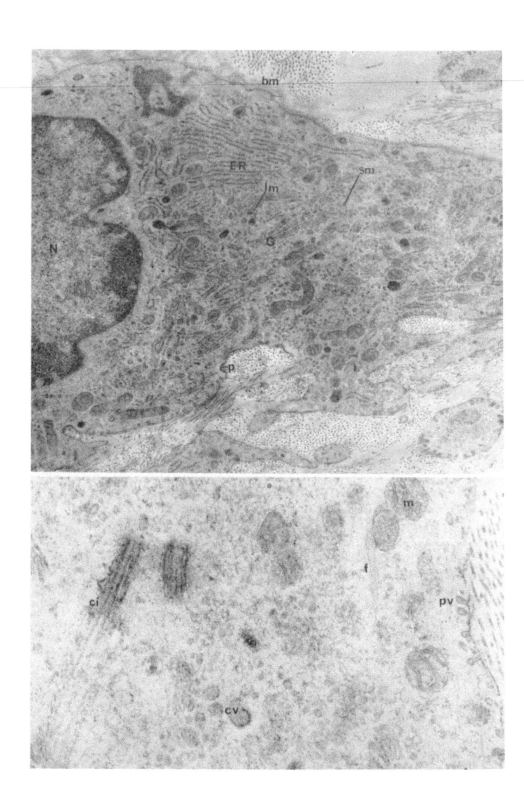

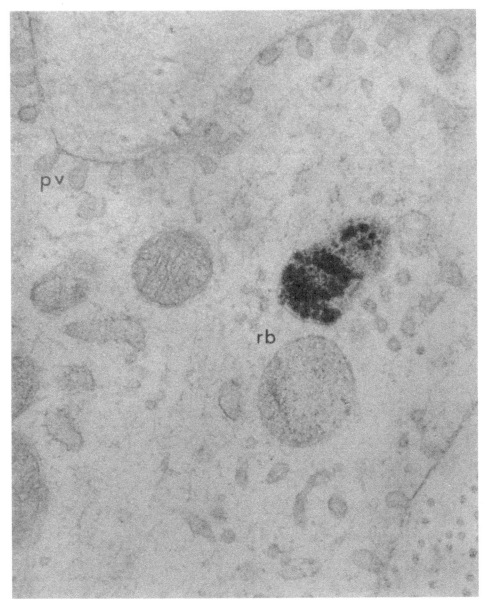

Fig. 5. Round bodies (rb), completely or partially surrounded by a limiting membrane and slightly larger than mitochondria, contain granules of various sizes and electron densities. Numerous pinocytotic vesicles (pv) contain moderately electron-dense basement membrane-like material. Magnification, 57,480×.

Fig. 3 (*top*). Synovial cell intermediate between cell type A and cell type B. It contains a well-developed rough-surfaced endoplasmic reticulum (ER) and Golgi complex (G). The nucleus (N) is undulated. Large (lm) and small (sm) microbodies are seen in close proximity to Golgi complex, which is composed of lamellae and saccules. Numerous pinocytotic vesicles and an occasional "pit" (p) are seen at the cellular membrane. An incomplete basement membrane (bm) surrounds the cell. Numerous mitochondria and occasional "coated" vesicles and round bodies are also seen. Magnification, 11,000×.

Fig. 4 (*bottom*). Synovial cell contains cilia (ci); pinocytotic vesicles (pv), "coated" vesicles (cv), mitochondria (m), and fine cytoplasmic filaments (f) are also seen. Magnification, 36,600×.

basement membrane-like material, but there is usually some electron-lucency in its core (Figs. 1, 3, 4). At times this "coated" vesicle is fused partly or entirely with the cellular membrane, and in the latter instance it forms a deep "pit" at the level of the cellular membrane (Figs. 1–3).

Our studies of normal guinea pig synovium are largely in agreement with the observations made on synovium in other species (2–6). Thus, the cells possessing abundant rough-surfaced endoplasmic reticulum correspond to the human synovial type B cell of Barland et al. (2). They are considered to be involved in protein synthesis, but they are not numerous in our material. The type A cell (2) with a prominent Golgi complex was more frequently observed. Evidence that Golgi complex is involved in the manufacturing and secretion of complex carbohydrates was provided by radio-autographic studies with injected titrium-labelled glucose (8). The radioactivity appeared first in the Golgi zone and subsequently in the secretions of the cells concerned (8). Since the synovial fluid has a high content of hyaluronic acid, it is reasonable to assume from the above that this complex mucopolysaccaride is secreted by the type A synovial cell and added to the dialysate from the subsynovial vessels on its way to the synovial cavity. Other experimental data with incubated tissue slices (9) and cultured synovial cells (10), as well as the presence of small cytoplasmic microbodies in the present and other (4, 11) studies, support the contention that the synovial cells secrete hyaluronic acid.

The presence of both pinocytotic and "coated" vesicles indicates that the synovial cells are also sampling the extracellular substances as it was shown that the former is involved in "ingestion" of macromolecules in amoeba (12) and the latter (via the "pit") is concerned with protein uptake (13, 14).

The presence of cilia in synovial cells would indicate that these cells have, in addition, a chemoreceptive function (15).

REFERENCES

1. WYLLIE, J. C., HAUST, M. D., and MORE, R. H. The fine structure of synovial lining cells in rheumatoid arthritis. Lab. Invest. 15: 519 (1966).
2. BARLAND, P., NOVIKOFF, A. B., and HAMERMAN, D. Electron microscopy of the human synovial membrane. J. Cell Biol. 14: 207 (1962).
3. COULTER, W. H. The characteristics of human synovial tissue as seen with the electron microscope. Arth. & Rheum. 5: 70 (1962).
4. LEVER, J. D., and FORD, E. H. Histological, histochemical, and electron microscopic observations on synovial membrane. Anat. Rec. 132: 525 (1958).
5. LUSE, S. A. A synovial sarcoma studied by electron microscopy. Cancer, 13: 312 (1960).
6. LANGER, E., and HUTH, F. Untersuchungen über den submikroskopischen Bau der Synovialmembran. Ztschr. Zellforsch. 51: 545 (1960).
7. WYLLIE, J. C., MORE, R. H., and HAUST, M. D. The fine structure of normal guinea pig synovium. Lab. Invest. 13: 1254 (1964).
8. PETERSON, M., and LEBLOND, C. P. Synthesis of complex carbohydrates in the Golgi region, as shown by radioautography after injection of labelled glucose. J. Cell Biol. 21: 143 (1964).

9. YIELDING, K. L., TOMKINS, G. M., and BUNIM, J. J. Synthesis of hyaluronic acid by human synovial tissue slices. Science, *125*: 1300 (1957).

10. CASTOR, C. W. Biosynthesis of mucopolysaccharides by normal human synovial cells in a simplified medium (Abstract). Ann. Rheum. Dis. *16*: 127 (1957).

11. JACKSON, S. F. Cytoplasmic granules in fibrogenic cells. Nature, *175*: 39 (1955).

12. BRANDT, P. W., and PAPPAS, G. D. An electron microscopic study of pinocytosis in ameba. 1. The surface attachment phase. J. Biophys. Biochem. Cytol. *8*: 675 (1960).

13. ROTH, T. F., and PORTER, K. R. Specialized sites on the cell surface for protein uptake. *In* Proceedings Fifth International Congress for Electron Microscopy, *edited by* S. S. Breese Jr. (Academic Press, Inc., New York, 1962), Vol. 2, p. ll-4.

14. ––– Membrane differentiation for protein uptake (Abstract). Fed. Proc. *22*: 178 (1963).

15. MUNGER, B. L. A light and electron microscopic study of cellular differentiation in the pancreatic islets of the mouse. Amer. J. Anat. *103*: 275 (1958).

The Fine Structure of
Rheumatoid Synovial Membrane*

JOHN C. WYLLIE,†
M. DARIA HAUST, and
ROBERT H. MORE

SPECIMENS of synovial membrane were obtained from four patients with rheumatoid arthritis and processed for electron microscopy as described in detail elsewhere (1).

The studies of Barland, Novikoff, and Hamerman (2) have shown that two types of cells can be identified in the lining cell layer of normal human synovium. The type A cell has numerous filopodia and large vacuoles; the type B cell has a well-developed rough-surfaced endoplasmic reticulum.

The synovial lining cells were enlarged and numerous in the rheumatoid synovia examined. Masses of fibrin were observed on the synovial membrane and between these cells (Fig. 1). The type A cells, which were superficially located, had numerous cytoplasmic extensions of filopodia and many vacuoles. Some of the vacuoles contained granular and fibrillar electron-dense material which resembled the fibrin in the intercellular space (Fig. 2). Large numbers of electron-dense round bodies or "residual bodies" were observed in some of these cells (Fig. 1).

The more prevalent type B cell was characterized by a well-developed rough-surfaced endoplasmic reticulum and a large Golgi complex (Fig. 3). The rough-surfaced endoplasmic reticulum was dilated and contained fibrillar material (Fig. 3). Numerous microbodies were noted in the vicinity of the Golgi complex. Small numbers of dense, round bodies, resembling those observed in the type A cells, were seen in these cells. The surrounding intercellular space contained fibrillar material in which collagen fibrils were identified (Fig. 4).

No structures resembling virus inclusions were observed in either cell type.

*From the Department of Pathology, Queen's University and Kingston General Hospital, Kingston, Ontario.

Supported by a grant-in-aid from the Canadian Arthritis and Rheumatism Society.

†Fellow of the Canadian Arthritis and Rheumatism Society.

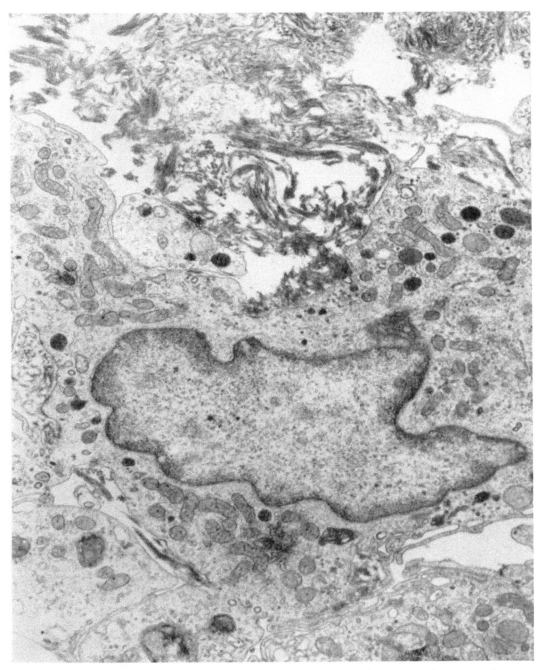

FIG. 1. Electron micrograph of rheumatoid synovium; tissue stained with uranyl acetate. There are deposits of fibrin in the intercellular space near a type A lining cell. Note dense round bodies within this cell. About 15,000×.

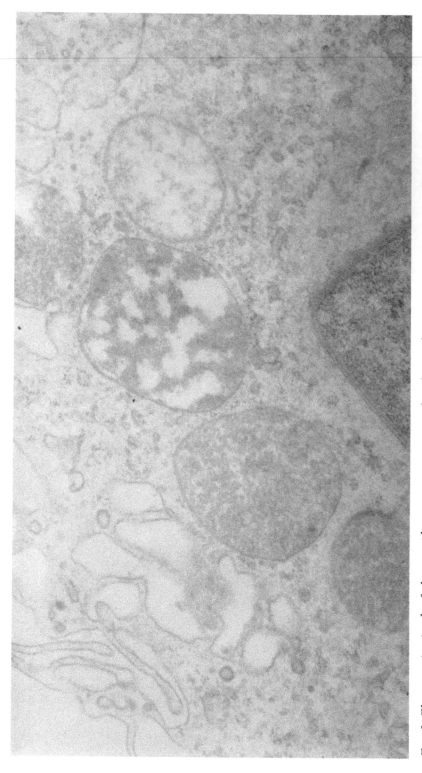

Fig. 2. Electron micrograph of rheumatoid synovium; tissue stained with uranyl acetate. A type A lining cell contains large vacuoles, partially filled with electron-dense granular and fibrillar material. About 30,000×.

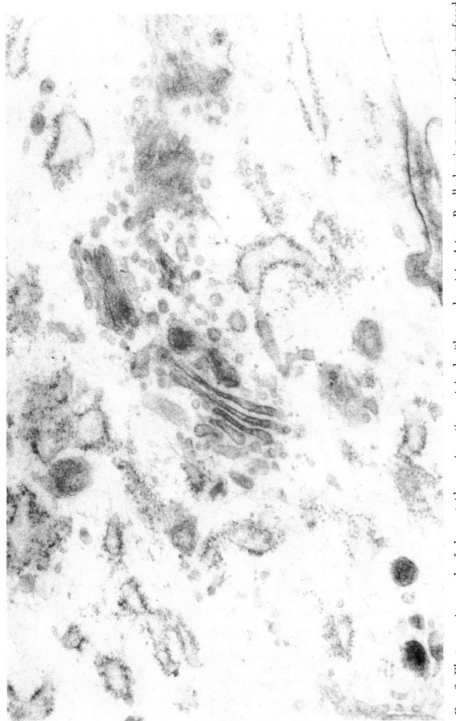

FIG. 3. Electron micrograph of rheumatoid synovium; tissue stained with uranyl acetate. A type B cell, showing segments of rough-surfaced endoplasmic reticulum and part of the Golgi complex (centre). The endoplasmic reticulum contains fibrillar material. About 32,000×.

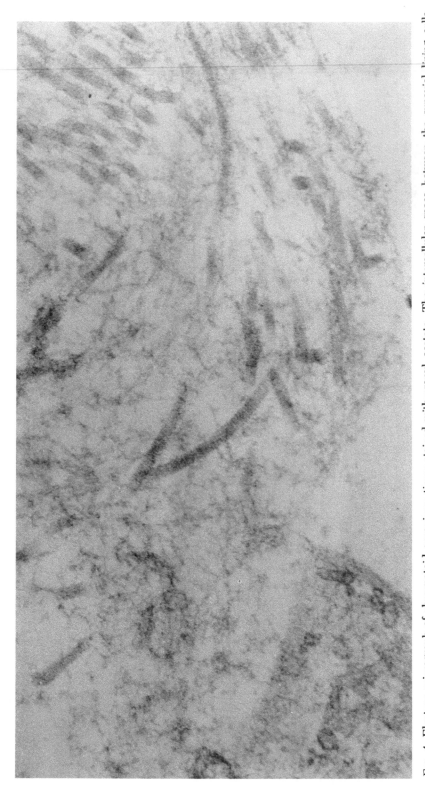

FIG. 4. Electron micrograph of rheumatoid synovium; tissue stained with uranyl acetate. The intercellular space between the synovial lining cells contains finely fibrillar material and collagen fibrils. About 60,000×.

The two cell types, designated A and B (2), of normal human synovium were distinguished on morphologic grounds. This distinction is maintained in rheumatoid arthritis as shown by Barland, Novikoff, and Hamerman (3). We have confirmed their findings. The two cell types appear to subserve different functions. Thus, the type A cell is actively engaged in phagocytosis and appears to remove fibrin from the intercellular space. On the other hand, the type B cell, with its rough-surfaced endoplasmic reticulum and Golgi complex, is equipped for synthesis and secretion. It is the probable source of the collagen fibrils observed in its vicinity. Collagen is not normally present around the lining cells in normal human synovium. The stimulus to its production in rheumatoid arthritis is not apparent. The deposition of fibrin and collagen in the intercellular space of the lining cell layer may well interfere with the diffusion nutrients from the subsynovial vascular bed to the joint cavity and hence contribute to cartilage damage. Barland, Novikoff, and Hemerman (3) observed structures resembling virus bodies within the lining cells; we did not note similar inclusions.

REFERENCES

1. WYLLIE, J. C., HAUST, M. D., and MORE, R. H. The fine structure of the synovial lining cell in rheumatoid arthritis. Lab. Invest. *15*: 519 (1966).
2. BARLAND, P., NOVIKOFF, A. B., and HAMERMAN, D. Electron microscopy of the human synovial membrane. J. Cell Biol. *14*: 207 (1962).
3. ——— Fine structure and cytochemistry of the rheumatoid synovial membrane, with special references to lysosomes. Am. J. Path. *44*: 853 (1964).

DISCUSSION

DR. R. C. MELLORS (*New York City*): As light-microscopy morphologists looking at rheumatoid synovitis, we originally had trouble in giving those surface cells a name. We called them endothelial cells and sometimes mesenchymal, and then the term synoviocyte was introduced. That was a good name that didn't mean too much. Now we are seeing the details of ultrastructure correlated with function.

However, I should like to turn to one dilemma. All the cells that exfoliate into synovial fluid—the polys, the macrophages, and the synoviocytes themselves—as you know, are present in synovial fluid in abundance in rheumatoid synovitis. When a macrophage has migrated and comes to lie right next door to the synoviocyte, what are the distinguishing features between such a macrophage and a synoviocyte, say a type A cell?

DR. MORRIS ZIFF (*Dallas, Texas*): The observation was made by Dr. Wyllie that lysosomes may contain fibrin and lipid, and this made me think about fibrinoid, which was mentioned by Dr. Mellors and by Dr. Wyllie.

Fibrinoid contains mostly fibrin and some lipid, with a little nuclear debris, at least in the rheumatoid subcutaneous nodules. I would wonder whether the fibrinoid in the subcutaneous nodule (which is surrounded by pallisaded cells resembling the proliferating rheumatoid synovial lining cells, which are also associated with fibrinoid in the rheumatoid synovial membrane) may not represent lysosomes that have been deposited by degraded phagocytic cells and left unabsorbed by the circulation.

Eventually this stuff piles up out of reach of enzymes and just collects as a sea of indigestible fibrin and lipid. This is actually what it looks like, I think, when you look at it in the electron microscope. It is just a collection of amorphous material, with many lysosomes.

CHAIRMAN: Which may explain its remarkable persistence, too.

DR. WYLLIE: First of all, with regard to distinguishing type A cells from macrophages, I agree that this is difficult. I have never seen such a development of a Golgi complex, though, in a macrophage or evidence of such a degree of secretion; so that one point that does help to distinguish would then be the presence of a fully developed Golgi complex. A second point is really just the location of the cell. *In situ* it looks as if it is placed among the other cells rather than being an infiltrating cell. I have seen macrophages infiltrating the synovium under the electron microscope, and they do look different from the type A cells.

The material that is in the intercellular space, usually called fibrinoid on the basis of light microscopy, may be made up of broken-down lysosomes, but morphologically it has the features of fibrin. It is a fibrous structure and it shows a characteristic axial periodicity exhibited by that particular fibrous protein. So, from my point of view, it is fibrin. It may have other things trapped in with it, but it is mainly fibrin.

DR. HAUST: One other distinguishing feature that I am sure Dr. Wyllie meant to say, too, is that the synovial cells have a basement membrane, whereas the macrophage never has a basement membrane. This is a very, very sure point on the basis of which these two cells can be distinguished, and we at no time felt that we were dealing with macrophages when we looked at these cells.

The Pathological Changes
in Articular Cartilage
Associated with
Persistent Joint Deformity:
An Experimental Investigation*

R. B. SALTER,
O. R. McNEILL, and
R. CARBIN

A VERY EFFECTIVE STIMULUS for experimental investigation is the clinical observation of a phenomenon for which there is as yet no satisfactory scientific explanation. The clinical observation that stimulated the present investigation was made on several occasions during the course of surgical operations on patients with persistent joint deformity. It was observed that in the presence of a long-standing and persistent joint deformity, the articular cartilage was grossly abnormal, and indeed sometimes completely absent, over the portion of the joint surface which, as a result of deformity, was no longer in contact with the opposing joint surface, but which was in fact in continuous contact with the synovial membrane.

We have made this observation on numerous occasions during the course of our orthopaedic work. Two examples are presented below.

A girl 17 years of age had paralytic poliomyelitis in early childhood as a result of which she had a residual problem with both thumbs. In her right thumb she had a 90-degree flexion deformity of the interphalangeal joint, which had been present for at least six years. This joint was painful. The interphalangeal joint of her left thumb was completely flail, and it was unstable. Arthrodesis of the interphalangeal joint of both thumbs was performed: on the right thumb to correct deformity and to relieve pain, and on the left thumb to provide stability. At the time of operation a striking difference was observed in the appearance of the articular cartilage of these two joints (Fig. 1). In the flail

*From the Division of Orthopaedic Surgery and the Research Institute of the Hospital for Sick Children, Toronto.

joint the articular cartilage of the head of the proximal phalanx looked perfectly normal. In the joint with the persistent flexion deformity, the part of the articular surface that was no longer opposing articular cartilage, but rather was in continuous contact with the synovial membrane, was completely devoid of cartilage.

A 14-year-old boy had paralytic poliomyelitis as a result of which he had a residual metatarsus elevatus, with a flexion deformity of the metatarsophalangeal joint (Fig. 2). Since this had been a persistent deformity of long duration, it is apparent that the dorsal portion of the articular cartilage of the head of the metatarsal would not have been in contact with the opposing surface of cartilage on the proximal phalanx but rather it would have been in continuous contact with synovial membrane. This boy's metatarsophalangeal joint was fused to correct deformity and to relieve pain. At the time of operation it was observed that the portion of articular cartilage that had been in continuous contact with only synovial membrane was grossly deficient (Fig. 3).

These observations and several similar observations stimulated the authors to seek an explanation. The hypothesis that we formulated to explain these clinical observations was as follows. When a joint is maintained in an extreme position, as it is in a persistent joint deformity, one portion of the joint surface is no longer in contact with the opposing joint surface, at any time; rather, it is in continuous contact with synovial membrane, which no longer glides freely over it. It was reasoned that under such circumstances the synovial membrane might become adherent to the underlying cartilage thereby obliterating the synovial space, in which case the cartilage would no longer have access to its main source of nutrition, namely, synovial fluid. Thus, deprived of its nutrition, the articular cartilage might undergo degenerative changes.

The purpose of the present investigation, therefore, was to elucidate the aetiology and pathogenesis of the pathological changes in articular cartilage that we had observed clinically, and to test the validity of our hypothesis.

Three series of experiments were designed, using a total of 62 rabbits. The first series of experiments in adult rabbits involved the production of a persistent joint deformity of the knee, by having the knee maintained in flexion for varying periods from three weeks to eight months (Fig. 4). Following the period of immobilization the animals were sacrificed and their knees were examined.

The second series was similar to the first, except that it was conducted in adolescent rabbits rather than adult rabbits.

The third series, which was conducted in adult rabbits, involved a study of remobilization after a period of immobilization, in order to determine the reversibility of the lesions, as well as their effect on the joint with subsequent function of the joint.

The lustre of the articular cartilage of the patellar groove of a control

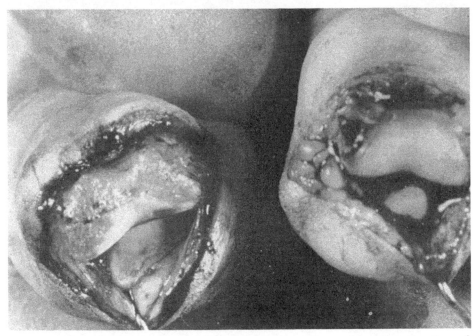

Fig. 1. The interphalangeal joint of the thumbs of a 17-year-old girl at the time of operation. Note the destruction of articular cartilage on the head of the proximal phalanx, the right thumb (left of figure), and the normal articular cartilage of the head of the proximal phalanx of the left thumb.

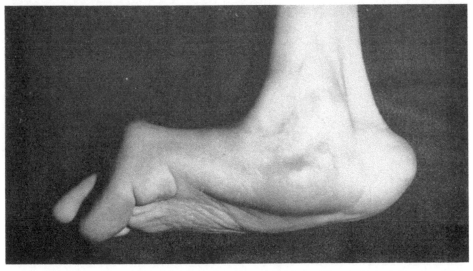

Fig. 2. Medial view of the right foot of a 14-year-old boy with paralytic deformity. Note the metatarsus elevatus and the associated flexion deformity of the first metatarso-phalangeal joint.

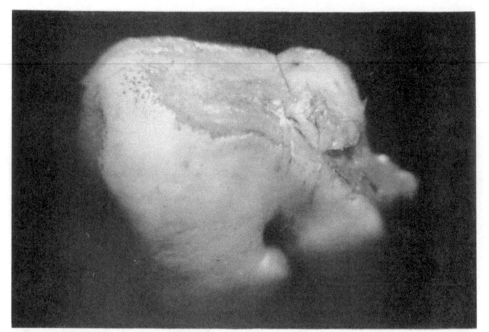

Fig. 3. Photograph of the joint surface of the head of the first metatarsal of the foot shown in Fig. 2. Note the destruction of articular cartilage on the dorsal portion of the joint (top of the figure).

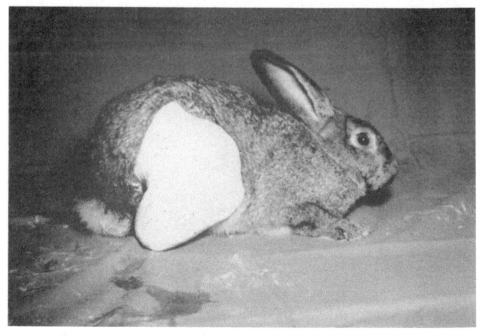

Fig. 4. Plaster immobilization of the right hind limb of a rabbit with the knee joint in a position of acute flexion.

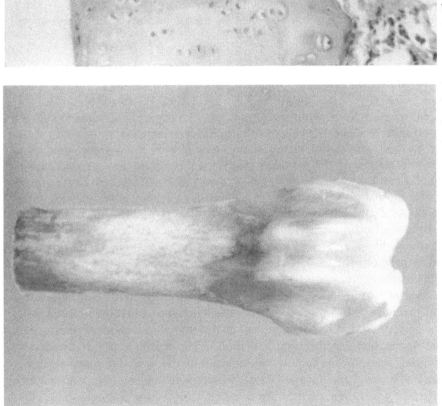

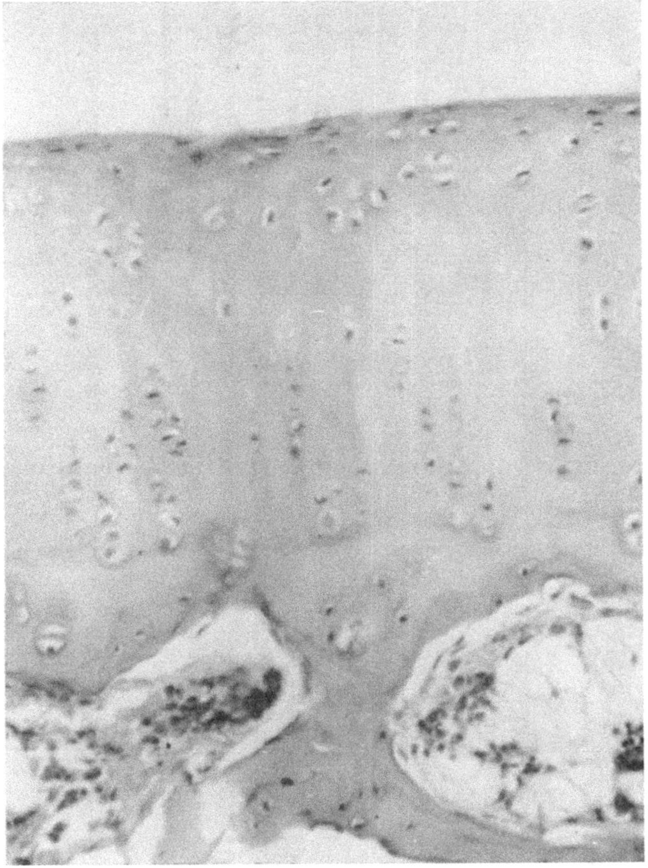

Fig. 6. Photomicrograph of the normal articular cartilage of the patellar groove of a control rabbit.

Fig. 5. Photograph of the anterior view of the distal end of the femur of a normal rabbit. Note the lustre of the normal articular cartilage of the patellar groove.

rabbit is seen in Fig. 5. In the rabbit a subsynovial fat pad exists immediately proximal to the cartilaginous surface of the patella. When the rabbit's knee is maintained in a position of acute flexion this suprapatellar fat pad overlies the middle area of the patellar groove.

The microscopic appearance of normal articular cartilage of the patellar groove of the rabbit is shown in Fig. 6.

The results of the first series of experiments revealed that all of the 42 joints in the adult animals that had been immobilized for a period of three weeks or longer demonstrated pathological changes in articular cartilage, varying from superficial necrosis (Grade I) to full thickness loss of cartilage (Grade III). However, in only half of the 20 joints in adolescent rabbits were there similar pathological changes, and these changes were not only less severe than in the adult animals, but they took a longer period of time to develop. From the third series of experiments it was found that the pathological changes were not reversible and that, furthermore, with subsequent use of the joint, these changes led to the development of degenerative arthritis.

The nature and extent of the lesions of articular cartilage seen in these experimental investigations may be seen in the photographs and photomicrographs from representative animals (Figs. 7 to 21).

DISCUSSION

The pathological changes demonstrated in these experiments develop slowly and would seem to be of the nature of a gradual degeneration.

Since the most important factor in the aetiology of the lesions appears to be local obliteration of the synovial space with resultant loss of nutrition to the articular cartilage, this lesion has been designated obliterative degeneration of articular cartilage. Normally, articular cartilage is subjected to both intermittent pressure and friction, both of which serve to aid the diffusion of the synovial fluid into the intercellular substance of the cartilage, which in turn behaves much like a sponge. Furthermore, during movement of the joint the synovial membrane glides freely over the joint surface.

In a previous experimental investigation (1), we showed that continuous compression of two articular cartilage surfaces interferes with cartilage nutrition and produces the lesion we have called pressure necrosis; this happens within a period of six days. In the present investigation, however, there is no pressure, nor is there any friction. Nutrition of the cartilage is interfered with by a different mechanism, namely, obliteration of the synovial space by adherence of the synovial membrane. Thus the synovial fluid can no longer reach the underlying cartilage, which, as a result, undergoes degeneration. This phenomenon would seem to be comparable with the effects of an adherent soft-tissue panus, as seen in rheumatoid arthritis and in tuberculous arthritis.

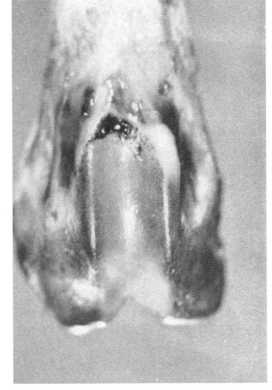

FIG. 7. Photograph of the distal end of the femur of an adult rabbit whose knee had been immobilized in flexion for a period of three weeks. Note the loss of lustre of the articular cartilage of the proximal position of the patellar groove and the destruction of cartilage in the proximal margin of the groove.

FIG. 8. Photomicrograph of a Grade I lesion of articular cartilage of the patellar groove of a rabbit. The chondrocytes have lost their staining power.

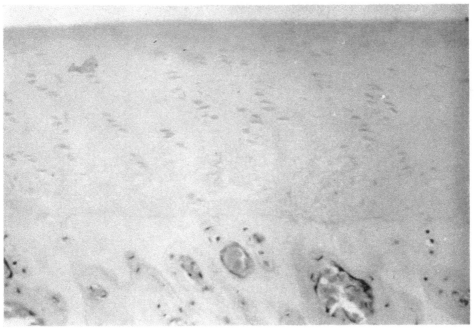

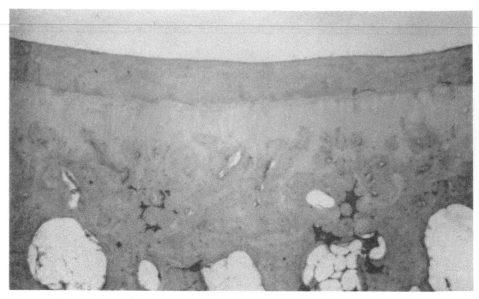

Fɪɢ. 9. Photomicrograph of a Grade II lesion of articular cartilage of the patellar groove of a rabbit. The superficial portion of the cartilage is necrotic but the deeper portion is still viable.

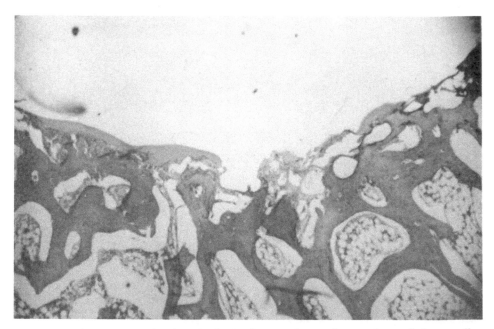

Fɪɢ. 10. Photomicrograph of a Grade III lesion of articular cartilage of the patellar groove of a rabbit. The full thickness of articular cartilage has disappeared and the underlying cancellous bone is exposed.

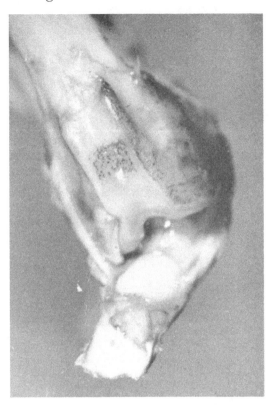

FIG. 11. Photograph of the lower end of the femur of a rabbit whose knee had been immobilized in flexion for 10 weeks. The patella and suprapatellar fat pad have been reflected distally. Note the lesion of articular cartilage in the middle third of the patellar groove. This area had been in continuous contact with the synovial membrane overlying the suprapatellar fat pad.

FIG. 12. Photomicrograph of the lesion of articular cartilage in the patellar groove of the rabbit shown in Fig. 11. Note the destruction of articular cartilage and the vascular infiltration from the underlying cancellous bone.

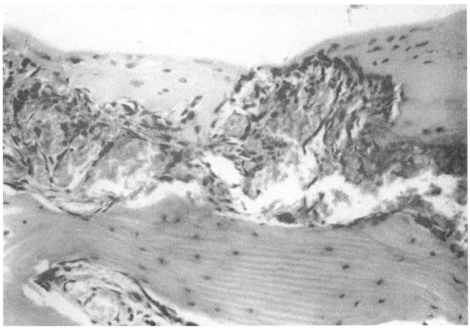

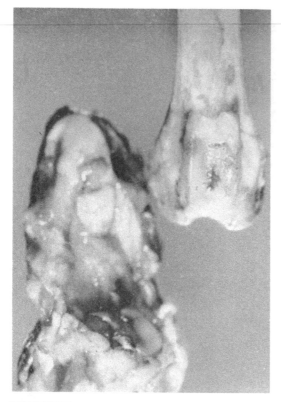

FIG. 13. Photograph of the lower end of the femur of a rabbit whose knee had been immobilized in flexion for 10 weeks. The patella and suprapatellar fat pad have been turned back (left of figure). Note the lesion of articular cartilage in the middle third of the patellar groove, the area that had been in continuous contact with the synovial membrane overlying the suprapatellar fat pad.

FIG. 14. Photomicrograph of the lesion of articular cartilage in the patellar groove of the rabbit shown in Fig. 13. Note the Grade III lesion of articular cartilage and the attachment of synovial membrane to the surface of the lesion.

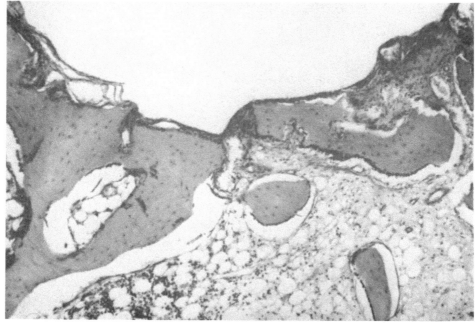

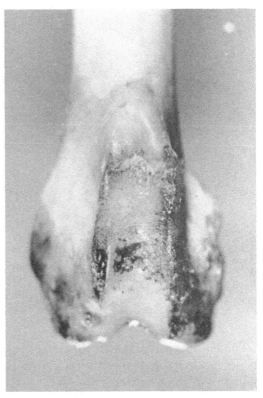

Fig. 15. Photograph of the lower end of the femur of a rabbit whose knee had been immobilized in flexion for a period of 12 weeks. Note the lesion of articular cartilage in the patellar groove and the additional lesions of cartilage along the margins of the groove. At these sites the synovial membrane had been adherent to the articular cartilage.

Fig. 16. Photomicrograph of the lesion of articular cartilage in the patellar groove of the rabbit shown in Fig. 15. Note the Grade III lesion of cartilage. At the extreme left of the figure synovial membrane is adherent to the surface of the lesion.

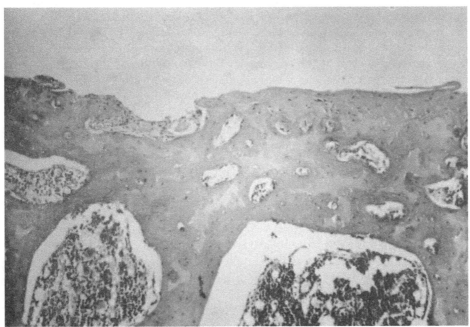

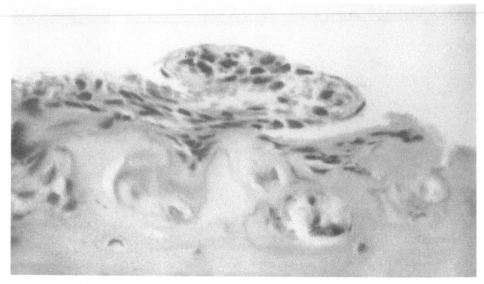

FIG. 17. High-power photomicrograph of the extreme left of the field shown in Fig. 16, showing the adherent synovial membrane.

The authors consider that the adherent synovial membrane in these experiments has acted as a mechanical barrier to the diffusion of synovial fluid by obliterating the synovial space. We have, therefore, chosen to designate the lesion "obliterative degeneration of articular cartilage." It is not simply a matter of loss of movement of the joint, since the other areas of the joint, also immobilized, did not show these changes. We do not believe that it is an aggressive action on the part of the synovial membrane, since we did not see any evidence of such action in our histological preparations.

The underlying cartilage gradually degenerates, is invaded by blood vessels, and is eventually absorbed. Attempts at healing are very limited indeed. Furthermore, with subsequent use of the joint, the lesion of obliterative degeneration of the cartilage leads to degenerative arthritis.

RELATION OF THE PRESENT INVESTIGATION TO CLINICAL PROBLEMS

The present investigation is related to clinical problems, first in the prevention of the lesion of obliterative degeneration and secondly in dealing with the lesion when it is already established.

Prevention of obliterative degeneration of cartilage involves prevention of deformity by maintaining a full range of movement in joints and by avoidance of very prolonged immobilization of a joint in an extreme position. Prevention

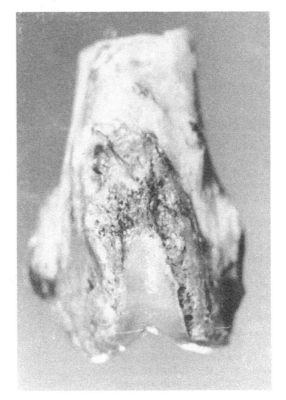

FIG. 18. Photograph of the lower end of the femur of a rabbit whose knee had been immobilized in flexion for a very prolonged period (8 months). Note the very marked destruction of articular cartilage.

FIG. 19. Photomicrograph of the lesion of articular cartilage in the patellar groove of the rabbit shown in Fig. 18. In addition to the Grade III lesion of articular cartilage there is marked disuse atrophy of the underlying cancellous bone.

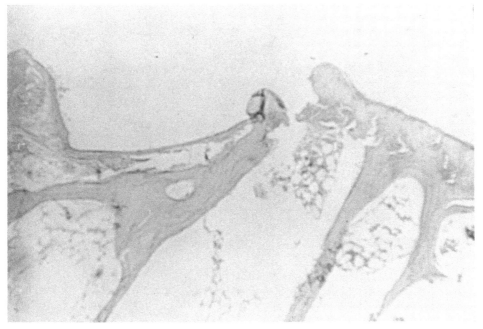

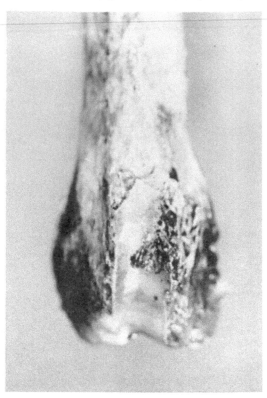

FIG. 20. Photograph of the lower end of the femur of a rabbit whose knee had been immobilized in flexion for a period of 12 weeks following which the rabbit had been allowed to run free for a period of 16 weeks (remobilization series of experiments). Note that the lesion of articular cartilage in the patellar groove is irreversible and that in addition there are lesions of degenerative osteoarthritis.

FIG. 21. Photomicrograph of the lesion of articular cartilage in the patellar groove of the rabbit shown in Fig. 20. There has been no regeneration of articular cartilage in the area of destruction. To the left of the figure there is hypertrophy of the cartilage at the margin of the lesion (chondrophyte formation).

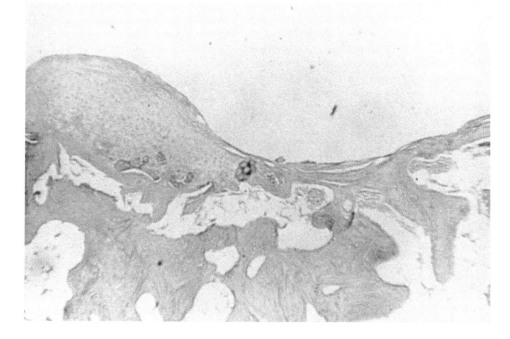

of the lesion also involves early correction of any existing joint deformity that is likely to persist. The prevention of the lesion in rheumatoid arthritis may well involve the early surgical removal of soft tissue panus and certainly involves the restoration or the maintenance of good range of movement.

Dealing with the already established lesion of obliterative degeneration necessitates only that this lesion be recognized and that its significance be appreciated, in order that it may be taken into consideration in deciding the best form of treatment for the deformity.

ACKNOWLEDGMENT

The authors wish to express their gratitude to the Canadian Arthritis and Rheumatism Society for the grant that has made this investigation possible.

REFERENCES

1. SALTER, R. B., and FIELD, P.   The effects of continuous compression on living articular cartilage. J. Bone & Joint Surg. *42-A*: 31 (1960).

The Effect of Papain in Predisposing to Suppurative Arthritis*

JOHN R. MARTIN, M.D.,
JOAN DE VRIES, M.D., and
SEAN MOORE, M.D.

THE OBSERVATION that joints severely damaged by rheumatoid arthritis (1) are liable to become the site of a suppurative arthritis has stimulated interest in the factors that predispose to bacterial arthritis. This susceptibility could be due to changes confined to the joints themselves, a reduction of the body's generalized mechanisms for dealing with infection, or a combination of local and systemic factors. Various aspects of these possibilities were studied by damaging the joints of rabbits and then injecting intravenously an organism which would normally be harmless and observing whether there was any predilection for infection to occur in the damaged joints. In other experiments of a similar nature cortisone was given intramuscularly to lower the animals' generalized resistance to infection.

METHOD AND MATERIAL

The agent used to damage the joint was papain, a proteolytic enzyme which splits chondroitin sulphate from chondromucoprotein in the matrix of cartilaginous structures (2). Its great advantage is that provided the dose is not too large the animal shows no ill effects. A 1 per cent solution was prepared in the manner described by Thomas by dissolving crude papain powder in isotonic saline and passing it through a Seitz filter (3). A freshly prepared supply kept refrigerated was used for each batch of animals.

Albino rabbits. weighing 700–1000 gm., were used since only the cartilage of young animals is susceptible to papain (3).

The organism selected for the production of the infective arthritis was *Escherichia coli* since 0.5–2 c.c. given intravenously does not produce suppurative arthritis in adult rabbits (4).

*From the Montreal General Hospital, Montreal.

RESULTS

It is necessary to stress the purely preliminary nature of this report and that further studies are in progress on the importance of local and general factors in the genesis of suppurative arthritis.

In the first three experiments the papain solution was given intravenously into one of the ear veins and 24 hours later the *E. coli* culture was also injected into one of the ear veins. The procedure and the results are summarized in Tables I to III. In the first experiment (Table I) the positive heart's blood and

TABLE I

2 c.c. 1 per cent papain solution given intravenously to rabbits 1, 2, and 3 only and 2 c.c. *E. coli* culture given intravenously 24 hours later to all rabbits (P, papain-injected animals; C, control animals; +, positive culture; −, negative culture)

Rabbit	Time sacrificed (in hours)	Heart's blood	Knee	Acetabulum
1 (P)	24	+	−	+
2 (P)	48 (died)	+	+ (pus)	
3 (P)	72	−	−	
4 (C)	24	+	+	+
5 (C)	72	−	−	

joint cultures in the papain-injected and control animals probably represent the residium of the bacteraemia arising from the injection of the organisms 24 hours previously. There is some support for this view because at 72 hours the papain-injected and control animals both showed negative heart's blood and knee cultures suggesting that they had been able to dispose of the organisms before they could obtain a foothold. It is of interest that the only example of gross pus in a joint was in a knee of the papain-injected animal that died 48 hours after receiving the *E. coli* inoculum. The same procedure was followed in the second experiment (Table II) but 1 c.c. of the *E. coli* culture was given instead of 2 c.c. The results seem to indicate that the bacteraemia persists for 24 to 48 hours. Since there was only one positive knee culture, it was thought that either the amount of *E. coli* given was insufficient or that the strain was insufficiently virulent. Consequently the experiment was repeated, but using a virulent strain of *E. coli* isolated from a severe human genito-urinary infection. The organisms were so lethal that there were no observable differences between the papain-injected and control animals (Table III).

Since papain by the intravenous route did not cause much destruction in the articular cartilages, it was thought that repeated daily injections of papain into one joint might produce more severe changes. Papain was injected into the right knee and, at the same time, isotonic saline into the left knee (Table IV). In this and subsequent experiments the *E. coli* culture was the same as that

TABLE II

2 c.c. 1 per cent papain solution given intravenously to rabbits
1, 2, 3, and 4 only and 1 c.c. *E. coli* culture given intravenously
24 hours later to all rabbits

Rabbit	Time sacrificed (in hours)	Heart's blood	Knee
1 (P)	24	—	—
2 (P)	24	+	—
3 (P)	48	—	—
4 (P)	72	—	—
5 (C)	24	+	—
6 (C)	24	+	—
7 (C)	48	+	+
8 (C)	72	—	—

TABLE III

2 c.c. 1 per cent papain solution given intravenously to rabbits
1, 2, and 3 only and 1 c.c. *E. coli* culture given intravenously
24 hours later to all rabbits

Rabbit	Time of death (in hours)	Heart's blood	Knee
1 (P)	24	+	+
2 (P)	24	+	+
3 (P)	48	+	+
4 (C)	24	+	+
5 (C)	25	+	+
6 (C)	24	+	+

TABLE IV

1 per cent papain solution injected intra-articularly into right
knee, 0.5 c.c. for 2 days and then 0.25 c.c. for 5 days; 0.85
per cent saline injected into left knee, 0.5 c.c. for 2 days and
then 0.25 c.c. for 5 days; 1 c.c. *E. coli* culture given 24 hours
after last dose of papain and saline

Rabbit	Time sacrificed (in hours)	Heart's blood	Knee Rt.	Knee Lt.
1	72	—	—	—
2	72	—	—	—

used in the first two experiments. The procedure followed was somewhat
similar to that described by Murray (5). A certain amount of the papain
escaped into the systemic circulation because the ears became slightly floppy
and remained so until the animals were sacrificed 72 hours after the injection
of the *E. coli*. The negative cultures could indicate that the organisms had
been destroyed before they could obtain a foothold; but it would be unwise

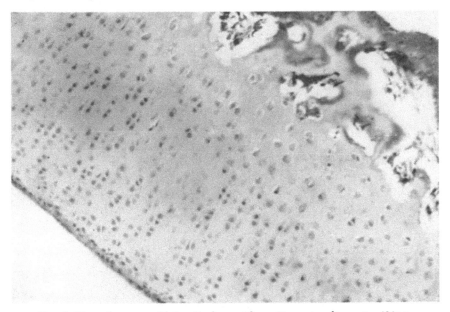

Fɪɢ. 1. Normal young rabbit articular cartilage. Haematoxylin-eosin. 400×.

to derive any conclusions from an experiment in which only two animals survived long enough to receive the *E. coli* inoculum. Sections of the papain- and saline-injected knees show the destructive effects of papain most markedly in the papain-injected knee (Fig. 2). The results of this experiment could indicate that papain injected intra-articularly did not injure the joint sufficiently or that the body's general systemic methods of dealing with infection were so strong that no organisms could obtain a foothold. It was therefore decided to give cortisone at the same time as the papain, which would enhance the animals' sensitivity to the effects of papain (3, 6) and at the same time lower the animals' systemic defences to infection. The procedures and results are summarized in Table V. There was a five-day gap between the last intra-articular injections and the administration of the *E. coli* so that any residual papain and saline would be absorbed from the joints. The dosage of the cortisone was halved after the *E. coli* was given with the hope of reducing the tendency of widespread dissemination of the infective organisms. The combination of intra-articular papain and intramuscular cortisone produced far more devastating effects than in previous experiments. The ears became just as floppy as when papain was given intravenously and the papain-injected knee became unstable with marked crepitus. There were several interesting findings:

1. The speed with which the *E. coli* reached the papain-injected knee in the animal that succumbed one hour after receiving the *E. coli* inoculum.

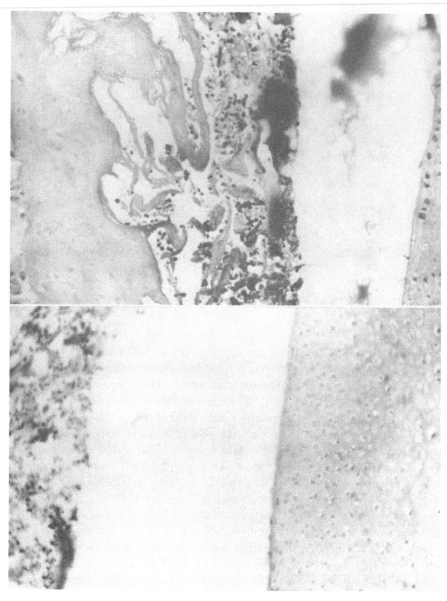

Fig. 2. Sections from the papain (*top*) and saline (*bottom*) injected knees showing loss of basophilia, some cartilaginous destruction as well as an acute inflammation reaction. The changes are more marked in the papain-injected knee. Haematoxylin-eosin. 400×.

TABLE V

1 per cent papain solution injected intra-articularly into right knee, 0.5 c.c. for 3 days and then 0.25 c.c. for 7 days; 0.85 per cent saline injected into left knee, 0.5 c.c., for 3 days and then 0.25 c.c. for 7 days; cortisone, 5 mg. intramuscularly, given daily concurrently for 2 weeks and then 2.5 mg. daily; 1 c.c. *E. coli* culture given intravenously 5 days after last dose of papain and saline

Rabbit	Time of death (in hours)	Heart's blood	Knee		Hip		Elbow		Shoulders		Miscellaneous
			Rt.	Lt.	Rt.	Lt.	Rt.	Lt.	Rt.	Lt.	
1	½	−	−	−							
2	1	+	+	−							
3	36	+	+	−							Septic pericarditis
4	48	+	Pus +	−	−	−	−	−	−	−	
5	60	+	Pus +	+	+						
6	84	−	−	−							
7	96	−	Pus +	−	−	−	Pus +	−	−		
8	96	+	Pus +	Pus +	−	−	Pus +	−	−		Liver abscess; pus in pleura

According to Shaffer it takes 13 hours for pneumococci administered intravenously to rabbits to reach the joint cavity (7).

2. The high percentage of positive heart's blood cultures—five of the eight animals.

3. Excluding the animal that died in half an hour, the higher incidence of positive cultures in the knees of animals injected with papain than in those injected with saline or in the control animals. There was also an impression that the largest amounts of pus were found in the papain-injected knee.

4. It is curious that the elbows of two animals were the only other joints where positive cultures were obtained. This might be ascribed to the fact that weight-bearing joints are the most sensitive to the effects of papain, and perhaps the elbows are more subject to mechanical stresses than the shoulders or hips. Slides from the papain- and saline-injected knees from rabbit 5 show extensive suppuration involving the synovium with pus in the articular cavity as well as marked destruction of the articular cartilages (Fig. 3).

To eliminate the possibility that these results could be due to cortisone alone, the previous experiment was repeated but omitting the papain. The procedure and results are summarized in Table VI. They show a lower incidence of joint infection than in the preceding experiment, indicating that the susceptibility of papain-injected joints to infection is due to the articular changes produced by the papain.

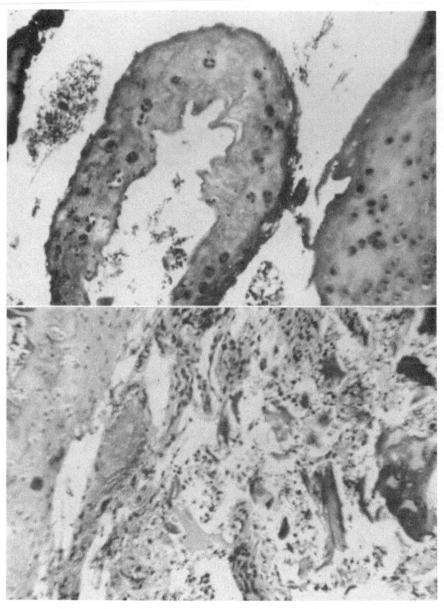

FIG. 3. Sections from the papain- (*top*) and saline- (*bottom*) injected knees demonstrating extensive suppuration in the synovium, pus in the articular cavity, and marked cartilagineous destruction. Haematoxylin-eosin. 400×.

TABLE VI

Cortisone, 5 mg. intramuscularly, given daily for the two weeks before giving *E. coli*, 1 c.c. intravenously. Cortisone then reduced to 2.5 mg. daily

Rabbit	Time sacrificed (in hours)	Heart's blood	Knee		Hip		Elbow		Shoulder		Miscellaneous
			Rt.	Lt.	Rt.	Lt.	Rt.	Lt.	Rt.	Lt.	
1	48	−	+	Pus −	−	−	Pus −	−	−	Pus +	Pleura +
2	72	−	−	−	−	−	−	−	−	−	
3	72	−	−	−	−	−	−	−	−	−	
4	72	−	−	−	−	−	−	−	−	−	
5	96	−	Pus +	−	−	+	−	−	−	−	
6	96	−	−	−	−	+	−	−	−	−	

CONCLUSIONS

1. Injuring a joint with papain does not make it more liable to develop suppurative arthritis.

2. Cortisone lowers the body's mechanisms for coping with infection and also prevents the reconstruction of articular cartilage. For both or one of these reasons, articular suppuration is more apt to occur when the animals are exposed to infection.

Further experiments are in progress to study the variables and to standardize the amounts of papain, cortisone, and *E. coli* which have to be given to produce these interesting results.

REFERENCES

1. KELLGREN, J. H., BALL, J., FAIRBROTHER, R. W., and BARNES, K. L. Brit. Med. J. *1*: 1193 (1958).
2. McCLUSKEY, R. T., and THOMAS, L. J. Exper. Med. *108*: 371 (1958).
3. THOMAS, L. J. Exper. Med. *104*: 245 (1956).
4. CECIL, R., ANGEVINE, D. M., and ROTHBAND, S. Am. J. Med. Sci. *198*: 463 (1939).
5. MURRAY, D. Arth. & Rheum. 7: 211 (1964).
6. McCLUSKEY, R. T., and THOMAS, L. Am. J. Path. *35*: 819 (1959).
7. SHAFFER, M. F., and BENNETT, E. B. J. Exper. Med. *70*: 293 (1939).

Experimental Production of Articular Lesions Resembling Those of the Shwartzman Reaction*

G. GABBIANI† and
R. B. MATHUR

LESIONS resembling those of the generalized Shwartzman reaction can be obtained in the rat by the intravenous administration of an eliciting substance (e.g., carbon particles, lead acetate, ferric chloride) following exposure to stress (1). Local thrombohaemorrhagic lesions are produced if simultaneously with these intravenous treatments adrenaline or noradrenaline is injected subcutaneously to localize the phenomenon at the injection site (2).

The resulting lesions are characterized by the formation of thrombi and haemorrhages in the target organs. Histologically, fibrin deposition can be seen in the glomerular capillaries of the kidneys, heart, lungs, and duodenum and at the site of topical catecholamine administration.

The question then arises whether it might be possible to localize these thrombohaemorrhagic changes in certain joints known clinically and experimentally to be frequent targets of similar phenomena. Forty 100-gm. rats were hence divided into four equal groups and treated as follows.

Group 1 received two consecutive i.v. injections, one of lead acetate (4.5 mg.) and one of ferric chloride (3.5 mg.), both in 1 ml. of water.

Group 2 received the same treatment and, in addition, one injection of noradrenaline (100 µg.) and one of 1 per cent NaCl solution, both in 0.1 ml. of water, in the cavity of the left and right knee joints.

Group 3 received two consecutive i.v. injections, one of cerium chloride (4.5 mg.) and one of ferric chloride (3.5 mg.), both in 1 ml. of water.

Group 4 received the same i.v. treatment as Group 3, plus noradrenaline and NaCl as in Group 2.

The day after the injections, the animals of Groups 1 and 3 appeared normal, while the condition of the animals of Groups 2 and 4 had deteriorated. Diffi-

*From the Institut de Médecine et de Chirurgie expérimentales, Université de Montréal, Montreal.
†Fellow of the Medical Research Council of Canada.

culty in walking due to haemorrhagic lesions in the region of the left knee was observed. The animals were sacrificed and, at autopsy, those of Groups 1 and 3 did not, whereas those of Groups 2 and 4 did, show thrombohaemorrhagic lesions in heart, kidneys, and (particularly pronounced) the left knee, where the quantity of synovial fluid was increased. No changes were observed in the right knee joint.

Histologically, the lesions were seen to be localized in the periarticular connective tissue and in the adjacent muscles, where thrombi, formed principally of fibrin and also of platelets, were noted together with the deposition of an alcian-blue-positive material, probably a mucopolysaccharide.

We can conclude that the joints are particularly sensitive to the production by our experimental means of thrombohaemorrhagic lesions similar to those of the Shwartzman reaction.

ACKNOWLEDGMENT

This work was supported by the Canadian Arthritis and Rheumatism Society.

REFERENCES

1. GABBIANI, G. Sensitization by stress for renal lesions resembling those of generalized Shwartzman phenomenon. Med. exp. (Basel), *11*: 209 (1964).
2. SELYE, H., and TUCHWEBER, B. Ein durch verschiedene Agenzien erzeugbares thrombohemorrhagisches Syndrom. Allergie u. Asthma *10*: 335 (1964).

PART II

The Immunoglobulins

Chairman: Dr. H. A. Smythe, Toronto

Enzymic Fragments of
Human Immunoglobulin*

G. E. CONNELL and
R. H. PAINTER

THE RULES OF NOMENCLATURE to be followed in describing some of our recent studies on human immunoglobulin are shown in Table I. This summary is based mainly on proposals of a committee of the World Health Organization (1) which have already been widely accepted by workers in the field. The term *immunoglobulin* and the abbreviation Ig are used here to describe the whole group of antibody-related proteins, although *gamma* is equally acceptable. The choice of the term immunoglobulin avoids any implication regarding electrophoretic mobility and confusion with earlier systems of nomenclature.

TABLE I

| | | Subunits | |
	Synonyms	Heavy chains	Light chains
HUMAN IMMUNOGLOBULINS			
IgG—Immunoglobulin G	γ_2-globulin, 7S gamma	γ	
IgA—Immunoglobulin A	γ_1A, β_2A	α	κ or λ
IgM—Immunoglobulin M	γ_1M, β_2M	μ	
(IgD)—Immunoglobulin D		δ	
PAPAIN FRAGMENTS			
Fab	S		
Fc	F		

The terms IgG, IgA, IgM, and IgD represent the four principal categories of human immunoglobulins. The last-named, IgD, has been described in two recent publications by Rowe and Fahey (2, 3), and there seems to be little doubt that it should be added to the family as a recognized member. The others, IgG, IgA, and IgM, which were formerly known as γ_2, γ_1A, and γ_1M (among other synonyms), are rather better known. IgG constitutes 80

*From the Department of Biochemistry and Connaught Medical Research Laboratories, University of Toronto, Toronto.

or 85 per cent of the total immunoglobulin of human serum, and has a sedimentation constant of 7S. IgM is the normal macroglobulin, the 19S antibody of normal serum.

The immunoglobulins can be separated into their constituent polypeptide chains by reductive cleavage, and two different kinds of polypeptide chains can be recognized. These are commonly called the heavy chains and the light chains. The different families of immunoglobulins are distinguished fundamentally by the differences in their heavy-chain constitutents, and these have been given a Greek letter corresponding to the name of the parent immunoglobulin, γ for G, α for A, μ for M, and δ for D. There are two kinds of light chains, κ and λ, which are found in all four of the immunoglobulin families.

Human gamma globulin can be split into two kinds of fragments by incubation with papain and a sulphydryl reagent. The fragments were formerly known as S for slow and F for fast, indicating their electrophoretic mobility in agar gel. These are now being called Fab and Fc. Fab can then be taken to mean "Fragment, antigen binding," because this fragment retains the antigen-binding properties of the parent immunoglobulin. Fc can be taken to mean "Fragment, crystallizable," because this fragment crystallizes readily at low ionic strength near neutrality.

The work which is the object of this presentation began about a year and a half ago with an observation that some preparations of immune serum globulin for clinical use* showed instability on prolonged storage. Immune serum globulin is prepared from human serum, by the cold ethanol fractionation procedure of Cohn and his associates (4, 5). It is, in fact, Cohn Fraction II redissolved to give a solution of 16.5 per cent protein in glycine buffer. It is normally stored in solution at 2° C. prior to use, and if this storage is continued for a very long time, one can observe changes in the electrophoretic patterns or, in extreme cases, the formation of a white precipitate. Similar observations have been made by a number of authors, notably Skvaril (6, 7), who used the ultracentrifuge and immunoelectrophoretic techniques to demonstrate the similarity between these changes and those brought about by the action of proteolytic enzymes on immunoglobulin preparations.

The changes in the starch-gel electrophoretic pattern are shown in Fig. 1. At the lower right is a photograph of the pattern after starch-gel electrophoresis in borate buffer at pH 8.6. The upper channels are fresh preparations of immune serum globulin showing the normal distribution of immunoglobulin G. The lowest channel shows a sample after prolonged storage; the pattern becomes extended in the cathode region, and in the anode region one can detect a number of distinct zones. If an acidic buffer at pH 3.6 containing 8M urea is used, quite a different pattern is obtained (upper right). The fresh preparation in the upper channel migrates slowly to the cathode in a

*Prepared by Connaught Medical Research Laboratories, University of Toronto.

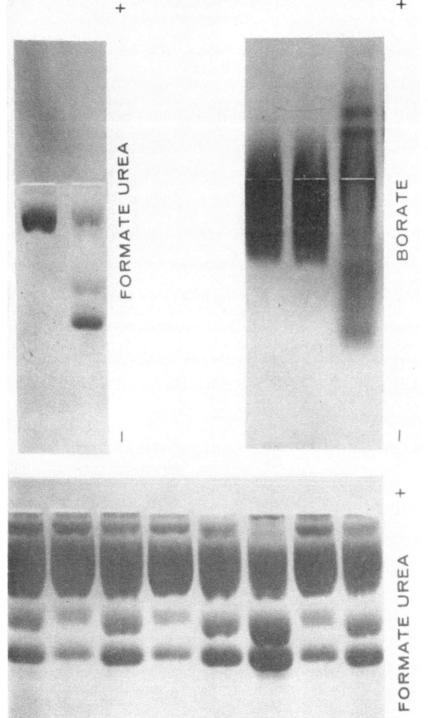

FIG. 1. Starch-gel patterns of fresh and aged immune serum globulin (for details refer to text).

broad zone. The altered preparation shows some residual material at this position, but shows two new zones moving much faster to the cathode.

It was possible to show subsequently that the faster of the two zones corresponds to material moving in the cathode region in the borate gel, and that the slower zone corresponds to the multiple zones in the anode region of the borate gel. The faster component in acid–urea gels is very much like the Fab fragment obtained by papain digestion, while the slower is very much like Fc. It is, in fact, this slower material that forms the precipitate in aged preparations as it crystallizes out of solution. It is proposed that the components of the aged preparation be called N-Fab and N-Fc to indicate their relationship to the papain fragments.

The acid–urea patterns of eight different preparations of immune serum globulin stored for various lengths of time are shown on the left of Fig. 1, and in each sample the two characteristic zones can be seen. In any given preparation the amount of these components can be correlated with age, but the effect of aging is variable from one preparation to the next.

The purification of these two components was undertaken and it was found that the two faster components could be separated from the parent material by gel filtration. On Sephadex G-100 in $0.5M$ NaCl the unaltered IgG was eluted first, and the N-Fab and N-Fc were eluted together in the second peak. The two components were separated from each other by ammonium sulphate fractionation. Fc was precipitated at a saturation of 33 per cent, while Fab was recovered mainly in a fraction between 41 and 60 per cent saturation with ammonium sulphate. The starch-gel electrophoretic patterns of the purified products are shown in Fig. 2.

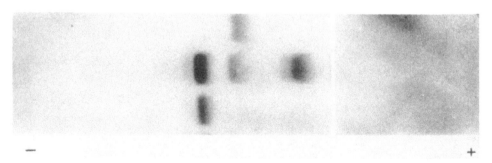

—   +

FIG. 2. Urea–formate starch-gel patterns of aged immune serum globulin (centre) and purified fragments; Fc (upper), Fab (lower).

Speculation at this stage on the cause of the instability resulted in a decision to examine the effect of a number of enzymes, particularly those that might be expected to appear in plasma fractions, to see if they might form similar products. Figure 3 shows what happened when immune serum globulin was incubated at 37° for 24 hours. With no added enzymes present, there was

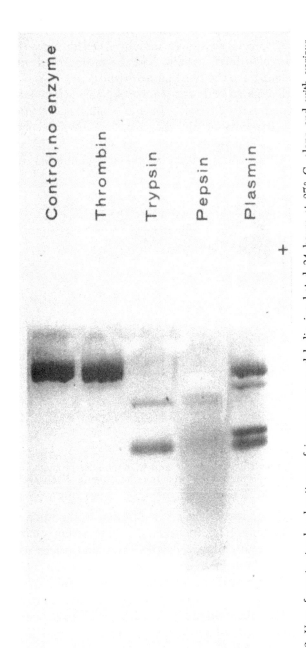

Fig. 3. Urea–formate starch-gel patterns of immune serum globulin incubated 24 hours at 37° C. alone and with various enzymes.

very little change. In the presence of thrombin, again there was no change. Trypsin gave just one of the zones in which we were interested (corresponding to Fab) and another zone of slower mobility. Pepsin, under these conditions, digested IgG much farther than had been observed in the stored preparations; but plasmin gave the two characteristic zones.

Figure 4 shows what happened in a time sequence when immune serum globulin was incubated with plasmin. In the control incubation, with no added plasmin, after four days at 37° the two zones N-Fab and N-Fc were just visible. The same components (called P-Fab and P-Fc) were present in abundance after a few hours with plasmin and could be detected after just one minute.

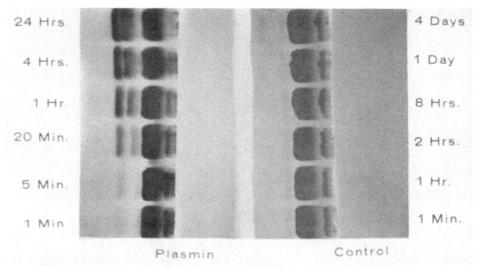

Fig. 4. Urea-formate starch-gel patterns of sequential samples of immune serum globulin incubated at 37° C. in the presence (left) and the absence (right) of plasmin.

A 24-hour plasmin digest was taken and submitted to the same fractionation procedure that had been used for the aged immune serum globulin. In Fig. 5 the fragments isolated after plasmin digestion and those isolated from aged immune serum globulin are compared by starch-gel electrophoresis. P-Fab proved to be identical in mobility with N-Fab, and P-Fc was identical with N-Fc. These fragments have been characterized by other means as well, including ultracentrifugal analysis, molecular-weight determination, amino-acid analysis, antibody activity, and so on, and by all of these methods they appear to be indistinguishable.

The investigation was extended to include the papain fragments. Fab and Fc were isolated by the same procedure that had been used for the other fragments, and were compared with the plasmin material and the material recovered from aged immune serum globulin. In the case of the Fab fragment, it has not been possible to demonstrate any differences between the papain product, the plasmin product, and the aged product. However, the Fc preparations from plasmin and papain digests do differ in their starch-gel electrophoretic patterns at pH 8.6 in the absence of urea (Fig. 6). N-Fc (not shown) and P-Fc show the same series of electrophoretic zones with identical mobilities, but in the pattern produced by the papain Fc material the multiple zones are stepped down in mobility, the slowest zone being absent and at least one extra zone of faster mobility being present.

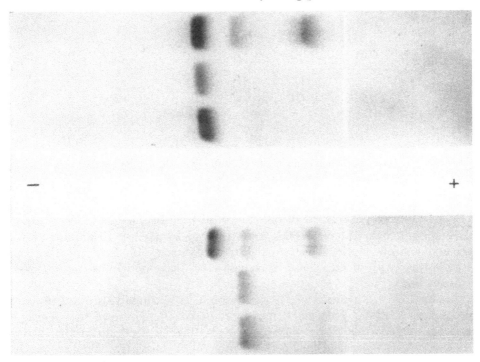

FIG. 5. Comparison of urea–formate starch-gel patterns of natural and plasmin-produced fragments from immune serum globulin. Upper gel: top channel, aged immune serum globulin; centre channel, N-Fab; lower channel, P-Fab. Lower gel: top channel, aged immune globulin; centre channel, N-Fc; lower channel, P-Fc.

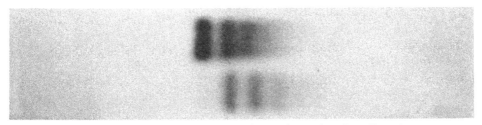

FIG. 6. Borate starch-gel pattern of P-Fc (upper) and Fc (lower).

This then is preliminary evidence that the Fc products from plasmin and from aged immune serum globulin are not identical with the papain fragment. At the present time it is thought that all the Fab fragments are identical.

This may now be put into context with what is known about the structure of IgG. Figure 7 presents a model that is based on several proposals in the current literature (8–10). IgG is equivalent hydrodynamically to a rod-shaped molecule 240 Å long, and elliptical in cross-section, with axes of 57 Å and 19 Å. The molecule consists of two identical halves, with an antigen-combining site on each half, and there is evidence that these two sites are identical in specificity.

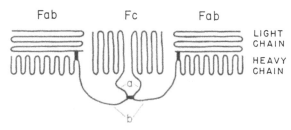

FIG. 7. Schematic model of IgG. Interchain disulphide bonds are represented by short, black bars.

Each half-molecule consists of one heavy polypeptide chain (M.W. 50,000) and one light chain (M.W. 20,000) held together by a single disulphide bond and non-covalent forces. The two half-molecules are also held together by a single disulphide bond. These interchain disulphide bonds are represented by heavy lines.

Putnam (11) has pointed out that γ-globulin is sensitive to several proteolytic enzymes, all of which yield similar products. The nature of the cleavage products suggests that in the native molecule there is a region of the heavy chain which is extremely sensitive to proteolytic enzymes. This region is indicated schematically in the model as an extended region near the middle of the heavy chain in the region of the interchain disulphide bond.

The weight of the evidence suggests that the bonds most sensitive to papain and pepsin are near the point marked *a*, so that cleavage by these enzymes in the absence of a reducing agent would leave the two Fab fragments linked by a disulphide bond. On the other hand, treatment with plasmin (or trypsin) in the absence of a reducing agent generates univalent Fab fragments. This suggests that the latter enzymes must cleave the heavy chain near point *b*, or possibly at both *a* and *b*. This difference between papain and plasmin in the site of attack might be one explanation of the observed differences between Fc and P-Fc.

ACKNOWLEDGMENT

This work was supported in part by grants from the Medical Research Council of Canada and from the Canadian Arthritis and Rheumatism Society.

REFERENCES

1. W.H.O. Bull. *30*: 447 (1964).
2. Rowe, D. S., and Fahey, J. L.   J. Exper. Med. *121*: 171 (1965).
3. ——— J. Exper. Med. *121*: 185 (1965).
4. Cohn, E. J., Strong, L. F., Hughes, W. L. Jr., Mulford, D. F., Ashworth, J. N., Melin, M., and Taylor, H. L.   J. Am. Chem. Soc. *68*: 459 (1946).
5. Oncley, J. L., Melin, M., Richert, D. A., Cameron, J. W., and Gross, P. M. Jr. J. Am. Chem. Soc. *71*: 541 (1949).
6. Skvaril, F. Nature, *185*: 475 (1960).
7. ——— Folio microbiologica (Prague), *5*: 264 (1960).
8. Cohen, S., and Porter, R. R.   Advances Immunol. *4*: 287 (1964).
9. Edelman, G. M., and Gally, J. A., Proc. Nat. Acad. Sci. *51*: 846 (1964).
10. Noelken, M. E., Nelson, C. A., Buckley, C. E. III, and Tanford, C., J. Biol. Chem. *240*: 218 (1965).
11. Putnam, F. W., Easley, C. W., and Lynn, L. T.   Biochem. et biophys. acta *58*: 279 (1962).

Serum and Urinary Gamma Globulins in Rheumatoid Arthritis[*]

DUNCAN A. GORDON,[†]
ARTHUR Z. EISEN,[‡] and
JOHN H. VAUGHAN[§]

THREE and probably four major classes of serum globulins with antibody activities known as immunoglobulins are now recognized in blood serum (1). Approximately 80 per cent of them are 7S γ_2 globulins or γG globulins. Edelman (2) and Fleishman (3) have shown that 7S γG globulins are composed of two types of polypeptide chains which Edelman has called heavy or H chains and light or L chains. The four classes of serum immunoglobulins now termed γG-, γA-, γD-, and γM-globulins[¶] resemble each other in containing antigen configurations corresponding to L chains. It is interesting that normal urinary gamma globulins for the most part have a small molecular weight, and properties like those of the L chains (4). We have been interested in studying these urinary gamma globulins in patients with rheumatoid arthritis (5, 6). The urines of all patients studied have failed to reveal protein by the usual clinical test with suphosalicylic acid.

The method employed by us to isolate urinary gamma globulins has been that of ion-exchange chromatography to absorb protein from urine onto carboxymethylcellulose columns and then to elute selectively the gamma globulins from diethylaminoethylcellulose columns (6).

The electrophoretic properties of isolated urinary material revealed the

[*]From the Department of Medicine, University of Rochester School of Medicine and Dentistry, Rochester, New York. Supported by grants AM 2443 and 8M01 FR-44-03 from the National Institutes of Health.

[†]Medical Research Fellow, Canadian Arthritis and Rheumatism Society. Present address: Wellesley Hospital, Rheumatic Disease Unit, Toronto.

[‡]Buswell Fellow in Medicine, 1961–62; present address: Biology Laboratory, Massachusetts General Hospital, Boston, Mass.

[§]Recipient of Career Research Award, National Institutes of Health.

[¶]Synonyms for the immunoglobulins designated as γG-, γA-, γD-, and γM-globulin in this paper are as follows: γG corresponds to IgG, γ_2, γ_{ss}, or 7S γ globulins; γA corresponds to IgA, γ_1A, or β_2A globulins; γD corresponds to IgD; γM corresponds to IgM, γ_1M, β_2M, or 19S γ globulins.

same broad mobility as normal serum gamma globulin, in contrast with the narrow electrophoretic bands characteristic of Bence-Jones proteins.

Immunoelectrophoresis of the isolated urinary protein revealed a main double arc of precipitation, which corresponded to the gamma-globulin components resembling L chains. A faintly doubled arc, due to a small amount of protein having the immunochemical characteristics of 7S γG-globulin or of free H chains, was also seen. It was possible to isolate urinary L chains free from 7S or H chains by chromatography on Sephadex G-100 in distilled water or in 1N acetic acid. Immunodiffusion of this sephadexed material (γ-u) is illustrated in Fig. 1. Anti-γ G is in the centre well and two bands are revealed, one of which shares antigenic determinants with Bence-Jones type 1 (kappa) protein and the other with Bence-Jones type 2 (lambda) protein. The fusion and spurring of the urine gamma globulins with 7S gamma globulin is in keeping with the fact that L chains have some, but not all, of the antigenic configurations present in whole 7S gamma globulins.

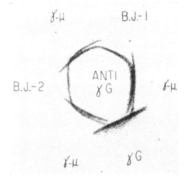

Fɪɢ 1. Immunodiffusion of urinary L Chains (γ-u) from Sephadex G-100 chromatography in distilled water with γ G-globulins and with types 1 and 2 Bence-Jones proteins.

Chromatography of the urinary gamma globulins on Sephadex G-100 in dilute salt gave the separation exhibited in Fig. 2. The late peak did not have the spectrophotometric properties of proteins or nucleic acids and is probably due to urinary pigment. The nature of the material present in the early and peak portions of the major peak is shown in Fig. 3. Anti-γ G is in both centre wells. On the right, a pattern indicating that the forerunning shoulder of the chromatogram was 7S γG-globulin is seen. Material from the height of the major peak exhibited heavy lines having partial identity with 7S gamma globulin. These heavy lines failed to appear in a diffusion with an antiserum reacting with H chains and are, therefore, what would be expected of L chains.

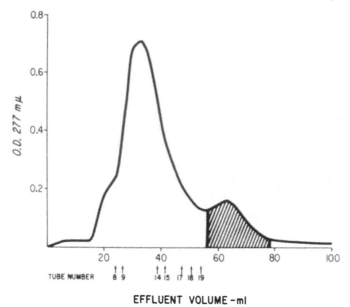

FIG. 2. Gel filtration on Sephadex G-100 of urinary γ-globulin in 0.15M NaCl.

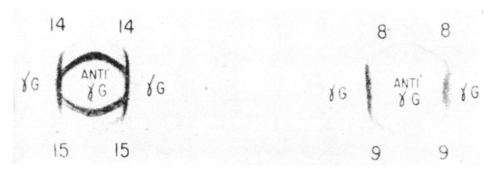

FIG. 3. Immunodiffusion of early and middle zone fractions obtained from Sephadex G-100 chromatography of urinary γ-globulins (Fig. 2).

Interest in the metabolic significance of the urinary gamma globulins has centred on whether they are a reflection of gamma-globulin synthesis or gamma-globulin breakdown. When Franklin administered I[131]-labelled 7S gamma globulin intravenously, he obtained data suggesting that most of the urinary gamma globulin with small molecular weight could be accounted for on the basis of 7S gamma-globulin breakdown (7). Stevenson, using I[131] 7S gamma globulin and immunochemical precipitation of urine protein, thought rather that the small urinary gamma globulin was an anabolic product in gamma-globulin metabolism (8). This uncertainty led us to analyse the question independently by *in vivo* administration of C¹⁴-labelled amino acid, tracing its incorporation into urine and serum components, much as Putnam had with Bence-Jones and myeloma proteins (9).

Our study was performed on identical 51-year-old twins. The rheumatoid twin had had arthritis for many years, while the normal twin was in good health. They were identical by many blood groupings and two years before the study the arthritic twin had accepted a skin graft from her sister.

Each twin received 100 μc. of C¹⁴ L-leucine intravenously (Fig. 4 demonstrates the incorporation of amino acid into the urine and serum gamma-globulin components). The specific activity is expressed as disintegrations per minute per optical density of protein (DPM/O.D.). The urine specific activity appears earlier, is greater, and falls off more rapidly compared with the appearance in serum 7S gamma globulin. The arthritic twin and the normal twin had the same patterns, but there was generally a higher level of activity in the proteins of the arthritic than in her sister.

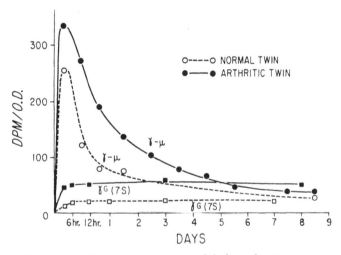

Fig. 4. Radioactivity in gamma globulins after intravenous administration of labelled amino acid to normal and arthritic twins.

In two other patients with rheumatoid arthritis, it was possible by Sephadex separation in distilled water, and in another by using 1N acetic acid, to show during the 6-hour and 12-hour intervals that the L-chain component of the urinary gamma globulins contained most, but not all, of the radioactivity.

The data from these experiments indicate that urinary gamma globulins are probably not generally degradation products of 7S gamma globulin, thus supporting the view that urinary gamma-globulin components represent some phase in the anabolism of 7S gamma globulins and may be a reflection of the over-all rate of gamma-globulin synthesis by the body. A survey was, therefore, made of the amounts of gamma globulin excreted in 24-hour urine collections from a variety of persons. In no case was enough urine protein present to be detectable by the sulphosalicylic acid test. Quantitation of urinary gamma globulin was obtained by recording the total optical density recovered in the chromatographic isolation method. The amount of gamma globulin recovered in the urine for 24-hour periods in normal subjects ranged from 1.5 to 7.0 optical density (O.D.) units, which corresponds approximately to 1–5 mg. of protein per 24 hours.

Figure 5 gives the value of the gamma-globulin excretion in 24 hours for a number of individuals. The values from normal persons are on the left, those from patients with rheumatoid arthritis (R) are in the centre, and those from patients with asthma (A), osteomyelitis (O), and serum sickness (S) are on the right.

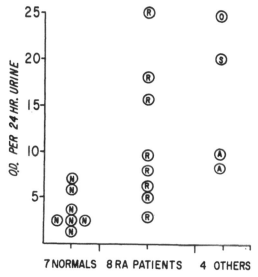

Fig. 5. Amounts of urinary γ-globulin excretion from a variety of persons.

Three pairs of twins discordant for rheumatoid arthritis were available for study. It can be seen in Fig. 6 that the arthritic member of the pair in each instance exhibited a larger value for gamma-globulin excretion in 24 hours than did the normal twin. The pair with the greatest difference was the one studied by radioleucine. In the twins with the least difference in total urinary gamma globulins, the clinical activity of the arthritic twin was minimal.

Thus, there is an increased 24-hour excretion of gamma globulins in patients with rheumatoid arthritis and certain other conditions, even though this increased excretion is not detectable by the clinical laboratory methods usually used for the demonstration of proteinura. The serum gamma-globulin level was elevated in only one of the foregoing patients, the one with osteo-myelitis.

The patient with the highest urinary level was a 51-year-old farmer's wife (L.Ro.) with rheumatoid arthritis of 4 years' duration. She was admitted to the hospital because of pain and bilateral foot and wrist nerve palsies. A calf-muscle biopsy showed flagrant arteritis. The latex titre was elevated, but lupus-erythematosus (LE) and antinuclear-factor (ANF) tests were negative.

On January 6, therapy with 6-mercaptopurine (6-MP) was initiated to suppress gamma-globulin production (see Fig. 7). High initial urinary gamma-globulin values underwent a prompt but moderate decrease with 6-MP therapy. The administration of 6-MP was discontinued because of leucopenia, and a rise in urinary gamma globulin was observed. On January 28 the dose

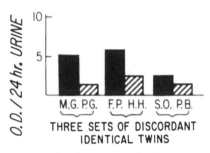

Fig. 6. Amounts of urinary γ-globulin excretion from three pairs of identical twins discordant for rheumatoid arthritis.

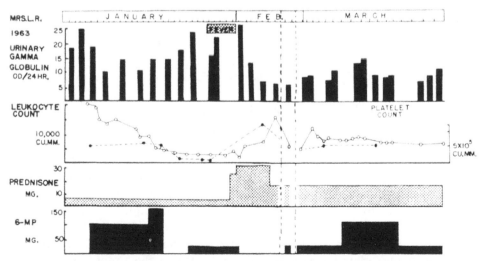

Fig. 7. Effect of 6-mercaptopurine (6-MP) and prednisone on quantity of urinary gamma globulins in a patient (L.Ro.) with rheumatoid arthritis complicated by vasculitis.

of prednisone was increased because of fever, and again a prompt but more profound drop in urinary gamma globulin was seen. A maintenance dose of 6-MP and an increased dose of prednisone were then instituted. A gradual escape was noted. Increased 6-MP again resulted in decreased urinary gamma globulin. The patient was discharged, with a continuation of 6-MP and prednisone prescribed. Thereafter she remained improved at home for the next five months until a rise in the serum transaminase level forced discontinuance of the 6-MP. At no time was her normal serum gamma-globulin level or elevated latex titre appreciably altered by therapy.

The second patient (D.We.) was a 54-year-old woman who had rheumatoid arthritis for 13 years. Her arthritis was complicated by progressive episcleritis and scleromalacia, recurrent pleural effusions, nail fold thrombi, small vasculitic nodules on the fingers, and sensory neuropathy. She had been taking a varying dosage of cortisone for 10 years and was receiving prednisone, 20 mg. daily, and salicylates, 2.0 G. daily, at the time of admission to the metabolic

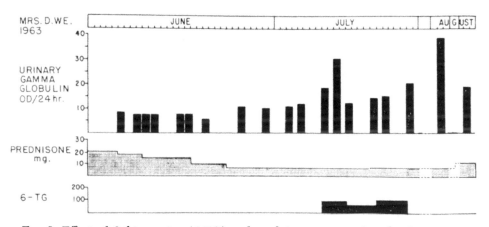

FIG. 8. Effect of 6-thioguanine (6-TG) and prednisone on quantity of urinary gamma globulins in a patient (D.We.) with rheumatoid arthritis complicated by vasculitis.

ward. Her latex titre had been 1:640. LE and ANF tests were negative. She was treated in the same manner as the previous patient (see Fig. 8). Her prednisone dosage was gradually decreased so that after 18 days she was taking 7.5 mg. daily. An increase in urine gamma globulin from 6–10 O.D. units to 30 O.D. units was observed with this reduction in corticosteriod dosage. When 100 mg. daily of 6-thioguanine (6-TG) was initiated, a decrease in urine gamma globulin to 12–14 O.D. units occurred. Although the white blood count and platelets were unaffected by 6-TG, this drug had to be discontinued because of gastro-intestinal symptoms. Two weeks after discontinuation of 6-TG, the urine gamma globulin was 28 O.D. units. When the prednisone dosage was increased to 10 mg. daily, a decrease in urine gamma globulin was again noted.

The concept that urinary L chains reflect some phase of gamma-globulin synthesis is supported by this study. While it is possible that some L chains are formed from gamma-globulin breakdown, it is unlikely that this can account for a very large proportion of the total excretion. One of our patients (F.Fl.) with agammaglobulinaemia was on replacement therapy with gamma globulin and had 7S γ G-globulin demonstrable in his urine, but no detectable free L chains. The finding, therefore, of small amounts of free L chains in normal serum (as well as in cerebrospinal fluid) permits one to consider that the urinary L chains are derived from the serum, probably by normal glomerular filtration.

Work by Edelman and Gally (10) suggests that L chains and H chains are manufactured separately in the cell and then assembled to form variously γG-, γA-, γD-, or γM-globulins. It also seems possible that L chains may escape from the assemblage process and appear in the serum and then in the urine. If this were the case, urinary L chains might have significance as a reflection of over-all gamma-globulin synthesis. Nevertheless, increased gamma-globulin excretion may reflect not only increased synthesis, but also any physiological or pathological increase in permeability of the kidneys to proteins in general.

Current studies with quantitative immunodiffusion techniques in Dr. Vaughan's laboratory indicate that even in patients with apparently normal kidneys there is often a significant increase in albuminuria concomitant with increased gamma globulinuria (11). Consequently, the hope that measurement of the quantity of L chains in the urine can be used as a reflection of the over-all rate of gamma-globulin synthesis seems unlikely to be fulfilled.

In conclusion, we believe that the foregoing observations support the notion that gamma globulins of small molecular weight in the urine are a reflection of some phase of gamma-globulin synthesis. Whether the change in the quantity of gamma globulinuria reflects a change in the rate of synthesis of the gamma globulins, or of the permeability of the kidney to proteins in general, is not entirely clear.

REFERENCES

1. Editorial, The immunoglobulins. New England J. Med. *272:* 376 (1965).
2. Edelman, G. M., and Benaceraff, B. On structural and functional relations between antibodies and proteins of the gamma system. Proc. Nat. Acad. Sci. *48:* 1035 (1962).
3. Fleishman, J. B., Pain, R. H., and Porter, R. R. Reduction of gamma globulin. Arch. Biochem., suppl. *1:* 174–80 (1962).
4. Berggard, I., and Edelman, G. M. Normal counterparts to Bence Jones proteins: Free L. polypeptide chains of human gamma globulin. Proc. Nat. Acad. Sci. *49:* 330 (1963).

5. GORDON, D. A., EISEN, A. Z., and VAUGHAN, J. H.   Serum and urinary gamma globulins in rheumatoid arthritis. Tr. A. Am. Physicians, 76: 222 (1963).

6. GORDON, D. A., EISEN, A. Z., and VAUGHAN, J. H.   Studies on urinary γ-globulins in patients with rheumatoid arthritis. Arth. & Rheum. 9: 579 (1966).

7. FRANKLIN, E. C.   Physicochemical and immunological studies of gamma globulin of normal human urine. J. Clin. Invest. 38: 2159 (1959).

8. STEVENSON, G. T.   Further studies of the gamma related proteins of normal urine. J. Clin. Invest. 41: 1190 (1962).

9. PUTNAM, F. W., and MIYAKE, A.   Proteins in multiple myeloma, VIII. Biosynthesis of abnormal proteins. J. Biol. Chem. 231: 671 (1958).

10. EDELMAN, G. M., and GALLY, J. A.   A model for the 7S antibody molecule. Proc. Nat. Acad. Sci. 51: 846 (1964).

11. VAUGHAN, J. H., and MARCHETTI, W. J.   Heavy chains components in urinary gamma globulins (in press).

Evidence of Abnormalities in the General Metabolism of Amino Acids in Rheumatoid Arthritis and Ankylosing Spondylitis*

JOSEPH J. B. ARMSTRONG,†
DOUGLAS BOCKING, and
JOHN B. DERRICK

NUMEROUS REPORTS in the literature have indicated that there may be differences in the amino-acid metabolism between normal individuals and those with rheumatoid arthritis (1–15). Much of the work, however, including some of our own (16, 17), has been incomplete because of the lack of accurate, rapid techniques for the separation and quantitative estimation of the amino acids present in biological fluids. With the availability of improved ion-exchange chromatographic techniques for the determination of all of the nin-hydrin-reactive compounds present in plasma and urine (18–20) it has become possible to re-evaluate previous findings and to investigate the problem further.

The present investigation was undertaken in an attempt to establish firmly such qualitative or quantitative differences as may exist between normal individuals and those with rheumatoid arthritis in their plasma levels of all the individual free amino acids and in their urinary levels of all the individual amino acids, in both the free and the bound forms.

As far as we are aware, no reports have appeared to date on the meta-bolism of amino acids in ankylosing spondylitis, a disease considered by some

*From the Departments of Biochemistry and Medical Research, Faculty of Medicine, University of Western Ontario and Westminster Hospital, Department of Veterans' Affairs, London, Ontario.

Based on a thesis submitted for the degree of Doctor of Philosophy by J.J.B.A. to the Department of Biochemistry, Faculty of Medicine, University of Western Ontario.

This work was supported by a grant from the Canadian Arthritis and Rheumatism Society.

†Present address: Department of Biochemistry, University of Toronto, Toronto.

investigators as a variant of rheumatoid arthritis, and by others as a separate entity (21). In view of these facts, an investigation has also been undertaken to determine whether any qualitative or quantitative differences exist between normal individuals and those with ankylosing spondylitis in their plasma levels of free amino acids or in their urinary excretion patterns of amino acids in both the free and the bound forms. Also, it was felt that a comparison of the amino-acid levels in persons with rheumatoid arthritis and ankylosing spondylitis would be of interest.

METHODS

The groups studied consisted of six normal males with no arthritic involvement (average age, 36 years), six males with clinically diagnosed rheumatoid arthritis (average age, 52 years), and six males with ankylosing spondylitis (average age, 42 years). The subjects were ambulant and they were encouraged to pursue their regular daily routine of activity. The dietary histories of all subjects were reviewed by a dietitian for adequacy with regard to protein, carbohydrate, and vitamin intake and the subjects were carefully screened with respect to their dietary habits. Only individuals conforming to a normal dietary pattern were chosen for the study.

The arthritic patients investigated had clinically active disease and, prior to the collection of urine specimens, had received no anti-inflammatory drugs for a period of at least three days. Twenty-four-hour urine collections were made commencing at 11.30 A.M. The urine was refrigerated during the collection period, and 6 ml. of toluene and 6 ml. of chloroform were put in the container as preservatives. Heparanized venous blood samples were taken 3½ hours post-prandially (i.e., 11.30 A.M.) on the morning that the urine collection was completed.

The blood was centrifuged and the plasma removed and processed within 30 minutes after withdrawal. The plasma was deproteinized with picric acid and subsequently processed by the method of Stein and Moore (22). Urine specimens were treated to remove excess ammonia (23), were quick-frozen, and stored at $-20°$ C. until analysed. Hydrolysis of urine samples was carried out by the procedure of Block (24), using formic and hydrochloric acids.

The amino-acid analyses were performed, using the cation-exchange resin and the automatic recording apparatus of Spackman, Moore, and Stein (18, 19), as modified by Piez and Morris (20).* Twenty-five amino acids and ninhydrin-reactive compounds could be resolved and estimated in the plasma. Lysine and 1-methylhistidine elute together and appear as a single peak. In plasma, however, the concentration of 1-methylhistidine is negligible compared with that of lysine (22), and, therefore, the single peak was calculated as lysine. Glutamine is largely decomposed to glutamic acid (85%) under

*Technicon Chromatography Corporation, Chauncey, New York.

the conditions of this method, probably as a result of the high starting temperature (60° C.) of the column. Therefore, the glutamic-acid levels determined
here actually represent this amino acid plus 85 per cent of the glutamine
present.

Urine samples were analysed for both "free" and "bound" amino acids. The
level of an amino acid following hydrolysis of the urine minus the
level in unhydrolyzed urine is referred to hereafter as the "bound" level
of the particular amino acid, i.e., the amount of the amino acid excreted in
conjugated form or in the form of peptides and/or proteins. Thirty-five
identifiable amino acids and other ninhydrin-reactive compounds could be
resolved. In the case of the urine analyses, the concentrations of lysine and
1-methylhistidine had to be expressed as the sum of two compounds, since,
unlike the situation in plasma, the level of 1-methylhistidine is not negligible in
urine (23, 25, 26). On the other hand, conversion of glutamine to glutamic
acid is of less importance in the urine analysis since glutamine excretion is
usually very low (23).

RESULTS

RHEUMATOID ARTHRITIS

Table I shows the comparative concentrations of 25 amino acids and ninhydrin-reactive compounds present in the plasma of normal subjects and
those with rheumatoid arthritis. While no qualitative differences between the
two groups were evident, significant differences ($P = 0.05$ or less) were
apparent in the concentration of seven amino acids in the plasma of the two
groups. The subjects with rheumatoid arthritis had significantly more aspartic acid and taurine, and significantly less threonine, methionine, histidine,
3-methylhistidine, and arginine in their plasma than did the normal subjects.
Glutamic acid, cystine, and ornithine levels were generally above normal in
the plasma of subjects with rheumatoid arthritis and lysine (plus 1-methylhisti-
dine), alanine, glycine, and serine levels were lower. Although some of the
observed differences are not statistically significant, they are, in our opinion,
sufficiently great to be of interest and to warrant comment. Throughout this
study, where such differences are apparent, they will, therefore, be com-
mented upon.

In Table II the urinary excretions of 31 amino acids and ninhydrin-reactive
compounds by the two groups are compared. Again no qualitative differences
between normal subjects and those with rheumatoid arthritis were evident. Of
the nine free amino acids and other ninhydrin-reactive compounds in which
the quantities excreted differed significantly from normal, aspartic acid and
glutamic acid were excreted in greater amounts by the group with rheumatoid
arthritis and threonine, serine, alanine, cystine, valine, lysine, and 1-methyl-
histidine, histidine, and 3-methylhistidine were excreted in small quantities.
As in the plasma, trends differing from the normal were also apparent for

TABLE I

THE PLASMA CONCENTRATIONS OF FREE AMINO ACIDS IN NORMAL SUBJECTS AND SUBJECTS WITH RHEUMATOID ARTHRITIS (MG./100 ML.)

Amino acid	Normal subjects	Subjects with rheumatoid arthritis	P
Taurine	0.67±0.033*	1.14±0.143	<0.010†
Hydroxyproline	0.02±0.009	0.01±0.005	
Aspartic acid	0.03±0.007	0.41±0.095	<0.005
Threonine	1.92±0.180	1.07±0.233	<0.020
Serine	0.88±0.028	0.74±0.097	
Glutamic acid	3.56±0.806	6.80±1.470	
Citrulline	0.32±0.039	0.26±0.020	
Proline	2.36±0.256	2.10±0.479	
Glycine	1.54±0.084	1.35±0.053	
Alanine	4.01±0.314	2.92±0.427	
Cystine	0.72±0.224	1.09±0.123	
α-NH$_2$-n-butyric acid	0.14±0.015	0.10±0.031	
Valine	2.23±0.099	2.41±0.227	
Methionine	0.14±0.022	0.06±0.023	<0.050
Isoleucine	0.58±0.054	0.67±0.087	
Leucine	1.08±0.048	1.24±0.148	
Tyrosine	0.78±0.068	0.75±0.113	
Phenylalanine	0.68±0.061	0.86±0.105	
β-NH-isobutyric acid	0.14±0.109	0.01±0.001	
Ethanolamine	0.02±0.005	0.02±0.007	
Ornithine	0.63±0.065	0.77±0.108	
Lysine	1.83±0.288	1.35±0.160	
Histidine	1.14±0.143	0.50±0.241	<0.050
3-Methylhistidine	0.05±0.008	0.04±0.010	<0.050
Arginine	0.92±0.156	0.39±0.097	<0.024
TOTAL	26.12±1.24	27.05±2.26	

*Mean plasma concentration ± standard error of the mean.
†P value for comparison of levels between normal and rheumatoid arthritic subjects.

several other amino acids. More taurine, ornithine, β-alanine, β-NH$_2$-isobutyric acid (BAIB),* and arginine are excreted by the group with rheumatoid arthritis and less methionine and glycine.

The pattern of differences for the free amino acids in the urines of the two groups is reflected in the total excretion of each of the amino acids, determined after hydrolysis of the urine. Possible exceptions are glutamic and aspartic acids, in which the total excretions by the rheumatoid arthritics were lower, although not significantly so, in spite of the fact that significantly more of these amino acids were excreted in the free state by these individuals than by the normal subjects.

The urinary excretion of the individual "bound" (hydrolysed minus free) amino acids by the normal subjects and those with rheumatoid arthritis was calculated. The only apparent significant difference was a lower excretion of

*The higher average excretion of BAIB by those with rheumatoid arthritis is due to the fact that one of the patients is a "BAIB-excreter." Some 10 per cent of the population excrete large amounts of this amino acid (26).

TABLE II

Comparison of the Urinary Excretion of Free and Total Amino Acids by Normal Subjects[*] and Subjects with Rheumatoid Arthritis[†]
(MG./24 HR.)

Amino acid	Free			Total		
	Normal subjects	Subjects with rheumatoid arthritis	P	Normal subjects	Subjects with rheumatoid arthritis	P
Taurine	148±37.4‡	186±42.6		128±18.1	189±51.2	
Hydroxyproline	0±0.0	0±0.0		24±5.4	37±4.7	
Aspartic acid	3±0.7	7±1.0	<0.005§	237±42.2	185±29.5	
Asparagine + glutamine	76±11.7	53±12.9		0±0.0	0±0.0	
Threonine	44±4.3	14±2.3	<0.001	61±5.0	43±8.9	
Serine	56±1.3	20±4.0	<0.001	79±4.5	42±7.2	<0.005
Glutamic acid	12±2.8	30±4.5	<0.010	574±48.2	484±43.3	
Citrulline	2±0.5	1±0.5		4±0.7	1±0.3	<0.050
α-NH$_3$-adipic acid	3±1.0	1±0.4		8±2.3	3±0.9	
Proline	0±0.0	0±0.0		75±4.1	81±7.3	
Glycine	151±14.5	115±18.2		830±92.6	585±92.0	
Alanine	48±5.1	31±5.0	<0.050	109±10.1	80±8.4	
Cystine	37±3.9	21±3.8	<0.025	75±14.1	68±9.6	
α-NH$_2$-n-butyric acid	6±2.0	3±0.6		9±1.5	3±0.4	<0.005
Valine	6±0.4	5±0.3	<0.025	33±3.9	35±4.5	
Methionine	6±1.2	3±0.8		6±0.6	3±0.7	<0.005
Isoleucine	8±1.6	7±0.7		14±1.1	13±1.4	
Leucine	6±0.6	5±0.7		31±3.9	32±5.4	
Tyrosine	29±4.0	24±1.9		54±5.2	51±5.4	
Phenylalanine	17±2.6	16±2.5		25±1.6	24±2.3	
β-Alanine	6±2.6	7±2.0		20±5.0	15±2.8	
β-NH$_2$-isobutyric acid	12±2.0	32±14.2		13±2.0	31±13.4	
γ-NH$_2$-n-butyric acid	2±0.7	1±0.3		15±1.6	13±1.9	
Ethanolamine	24±3.3	20±2.9		25±4.0	24±3.1	
Ornithine	7±2.3	16±5.7		12±4.4	18±4.3	
Lysine + 1-methylhistidine	135±12.6	69±10.5	<0.005	186±13.2	114±21.2	<0.020
Histidine	280±23.8	180±77.4	<0.025	314±21.2	218±32.4	<0.050
3-Methylhistidine	59±4.6	32±1.7	<0.001	134±36.2	67±7.1	<0.050
Arginine	14±5.2	21±6.8		40±4.9	31±6.5	
TOTAL	1195±51.2	920±41.4	<0.005	3129±198.4	2486±167.6	<0.050

*Total nitrogen excretion by the normal subjects (gm./24 hr.) = 9.91 ± 1.02.
†Total nitrogen excretion by rheumatoid arthritic subjects (gm./24 hr.) = 9.72 ± 0.95.
‡Mean 24-hour excretion level ± standard error of the mean.
§P value for comparison of levels between normal and rheumatoid arthritic subjects.

arginine in the bound form. The sum total excretion of bound amino acids is not significantly different in the two groups, although there does appear to be a tendency towards lower total excretion levels by the group with rheumatoid arthritis.

The differences between the two groups are summarized in Table III, where the amino acids have been grouped according to whether the levels were above or below normal. In the majority of cases, when an amino-acid concentration is different from the normal in the plasma, the urine content of the

TABLE III

SUMMARY OF QUANTITATIVE DIFFERENCES FROM NORMAL IN THE AMINO ACIDS OF THE PLASMA AND URINE OF SUBJECTS WITH RHEUMATOID ARTHRITIS

| | Urine | |
Plasma	Before hydrolysis	After hydrolysis
BELOW NORMAL		
Threonine*	Threonine	Threonine
Histidine	Histidine	Histidine
3-Methylhistidine	3-Methylhistidine	3-Methylhistidine
Methionine	Methionine	Methionine
Lysine +	Lysine +	Lysine +
1-methylhistidine	1-methylhistidine	1-methylhistidine
Alanine	Alanine	Alanine
Glycine	Glycine	Glycine
Serine	Serine	Serine
	Valine	
	Cystine	Cystine
Arginine		
	α-NH$_2$-butyric acid	α-NH$_2$-n-butyric acid
ABOVE NORMAL		
Cystine		
Taurine	Taurine	Taurine
Aspartic acid	Aspartic acid	
Glutamic acid	Glutamic acid	
Ornithine	Ornithine	Ornithine
		Hydroxyproline

*Amino acids that are underlined are those that are significantly different from normal ($P < 0.050$); the remainder show marked trends from normal.

amino acid (either free, total, or both) also differs from the normal in the same direction. Cystine is the noteworthy exception in that it tends to be above the normal level in the plasma of rheumatoid arthritics and to be excreted by them in the free state in amounts significantly less than normal.

ANKYLOSING SPONDYLITIS

The concentrations of 25 amino acids and ninhydrin-reactive compounds present in the plasma of normal subjects and those with ankylosing spondylitis are listed in Table IV. No qualitative differences between the two groups were observed in the chromatographic profiles. However, statistically significant quantitative differences ($P = 0.05$ or less) were observed in the concentrations of nine amino acids in the plasma of the two groups; the levels of taurine, hydroxyproline, aspartic acid, glutamic acid, isoleucine, leucine, tyrosine, and phenylalanine were significantly higher in the plasma of the

TABLE IV

PLASMA LEVELS OF FREE AMINO ACIDS IN NORMAL SUBJECTS AND THOSE WITH
ANKYLOSING SPONDYLITIS (MG./100 ML.)

Amino acid	Normal subjects	Spondylitics	P
Taurine	0.67±0.033*	1.26±0.126	<0.001†
Hydroxyproline	0.02±0.009	0.29±0.110	<0.050
Aspartic acid	0.03±0.007	0.40±0.032	<0.001
Threonine	1.92±0.180	1.56±0.092	
Serine	0.88±0.028	1.00±0.087	<0.020
Citrulline	0.32±0.039	0.48±0.071	
Proline	2.36±0.256	2.57±0.349	
Glycine	1.54±0.084	1.30±0.145	
Alanine	4.01±0.314	2.73±0.200	<0.010
Cystine	0.72±0.224	0.87±0.130	
α-NH$_2$-n-butyric acid	0.14±0.015	0.19±0.022	
Valine	2.23±0.099	2.57±0.170	
Methionine	0.14±0.022	0.15±0.075	
Isoleucine	0.58±0.054	0.81±0.059	<0.020
Leucine	1.08±0.048	1.47±0.102	<0.010
Tyrosine	0.78±0.068	1.10±0.059	<0.010
Phenylalanine	0.68±0.061	0.91±0.084	<0.050
β-NH$_2$-isobutyric acid	0.14±0.109	0.21±0.205	
Ethanolamine	0.02±0.005	0.04±0.019	
Ornithine	0.63±0.065	0.86±0.144	
Lysine	1.83±0.288	1.93±0.276	
Histidine	1.14±0.143	1.10±0.228	
3-Methylhistidine	0.05±0.008	0.05±0.008	
Arginine	0.92±0.156	0.84±0.132	
TOTAL	26.12±1.24	31.64±1.56	<0.025

*Mean plasma concentration ± standard error of the mean.
†P for comparison of levels between normal and spondylitic subjects.

spondylitic subjects, while the level of alanine was significantly lower. The levels of the remaining amino acids were essentially comparable in the two groups. The total plasma level of amino acids was significantly greater in the spondylitic than in the normal individuals.

In Table V the urinary excretion of 31 amino acids and ninhydrin-reactive compounds by the two groups has been compared. Again, no qualitative differences between the normal and the spondylitic groups were observed.

TABLE V

Comparison of the Urinary Excretion of Free, Total, and Bound Amino Acids by Normal Individuals and Those with Ankylosing Spondylitis (mg./24 hr.)

Amino acid	Free (before hydrolysis)			Total (after hydrolysis)			Bound (total − free)		
	Normal subjects	Spondylitics	P†	Normal subjects	Spondylitics	P	Normal subjects	Spondylitics	P
Taurine	148±37.4*	111±33.6		128±18.1	133±35.1		—	21±22.3	
Hydroxyproline	0±0.0	0±0.0		24±4.5	54±13.6		24±5.4	54±13.6	
Aspartic acid	3±0.7	6±3.2		237±42.2	180±22.0		234±42.0	174±21.3	
Asparagine + glutamine	76±11.7	57±3.6		0±0.0	0±0.0				
Threonine	44±4.3	30±4.9		61±5.0	42±4.8	<0.025	18±4.3	12±3.5	
Serine	56±1.3	36±6.7	<0.020	79±4.5	52±6.5	<0.020	22±4.2	17±3.8	
Glutamic acid	12±2.8	23±9.9		574±48.2	475±41.6		563±49.3	452±36.6	
Citrulline	2±0.5	1±0.7		3±0.7	1±0.1		1±0.9	1±0.6	
α-NH₂-adipic acid	3±1.0	3±0.5		8±2.3	4±1.4		4±2.1		
Proline	0±0.0	0±0.0		75±4.1	71±7.7		75±4.1	71±7.7	
Glycine	151±14.5	150±40.8		830±92.6	660±77.6		680±93.9	510±69.1	
Alanine	48±5.1	29±3.4	<0.020	109±10.0	60±5.1	<0.005	61±7.2	32±3.6	<0.005
Cystine	37±3.9	21±3.5	<0.020	75±14.1	53±5.7		38±11.5	32±6.4	
α-NH₂-n-butyric acid	6±2.0	3±0.5		9±1.5	6±0.4		2±1.9	3±0.5	
Valine	6±0.4	6±0.8		33±3.9	22±1.2	<0.050	26±4.0	16±1.3	<0.050
Methionine	6±1.2	4±1.0		6±0.6	7±1.5		0±0.0	3±1.0	
Isoleucine	8±1.6	8±1.1		14±1.1	13±1.8		6±1.6	6±1.2	
Leucine	6±0.6	5±0.5		31±3.9	24±2.2		25±3.9	19±2.3	
Tyrosine	29±4.0	24±4.2		54±5.2	50±5.5		25±3.8	26±5.1	
Phenylalanine	17±2.6	15±1.8		25±1.6	32±4.2		8±1.6	17±3.4	<0.050
β-Alanine	6±2.6	4±1.8		20±5.0	36±2.3	<0.020	14±3.5	32±3.0	<0.005
β-NH₂-isobutyric acid	12±2.2	10±2.2		13±2.2	15±1.9		1±1.2	5±1.4	<0.050
γ-NH₂-n-butyric acid	2±0.7	2±0.5		15±1.6	10±0.8	<0.050	12±1.8	6±1.0	<0.020
Ethanolamine	24±3.3	24±4.3		25±4.0	24±3.4		1±1.5	1±3.8	
Ornithine	7±2.3	8±3.2		12±4.4	14±3.7		6±3.0	7±5.6	
Lysine + 1-methylhistidine	135±12.6	128±30.2		186±13.2	158±31.4		50±2.2	30±4.1	<0.005
Histidine	280±23.8	179±40.5		314±21.2	201±43.2	<0.050	34±5.4	22±7.0	
3-Methylhistidine	59±4.6	48±5.2		136±36.2	102±17.0		75±34.9	53±12.9	
Arginine	14±5.2	9±1.8		40±4.9	27±2.2	<0.050	26±4.0	19±1.5	
TOTAL	1195±59.2	943±134.3		3129±198.4	2528±222.6		2063±195.7	1587±123.1	

*Mean 24-hour excretion level ± standard error of the mean.
†P for comparison of levels between normal and spondylitic subjects.

The excretion of free serine, alanine, and cystine is significantly lower in the group with ankylosing spondylitis than in the normal subjects. There is a tendency towards a higher excretion of aspartic and glutamic acid and towards a lower excretion of taurine, threonine, and histidine. The mean total excretion of free amino acids by the spondylitic individuals appears to be lower than the normal level, but the difference is not statistically significant.

Levels of seven amino acids in the hydrolyzed urine (Table V) are significantly lower in the spondylitics than in the normal subjects, i.e., threonine, serine, alanine, valine, γ-NH$_2$-n-butyric acid, histidine, and arginine. On the other hand, the level of β-alanine is significantly higher in the spondylitics. The levels of several other amino acids are only slightly different from normal; hydroxyproline is increased and aspartic acid, glutamic acid, glycine, and cystine are decreased.

The excretion pattern of bound amino acids (Table V, hydrolysed minus free) by the group with ankylosing spondylitis is strikingly different from that of the normal subjects. The excretion of bound alanine, valine, γ-NH$_2$-n-butyric acid, and lysine plus 1-methylhistidine is significantly lower in the spondylitics, while the excretion of bound phenylalanine, β-alanine, and β-NH$_2$-isobutyric acid (BAIB) is significantly increased. The excretion levels of bound aspartic acid, threonine, serine, glutamic acid, α-NH$_2$-adipic acid, glycine, histidine, and 3-methylhistidine are slightly lower than normal, while the excretion of bound hydroxyproline appears to be greater. However, in spite of individual differences in the excretion of bound amino acids, there is no significant difference between the two groups in their total excretion of bound forms.

A summary of the differences in the amino acids of plasma and urine between the normal subjects and those having ankylosing spondylitis is shown in Table VI. Of particular interest is the finding that when the level of an individual's amino acid in the plasma differs from normal, this difference is not paralleled in the urine; in most cases, in fact, the changes in the urinary levels occur in the opposite direction.

DISCUSSION

RHEUMATOID ARTHRITIS

Comparison of the data accumulated on the group of normal adult males in this study shows good agreement with the values given for the plasma and urinary amino-acid levels of several other groups of normal males studied under generally similar conditions (22, 23, 25, 26). A criterion in this study was conformity of the individuals participating to a similarly normal and adequate diet, thus obviating the effects of undue disturbance of the regular dietary pattern such as can be the case in rigidly controlled dietary regimens. It is felt, therefore, that the quantitative differences from normal observed

TABLE VI

SUMMARY OF THE QUANTITATIVE DIFFERENCES FROM NORMAL IN THE
AMINO ACIDS OF THE PLASMA AND URINE OF SUBJECTS WITH
ANKYLOSING SPONDYLITIS*

| | Urine | |
Plasma	Before hydrolysis	After hydrolysis
BELOW NORMAL		
Threonine	Threonine	Threonine
	Serine	Serine
Alanine	Alanine	Alanine
	Cystine	Cystine
	Histidine	Histidine
		Valine
		Glycine
		α-NH$_2$-n-butyric acid
		Arginine
	Taurine	
		Aspartic acid
		Glutamic acid
ABOVE NORMAL		
Taurine		
Aspartic acid	Aspartic acid	
Glutamic acid	Glutamic acid	
Isoleucine		
Leucine		
Tyrosine		
Phenylalanine		
Hydroxyproline		Hydroxyproline
		β-Alanine

*The amino acids that are underlined are those that are significantly
different from normal; the remainder show marked trends.

in the amino acids of the plasma and urine of these subjects are not attributable
to dietary influences, since it is well established that neither the total quantity
nor the distribution of the amino acids in urine can be correlated with the
dietary intake of high-biological-value protein (28, 30).

In general, in so far as the direction of the differences is concerned, the
findings in the present study substantiate the observations of other investigators (1–6), although the ranges of quantitative values obtained using the
newer analytical technique sometimes vary considerably from earlier reports.
There are, however, some instances in which the present results do not substantiate previous findings. Further, since the present investigation embraced
the complete spectrum of amino acids, it was possible to demonstrate quantita-

tive differences not previously reported in some of the amino acids in the plasma and urine of the two groups. It will be noted that no qualitative differences were seen in the ninhydrin-reactive compounds in the plasma and urine of the two groups.

The findings of Borden and co-workers (5) that plasma concentrations of threonine, arginine, and histidine were significantly lower than normal in rheumatoid arthritics and of Devries and Alexander (1) that plasma glycine concentrations were also consistently below normal in these subjects have been substantiated in this study (Table I). However, the plasma concentrations of proline were not found to be significantly lower than normal, as had been reported by Trnavska and Sitaj (11). The significantly lower than normal plasma concentrations of methionine and 3-methylhistidine have not been observed previously.

Almost half of the free amino acids of the plasma of the subjects with rheumatoid arthritis were either significantly lower or showed some evidence of being lower than normal, but some of them were found to be present in above normal concentrations. Aspartic acid and taurine concentrations were significantly above normal, while cystine, glutamic acid, and ornithine showed marked but not statistically significant trends in this direction. In view of these differences, it is interesting that the total concentration of amino acids (expressed as mg. amino acids/100 ml. plasma) is essentially the same in the two groups.

In general, the excretion pattern of free amino acids by the subjects with rheumatoid arthritis is a reflection of the situation prevailing in the plasma (Table III). A lower plasma level of an individual amino acid in the rheumatoid than in the normal subjects is accompanied by a lower urinary excretion of the free amino acid. Similarly, a higher plasma concentration of an individual amino acid in the rheumatoids is accompanied by a high excretion level of the free amino acid. Exceptions to this generalization are the below-normal plasma concentration and above-normal excretion level of arginine and the reverse for cystine. Only in the cases of glutamic and aspartic acids did hydrolysis of the urine change the direction of the differences seen in the free amino acids.

Several conclusions can be drawn from these observations. The significantly lower excretion of amino acids by the subjects with rheumatoid arthritis, apparent following hydrolysis of the urine, is the result of a lower total excretion of both free and bound amino acids. The total level of free amino acids in the plasma is the same in the two groups and is accompanied by a significantly lower than normal excretion of free amino acids by the group with rheumatoid arthritis. Thus, it would seem that the plasma levels of free amino acids are actively maintained through reduced excretion by the kidneys. The lower excretion is not accounted for by a greater than normal excretion of bound forms of the amino acids. Intestinal malabsorption of particular, or of all, amino acids by the rheumatoid arthritic patients is a possibility, but there is no clinical or experimental evidence in support of it. It could be that amino-acid catabolism is accelerated in rheumatoid arthritics, although if this were the case, an increased level in the excretion of total nitrogen by the rheumatoid subjects should be evident: the total nitrogen excretion by the two groups is not significantly different; it is, in fact, almost identical (Table II). The further increase in non-amino-acid nitrogen excretion that might be expected should this condition prevail should, a priori, be accompanied by an increased urea excretion by the rheumatoids. Such does not appear to be the case (15).

Reports in the literature do lend indirect support to the possibility that amino acids in individuals with rheumatoid arthritis may be channelled into increased synthesis of nitrogenous compounds, probably mucopolysaccharides and certain proteins. The administration of either of the protein catabolic hormones, cortisone or ACTH (5, 15), has been shown not only to increase the relative excretion of free amino acids to a greater extent in individuals with rheumatoid arthritis than in normal subjects, but also in many instances to increase the absolute excretion levels to a greater extent. These relative and absolute increased excretions appear to persist as long as the hormone is administered. Borden et al. (5) have remarked that these findings must reflect intrinsic changes in protein metabolism, but they offer no suggestions as to what the qualitative nature of such changes may be.

Several authors have presented evidence indicating that there is increased mucopolysaccharide synthesis during inflammatory states, such as occurs in rheumatoid arthritis (31–35). Clinical studies have shown an increased total content of synovial hyaluronic acid in the inflamed joints (36, 37). Further, it has been shown that gold chloride, salicylate, phenylbutazone, and hydrocortisone have an inhibiting effect upon the enzyme transamidase; the function of this enzyme is to catalyse the synthesis of glucosamine-6-phosphate. It has been suggested that the inhibition of mucopolysaccharide synthesis might be a common reason for the therapeutic effectiveness of these various antirheumatic drugs (38). There may be a relationship between these observations and the excess of glutamic acid and/or glutamine accompanied by a lower than normal level of free amino acids found in subjects with rheumatoid arthritis in this study. It is well established that practically all of the amino acids can be converted to glutamic acid, either directly or by way of the TCA cycle. In this study it has been shown that in rheumatoid arthritis, during an exacerbation of the disease, even though the levels of most other amino acids may be lower than normal, the plasma and excretion levels of free glutamic acid and/or glutamine are always higher than normal. Thus, there is a possibility that a greater than usual proportion of the free amino acids is being channelled into the formation of glutamic acid and glutamine with a resultant increase in the synthesis of mucopolysaccharides, especially of hyaluronate proteins, during the course of the inflammatory reaction that accompanies an exacerbation of the disease. Alternatively, Nettlebladt and Sandell (15) have suggested that the high serum glutamic-acid levels seen in rheumatoid arthritis may reflect an incompetent ATP-dependent glutamine synthesis system in these patients.

It is improbable, however, that the conversion of free amino acids to glutamine could account entirely for the lower levels of free amino acids which have been shown to be present in the rheumatoid arthritics. A concomitant requirement for amino acids for the synthesis of certain proteins, probably abnormal, could also contribute to lowering of the amino-acid levels. The abnormal proteins involved could be those containing large amounts of basic amino acids, reported by Hamerman and Sandson (39) to be associated with the hyaluronic acid of synovial fluid in rheumatoid arthritis, and the serologically active gamma globulin, known as the rheumatoid factor (RF), which has been found in both the synovial fluid and the serum of a large percentage of individuals with rheumatoid arthritis (40). The possibility that the data on amino acids presented here might also be found in inflammatory conditions other than rheumatoid arthritis is obviated to some degree by the observations of Nettlebladt and Sandell (15) who did not find similar differences in the plasma amino acid levels of normal individuals and those with pneumonia or nephritis.

The large number of amino acids that show plasma and/or excretion levels which are different from normal in the present study (Table III) suggests that these differences probably represent a generalized abnormality of amino-acid metabolism in rheumatoid arthritis, possibly involving mechanisms such as those outlined above, rather than a specific abnormality in the metabolism of one or more particular amino acids. While previous evidence in the literature (8, 9, 12) has suggested that abnormalities in the metabolism of various individual amino acids may be seen in association with rheumatoid arthritis, it seems unlikely, in the light of the present findings, that individual metabolic lesions are of primary importance in the aetiology or pathogenesis of the disease.

ANKYLOSING SPONDYLITIS

The present report is believed to be the first investigation into the general metabolism of amino acids in ankylosing spondylitis. From the viewpoint of the plasma concentrations and urinary excretion levels of amino acids it has been shown that the metabolism of amino acids by patients with ankylosing spondylitis differs in many respects from that of normal subjects. In some instances these differences resemble those observed between rheumatoid arthritics and normal individuals, but in the other instances they do not.

The plasma concentrations of certain individual amino acids in both rheumatoid arthritic and spondylitic patients differ to the same degree as do those found in normal subjects; increased levels of taurine, aspartic acid, glutamic acid, and ornithine are found in both conditions. The spondylitic patients, like the rheumatoid arthritic paitients, showed lower than normal levels of threonine and alanine, but they did not have lower than normal plasma concentrations of glycine, serine, lysine, methionine, histidine, 3-methylhistidine, and arginine (Table IV). Plasma concentrations of hydroxyproline, isoleucine, leucine, tyrosine, and phenylalanine were significantly higher in the spondylitic than in the normal individuals, whereas these five amino acids were found to be present in the same concentrations in the plasma of rheumatoid arthritic and normal individuals. The total level of plasma amino acids was found to be signficantly higher in the spondylitic than in the normal subjects (Table IV), a situation which did not prevail in the comparison of rheumatoid arthritic and normal individuals.

Only the levels of free alanine and threonine are lower and only the levels of free aspartic acid and glutamic acid are higher than normal in both the plasma and urine of the spondylitic patients (Table VI). In the remainder of the amino acids in which there are demonstrable differences from the normal, the excretion levels of the free amino acids do not directly reflect the plasma concentration. In contrast to this situation, the plasma levels of 13 amino acids differ between rheumatoid arthritic and normal individuals, and these differences, as a general rule, are paralleled by similar differences in the excretion levels of these amino acids (Tables III and VI).

The mean total excretion level of bound amino acids by the spondylitic patients (Table V) is similar to that of rheumatoid arthritic subjects, but there is considerable variation between the two groups in their excretion levels of bound individual amino acids.

The total 24-hour excretion levels of free amino acids by the spondylitic individuals are lower than normal in spite of significantly higher than normal levels of free amino acids in the plasma. Allowing for maximum plasma volume in a given spondylitic individual (i.e., ca. 3000 ml), the higher than normal levels of plasma free amino acids in the spondylitic individuals are less than the deficit in urinary excretion levels of free amino acids by these individuals. This again suggests, as in the case of the subjects with rheumatoid arthritis, that the plasma levels of free amino acids are actively maintained through reduced excretion by the kidneys. It would seem that, along with the numerous clinical similarities existing between the two disease states, at least some of the underlying metabolic abnormalities could be the same as those postulated for rheumatoid arthritis: possible increased synthesis of mucopolysaccharides and abnormal proteins.

The differences from normal which have been discussed can be summarized as in Table VII.

There is considerable clinical controversy as to whether or not rheumatoid arthritis and ankylosing spondylitis are separate and distinct disease entities

TABLE VII

	Rheumatoid arthritis	Ankylosing spondylitis
Total plasma free amino acids	Unchanged	Significantly increased
Urinary excretion		
1. Free amino acids	Significantly decreased	Decreased
2. Bound amino acids	Decreased	Decreased
3. Total amino acids	Significantly decreased	Decreased

(21). The present investigation suggests that there are differences in the metabolism of individual amino acids in the two disease states, but the over-all situation does bear many similarities.

SUMMARY

The complete spectrum of amino acids and ninhydrin-reactive compounds present in the plasma and urine of normal males and of male patients with rheumatoid arthritis and ankylosing spondylitis has been determined.

1. Results of the assays on the normal group, maintained on their usual diet and routine, showed no significant differences from other studies on normal males.

2. No qualitative differences among the three groups were evident.

3. At least 5, and possibly more, of the 25 amino acids and ninhydrin-reactive compounds determined in the plasma were below normal concentration in the group with rheumatoid arthritis. The total plasma amino-acid concentrations, however, were similar in the two groups, principally as a result of greater than normal concentrations of aspartic acid, glutamic acid (or glutamine), and taurine.

4. The urine of the rheumatoid arthritic subjects showed below-normal excretion levels of at least nine, and possibly several more, free amino acids and ninhydrin-reactive compounds and above-normal excretion levels of free aspartic acid, free glutamic acid, and possibly of taurine and ornithine. The total excretion of free amino acids was significantly below the normal level.

5. In the patients with rheumatoid arthritis, the levels of individual amino acids (free plus bound) following hydrolysis of the urine showed trends generally similar to those observed in the excretion of free amino acids. The total level of amino acids in the hydrolysed urine was significantly below normal.

6. The results indicate that in the subjects with rheumatoid arthritis the

plasma levels of free amino acids are actively maintained through reduced excretion by the kidneys.

7. Since the concentration of a large number of amino acids in the patients with rheumatoid arthritis differs from the normal plasma and/or excretion levels in this study, it is suggested that this probably represents a generalized abnormality of amino-acid metabolism in these patients, rather than a specific metabolic abnormality of one or more particular amino acids.

8. The plasma levels of eight amino acids, namely taurine, aspartic acid, glutamic acid, isoleucine, leucine, tyrosine, phenylalanine, and hydroxyproline, were significantly higher in the spondylitic than in the normal group. The plasma levels of threonine and alanine were below normal. The total level of plasma free amino acids was significantly greater than normal in the spondylitic subjects.

9. The excretion levels of at least three, and possibly up to six, amino acids were lower than normal in the spondylitic subjects. The excretion of free aspartic acid and glutamic acid was found to be increased, while the total excretion level of free amino acids was found to be lower than normal in the spondylitic group of subjects.

10. The urinary excretion of amino acids by the spondylitic group following hydrolysis of the urine (i.e., free plus bound) showed trends similar to those observed in the free amino acids, with the exception of glutamic and aspartic acids. The total excretion of these two amino acids by the spondylitic individuals was less than normal. The total level of amino acids in the hydrolysed urine of these subjects was found to be lower than that observed in the normal group.

11. In individuals with ankylosing spondylitis the plasma levels of free amino acids are actively maintained through reduced excretion by the kidneys. It is of interest that the same situation prevails in rheumatoid arthritis.

12. In so far as the generalized metabolism of amino acids is concerned, this study suggests that there are many similarities between rheumatoid arthritis and ankylosing spondylitis.

ACKNOWLEDGMENTS

The authors are grateful for the valuable technical assistance of Mrs. J. MacDonald and the staff of the Clinical Investigation Unit at Westminster Hospital, and wish to acknowledge the advice of Dr. R. J. Rossiter and Dr. J. A. F. Stevenson throughout the course of this study.

REFERENCES

1. DeVRIES, A., and ALEXANDER, B. Studies of amino acid metabolism. II. Blood glycine and total amino acids in various pathological conditions, with observations on the effects of intravenously administered glycine. J. Clin. Invest. 27: 655 (1948).

2. BORDEN, A. L., WALLRAFF, E. B., BRODIE, E. C., HOLBROOK, W. P., HILL, D. F., STEPHENS, C. A. L., JR., KENT, L. T., and KEMMERER, A. R. Plasma levels of free amino acids in normal subjects compared with patients with rheumatoid arthritis. Proc. Soc. Exper. Biol. & Med. *75*: 28 (1950).

3. BRODIE, E. C., WALLRAFF, E. B., BORDEN, A. L., HOLBROOK, W. P., STEPHENS, C. A. L., JR., HILL, D. F., KENT, L. T., and KEMMERER, A. R. Urinary excretion of certain amino acids during ACTH and cortisone treatment in rheumatoid arthritis. Proc. Soc. Exper. Biol. & Med. *75*: 285 (1950).

4. STEPHENS, C. A. L., JR., WALLRAFF, E. B., BORDEN, A. L., BRODIE, E. C., HOLBROOK, W. P., HILL, D. F., KENT, L. T., and KEMMERER, A. R. Apparent free histidine plasma and urine values in rheumatoid arthritis treated with cortisone and ACTH. Proc. Soc. Exper. Biol. & Med. *74*: 275 (1950).

5. BORDEN, A. L., BRODIE, E. C., WALLRAFF, E. B., HOLBROOK, W. P., HILL, D. F., STEPHENS, C. A. L., JR., JOHNSON, R. B., and KEMMERER, A. R. Amino acid studies and clinical findings in normal adults and rheumatoid arthritic patients treated with ACTH. J. Clin. Invest. *31*: 375 (1952).

6. LEMON, H. M., CHASEN, W. H., and LOONEY, J. M. Abnormal glycine metabolism in rheumatoid arthritis. J. Clin. Invest. *31*: 993 (1952).

7. ZIFF, M., KIBRICK, A., DRESNER, E., and GRIBETZ, H. J. Excretion of hydroxyproline in patients with rheumatic and non-rheumatic diseases. J. Clin. Invest. *35*: 579 (1956).

8. NISHIMURA, N., YASIN, M., OKAMOTO, H., KANAZAWA, M., KATOKE, Y., and SHIBATA, Y. Intermediary metabolism of phenylalanine and tyrosine in diffuse collagen diseases. A.M.A. Arch. Dermat. *77*: 255 (1958).

9. McMILLAN, M. The identification of a fluorescent reducing substance in the urine of patients with rheumatoid arthritis. The excretion of 3-hydroxyanthranilic acid in this and other conditions. J. Clin. Path. *13*: 140 (1960).

10. MECHANIC, G., SKUPP, S. J., SAFIER, L. B., and KIBRICK, A. C. Isolation of two peptides containing hydroxyproline from urine of a patient with rheumatoid arthritis. Arch. Biochem. *86*: 71 (1960).

11. TRNAVSKA, Z., SITAJ, S. The changes of free amino acids in serum and urine in patients with rheumatoid arthritis. Ztschv. Rheumaforsch. *19*: 125 (1960). Cited from Chem. Abstr. *54*: 15627 (1960).

12. BETT, I. M. Metabolism of tryptophan in rheumatoid arthritis. Ann. Rheumat. Dis. *21*: 63 (1962).

13. KIBRICK, A. C., HASHIRO, C. O., and SAFIER, L. B. Hydroxyproline peptides in urine of arthritic patients and controls on a collagen-free diet. Proc. Soc. Exper. Biol. & Med. *21*: 79 (1962).

14. McCORMICK, J. N., ROBINSON, R., SMITH, P., and DAY, J. Tyrosyluria in rheumatoid arthritis. Ann. Rheumat. Dis. *21*: 79 (1962).

15. NETTLEBLADT, E., and SANDELL, B. Amino-acid content of serum in rheumatoid arthritis. Ann. Rheumat. Dis. *22*: 269 (1963).

16. DERRICK, J. B., HANLEY, A., and BOCKING, D. Amino acids in blood and urine of normal and arthritic subjects before and after a glycine load given with and without adreno-corticotrophin. Canad. J. Biochem. Physiol. *37*: 1005 (1957).

17. ARMSTRONG, J. J. B. Studies of the metabolism of amino acids in human subjects. M.Sc. Thesis, University of Western Ontario, London, Ontario (1959).

18. MOORE, S., SPACKMAN, D. H., and STEIN, W. H. Automatic recording apparatus for use in the chromatography of amino acids. Anal. Chem. *30*: 1190 (1958).

19. ——— Automatic recording apparatus for use in the chromatography of amino acids. Fed. Proc. *17*: 1107 (1958).

20. PIEZ, K. A., and MORRIS, L. A modified procedure for the automatic analysis of amino acids. Anal. Biochem. *1*: 187 (1960).

21. SCHULMAN, L. E., and BUNIM, J. J. Disorders of the joints. *In* Principles of Internal Medicine, 3rd ed., edited by T. R. Harrison, R. D. Adams, I. L. Bennett, W. H. Resnick, G. W. Thorn, and M. M. Wintrobe (McGraw-Hill Book Co., Inc. New York, 1958), chap. 265.

22. STEIN, W. H., and MOORE, S. The free amino acids of human blood plasma. J. Biol. Chem. 211: 915 (1954).
23. STEIN, W. H. A chromatographic investigation of the amino acid constituents of normal urine. J. Biol. Chem. 201: 45 (1953).
24. BLOCK, R. J., and WEISS, K. W. Amino Acid Handbook (Ryerson Press, Toronto, 1956).
25. EVERED, D. F. The excretion of amino acids by the human. A quantitative study with ion-exchange chromatography. Biochem. J. 62: 416 (1956).
26. SOUPART, P. Urinary excretion of free amino acids in normal adult men and women. Clin. chim. acta, 4: 265 (1959).
27. HARRIS, H. Family studies on urinary excretion of B-aminoisobutyric acid. Ann. Eugenics, 18: 43 (1953).
28. GREENSTEIN, J. P., and WINITZ, M. Chemistry of the Amino Acids, Vol. 1 (John Wiley and Sons, New York, 1961).
29. KIRSNER, J. B., SHIFFNER, A. L., and PALMER, W. L. Studies on amino acid excretion in man. III. Amino acid levels in plasma and urine of normal men fed diets of varying protein content. J. Clin. Invest. 28: 716 (1949).
30. NASSETT, E. S., and TULLY, R. H. Urinary excretion of essential amino acids by human subjects fed diets containing proteins of different biological value. J. Nutrition, 44: 477 (1952).
31. BUNTING, H. The distribution of acid mucopolysaccharides in mammalian tissues as revealed by histochemical methods. Ann. New York Acad. Sci. 52: 977 (1950).
32. BAOS, N. F., and FOLEY, J. B. The effects of growth, fasting and trauma on the concentrations of connective tissue hexosamine and water. Proc. Soc. Exper. Biol. & Med. 86: 690 (1954).
33. DIFERRANTE, N. Urinary excretion of acid mucopolysaccharides by patients with rheumatoid arthritis. J. Clin. Invest. 36: 1516 (1957).
34. DIFERRANTE, N., ROBBINS, W. C., and RICH, C. Urinary excretion of acid mucopoly-saccharides by patients with lupus erythematosus. J. Lab. & Clin. Med. 50: 897 (1957).
35. KERBY, G. P. The effect of inflammation on the hexuronate-containing polysac-charides of human plasma. Proc. Soc. Exper. Biol. & Med. 109: 473 (1962).
36. RAGAN, C., and MEYER, K. The hyaluronic acid of synovial fluid in rheumatoid arthritis. J. Clin. Invest. 28: 56 (1949).
37. BOLLET, A. J. The intrinsic viscosity of synovial fluid hyaluronic acid. J. Lab. & Clin. Med. 48: 721 (1956).
38. BOLLET, A. J. Inhibition of glucosamine-6-PO_4 synthesis by salicylates and other anti-inflammatory agents in vitro. Arth. & Rheum. 4: 624 (1961).
39. HAMERMAN, D., and SANDSON, J. A possible difference in the hyaluronate of normal and rheumatoid synovial fluids. Arth. & Rheum. 5: 110 (1952).
40. BLAND, J. H., and CLARK, L. G. Rheumatoid factor in serum and synovial fluid. Arth. & Rheum. 5: 102 (1962).

The Separation of
Soluble Antigen-Antibody
Complexes from Serum*

R. BAUMAL† and
I. BRODER‡

EXPERIMENTAL STUDIES relating to the possible role of soluble antigen–antibody complexes in the pathogenesis of disease have indicated that soluble complexes may produce the type of tissue damage found in glomerulonephritis and serum sickness (1–4). On the basis of the observations made in these animal studies, it has been suggested that a number of human diseases may also be caused by soluble antigen–antibody complexes (5–7). Among the suspect clinical disorders are serum sickness, glomerulonephritis, rheumatoid arthritis, and the collagen diseases. However, it has not been possible to study whether soluble antigen–antibody complexes are associated with human disease, as there has been no sensitive method for demonstrating their presence in serum.

A number of investigators have reported that soluble antigen–antibody complexes prepared in antigen excess may produce effects resembling those seen in anaphylaxis (8–12). We have found in the isolated perfused guinea-pig lung that an injection of soluble complexes into the pulmonary artery leads to the release of histamine and an increase in the air inflow pressure (13). The lungs are activated by as little as 1 to 2 μg. of antibody protein in the form of a soluble complex with antigen, and no activation is seen with antigen alone, antiserum alone, or antigen in normal serum.

We considered the possibility that the perfused guinea-pig lung might serve as a bioassay for detecting soluble antigen–antibody complexes in serum. However, the capacity of soluble complexes to activate the guinea-pig lung is inhibited by the simultaneous administration of a relatively large amount of serum (13). As this would preclude detection of a low concentration of complexes in serum, it was first necessary to develop a method for separating complexes from the inhibitory component(s) of serum.

*From the Department of Medicine, Toronto Western Hospital and University of Toronto, Toronto. Supported by the Canadian Arthritis and Rheumatism Society.
†Medical Research Fellow, Medical Research Council of Canada.
‡Medical Research Scholar, Medical Research Council of Canada.

In the present studies, it was found that soluble antigen–antibody complexes could be separated from their serum inhibitor(s) by gel filtration on Sephadex G-200. Using this fractionation procedure, a biologically active material with properties similar to those of soluble antigen–antibody complexes was demonstrated both in the serum of rabbits injected with a foreign protein, and in the serum of persons with rheumatoid arthritis.

MATERIALS AND METHODS

Crystalline bovine plasma albumin (Armour, BPA) was used in immunizing adult rabbits. We have found, as have others (14), that BPA contains a small amount of polymerized BPA; in the chromatographic studies described below, the BPA used had been freed of polymers by gel filtration on Sephadex G-200 (Pharmacia). Labelled BPA was prepared by conjugation with fluorescein isothiocyanate (15), and fluorescence was measured in a Turner model 110 flurometer. Soluble antigen–antibody complexes were formed either in the immune serum by adding a mixture of labelled and unlabelled BPA in an amount greater than that required for equivalence, or by adding excess antigen to the washed precipitate prepared at equivalence (13).

Gel filtration was performed on columns of Sephadex G-200, using as the eluent $0.1M$ trishydroxymethylaminomethane pH 8 in $1M$ sodium chloride (16). The optical density of the effluent was measured at 280 mμ in a Beckman DU-2 spectrophotometer. The fractions were concentrated by dialysis in polyethylene glycol (Carbowax, 20,000, Union Carbide) and then dialysed extensively against $0.15M$ sodium chloride containing $0.03M$ sodium phosphate pH 7.4 (buffered saline).

The isolated perfused guinea-pig lung system has been described in detail previously (13), and was used without modification. The pulmonary artery was perfused with warm Tyrode solution which drained through the left atrium and was collected in timed fractions. The trachea was perfused with a constant stream of air and the air inflow pressure was recorded continuously. Histamine bioassays were performed using a semi-automatic procedure (17), and were expressed in terms of the histamine base. The area of recorded alterations in the air inflow pressure was measured with a metric scale planimeter.

Quantitative precipitin tests (18), double diffusion in agar (19) and fractionation of soluble antigen–antibody complexes at 50 per cent saturation with ammonium sulphate (20) were all carried out using standard methods.

RESULTS

GEL FILTRATION OF SERUM AND SOLUBLE ANTIGEN–ANTIBODY COMPLEXES ON SEPHADEX G-200

Normal rabbit serum was arbitrarily divided into five fractions after passage through Sephadex G-200 (Fig. 1A). Flodin and Killander (16), using human serum, have shown that fraction 1 contains the macroglobulins, fraction 3 the globulins of lower molecular weight, and fraction 5 albumin. In agreement with this, we found that anti-BPA was present in fraction 3 of serum from rabbits immunized with BPA (Fig. 1B). Also fluorescein-labelled BPA appeared in fraction 5 when added to normal rabbit serum prior to gel filtration (Fig. 1C). Furthermore, when excess labelled BPA was added to

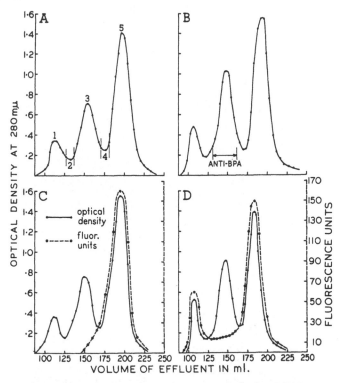

FIG. 1. Gel filtration of rabbit serum on Sephadex G-200.
A. 1 ml. normal rabbit serum.
B. 1 ml. of serum from a rabbit immunized with BPA. Each of the fractions was concentrated and tested for anti-BPA by double diffusion in agar against BPA.
C. A mixture of labelled and unlabelled BPA was added to 1 ml. of normal rabbit serum.
D. A mixture of labelled and unlabelled BPA was added to 1 ml. of anti-BPA serum, in an amount five times that required for equivalence.

immune serum forming soluble antigen–antibody complexes, the BPA appeared not only in fraction 5 but also in fraction 1, and antibody was no longer detected in fraction 3 (Fig. 1D). The disappearance of antibody from fraction 3 and the appearance of antigen in fraction 1 suggested that the soluble antigen–antibody complexes were present in fraction 1. In the following studies, we have confined our attention to fractions 1, 3, and 5.

BIOLOGICAL ACTIVITY OF FRACTIONS OBTAINED FROM SERUM CONTAINING SOLUBLE
ANTIGEN–ANTIBODY COMPLEXES

Fractions from serum containing soluble antigen–antibody complexes were
tested for biological activity in the perfused guinea-pig lung. Active fractions
produced both histamine release and an increase in the air inflow pressure
(Figs. 2–4). We have previously reported similar findings using known
preparations of soluble antigen–antibody complexes (13).

The lung-stimulating activity of serum containing soluble antigen–antibody
complexes was present mainly in fraction 1 (Fig. 2). In contrast, the fractions

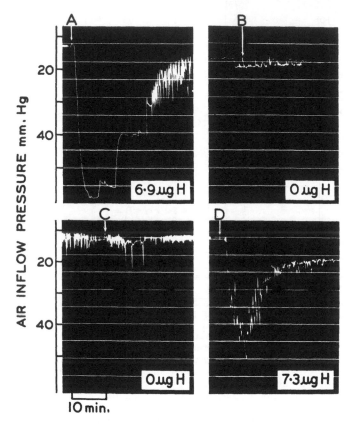

Fig. 2. Location of biological activity in Sephadex G-200
fractions of serum containing soluble complexes. BPA was
added to anti-BPA serum in an amount five times that required
for equivalence, and the fractions obtained after gel filtration
were tested for biological activity in a single perfused guinea-
pig lung. Each fraction was used in an amount proportional to
the volume in which it was eluted. At A and D, injections of
fraction 1 were given, and at B and C, fractions 3 and 5
respectively were given in amounts four times greater than
that of fraction 1.

of normal rabbit serum were inactive when injected in amounts 64 times greater than comparable amounts of fraction 1 from serum containing complexes in a concentration of 2.5 mg. of antibody protein per ml.

Several methods were used in characterizing the biologically active material found in fraction 1 obtained from serum containing soluble complexes. First, when fraction 1 was further fractionated at 50 per cent saturation with ammonium sulphate, there was no residual activity in the dialysed supernatant. Secondly, a precipitate was formed when fraction 1 was titrated with sheep anti-rabbit gamma globulin (Hyland), and the supernatant from a mixture in optimal proportions was inactive in the lung. Normal sheep serum added to fraction 1 produced no inhibition. Thirdly, the activity was inhibited if fraction 1 was mixed with an excess of normal rabbit globulin prior to injection. Fourthly, when fraction 1, obtained in the usual manner, was repassed through Sephadex G-200, using as eluent 0.1M glycine-HCl pH 3, the main fraction obtained on repassage was no longer biologically active. These characteristics of the biologically active material in fraction 1 of serum containing soluble antigen–antibody complexes are identical with those of known soluble antigen–antibody complexes.

CHARACTERIZATION OF THE SERUM INHIBITOR(s) OF SOLUBLE COMPLEXES

Normal rabbit serum was passed through Sephadex G-200, and the fractions obtained were tested for their capacity to inhibit either known soluble complexes or biologically active fraction 1 from serum containing soluble complexes (Fig. 3). Inhibition was observed only with fraction 3 of normal rabbit serum, while fractions 1 and 5 of normal rabbit serum failed to inhibit in amounts up to 30 times greater than fraction 3. Fraction 3 from serum containing soluble complexes was similar in its inhibitory activity to fraction 3 from normal rabbit serum.

These findings indicated that when serum containing soluble antigen–antibody complexes was fractionated on Sephadex G-200, the soluble complexes were found in fraction 1 and their inhibitor(s) was found in fraction 3. Gel filtration on Sephadex G-200 is, therefore, an effective method of separating soluble antigen–antibody complexes from the inhibitory fraction of serum.

SENSITIVITY OF THE BIOASSAY FOR DETECTING SOLUBLE ANTIGEN–ANTIBODY COMPLEXES IN SERUM

A series of studies was performed in which increasing concentrations of soluble complexes were added to normal rabbit serum and the serum was tested for biological activity in the isolated perfused guinea-pig lung before and after gel filtration on Sephadex G-200. In the case of serum containing 200 μg. of antibody protein per ml., no activity could be detected in a dose of the whole serum containing 50 μg. of antibody protein. However, when serum containing as little as 20 μg. of antibody protein per ml. was first fractionated

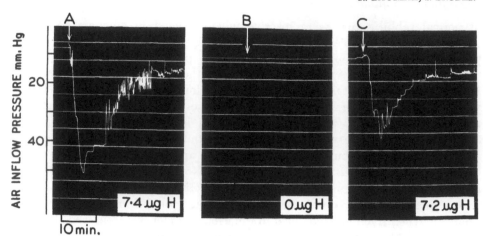

Fig. 3. Inhibition of the activity of soluble complexes by the fractions of normal rabbit serum obtained from Sephadex G-200. Equal aliquots of fraction 1 obtained from serum containing soluble antigen–antibody complexes were mixed prior to injection with fractions 1 (at A), 3 (at B), and 5 (at C) obtained from normal rabbit serum. The fractions from normal rabbit serum were used in equal amounts, proportional to the volume of effluent in which each fraction was respectively eluted. The responses shown were obtained from a single lung.

on Sephadex G-200, biological activity could be detected in fraction 1, using a dose calculated to contain 8 μg. of antibody protein (Table I). An increase in sensitivity of more than 60-fold is, therefore, achieved by fractionation on Sephadex G-200.

BIOLOGICAL ACTIVITY IN THE SERUM OF RABBITS INJECTED WITH BPA

Rabbits were injected intravenously with 250 mg. of fluorescein-labelled BPA per kg. body weight, and serum was collected on alternate days for

TABLE I

ENHANCED SENSITIVITY OF DETECTING SOLUBLE ANTIGEN–ANTIBODY COMPLEXES (SC) IN SERUM

(Gel filtration was carried out on Sephadex G-200 using on one column normal rabbit serum (NRS) alone, and on a second column NRS to which was added BPA–anti-BPA SC in five times antigen excess at a concentration of 20 μg. of antibody protein per ml. of serum. Comparable doses of fraction 1 from each column were injected into the same lung)

Preparation	Dose	Constriction (cm.^{2})	Histamine (μg)
1. NRS + SC G-200 Fr 1	8 μg. Ab	14.0	2.2
2. NRS G-200 Fr 1	Equiv. to 1 & 3	0	0
3. NRS + SC G-200 Fr 1	8 μg. Ab	9.6	1.8

measurement both of residual circulating antigen and of biological activity in the perfused guinea-pig lung. The conditions used in these experiments duplicated those described by Dixon and co-workers in their studies of experimental serum sickness (3). A biologically active material showing the properties of soluble antigen–antibody complexes was first detected seven days after antigen administration and reached a maximum level during the phase of immune elimination (days 9–12). These observations are in agreement with those made by Dixon and co-workers, who identified soluble complexes by a different technique; in their studies, the BPA was labelled with I^{131}, and complexes were considered to be present when fractionation of serum at 50 per cent saturation with ammonium sulphate yielded a radioactive precipitate. These investigators also carried out morphological studies, and were able to demonstrate a parallel relationship between the presence of circulating soluble complexes and the time course of serum sickness.

CLINICAL STUDIES

1. *Serum Sickness*

In view of the foregoing experimental findings, we examined the serum of persons who were suffering from serum sickness following a prophylactic injection of horse antitetanus serum. Of 10 acute-phase sera studied, none had biological activity in the perfused guinea-pig lung, either before or after fractionation on Sephadex G-200. This could not be explained on the basis that human antibody cannot activate the perfused guinea-pig lung, as we have shown in other studies that soluble antigen–antibody complexes prepared with human gamma-G antibody were active in this system. Therefore, our negative findings may be interpreted as indicating either that circulating soluble antigen–antibody complexes are not present in human serum sickness, or that they are present at too low a concentration for detection, or that they contain an immunoglobulin that is not biologically active in this system.

2. *Rheumatoid Arthritis*

The serum of some patients with rheumatoid arthritis has been shown to contain abnormal components having sedimentation coefficients ranging from approximately 9S to 22S (21, 22). Although the exact nature of these components has not been defined, it has been suggested that they may be complexes consisting of an auto-antibody in combination with 7S gamma globulin as the antigen (23).

In view of this suggestion, sera of patients with rheumatoid arthritis were tested for biological activity in the perfused guinea-pig lung. Of 33 sera tested following gel filtration on Sephadex G-200, more than 50 per cent contained a material in fraction 1 which activated the guinea-pig lung (Fig. 4). Fractions 3 and 5, however, were inactive. The biologically active component was no longer evident either in the supernatant obtained by fractionation at

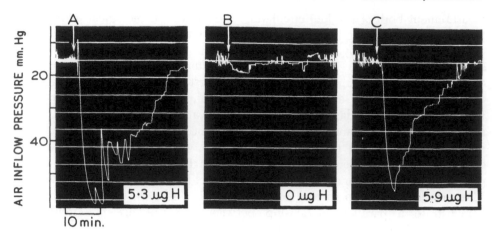

Fig. 4. Biological activity in serum from patient (E.J.) with rheumatoid arthritis. Equal injections of fraction 1 were given to a single lung at A, B, and C. At B, fraction 1 was mixed prior to injection with a proportional amount of fraction 3 obtained from the same serum.

50 per cent saturation with ammonium sulphate, or following the addition of an excess of human globulin to fraction 1, or if fraction 1 was obtained by gel filtration, using $0.1M$ glycine-HCl pH 3 as eluent. These characteristics are identical with those described above for known soluble antigen–antibody complexes. We have found no comparable biological activity in the Sephadex fractions of serum obtained from healthy individuals.

These studies have been concerned mainly with defining the characteristics, relative to those of soluble antigen–antibody complexes, of the biologically active material present in rheumatoid serum. It is not yet clear what relationship exists between this material and either the pathogenesis of rheumatoid arthritis or the serum protein abnormalities described in this disease.

CONCLUSIONS AND SUMMARY

Our aim in these studies has been to establish a method for detecting low levels of soluble antigen–antibody complexes in serum, based on the known capacity of complexes to activate a process resembling anaphylaxis in the perfused guinea-pig lung (13). As the activity of low levels of complexes is inhibited by a relatively high concentration of serum, it was first necessary to develop a technique for separating complexes from the inhibitor(s) present in the serum. This separation was achieved by gel filtration on Sephadex G-200, following which it was possible to detect antigen–antibody complexes originally present in the serum at a concentration as low as 20 μg. of antibody protein per ml. Criteria have been established by which materials biologically active in the perfused guinea-pig lung may be compared and identified with soluble antigen–antibody complexes.

We have identified a biologically active material which fulfils the criteria for antigen–antibody complexes, present both in the serum of rabbits following an injection of foreign protein and in the serum of persons with rheumatoid arthritis. Other investigators have proposed that soluble antigen–antibody complexes are responsible for the manifestations of serum sickness in rabbits (3). However, the significance of the biologically active material in the serum of persons with rheumatoid arthritis is not known at present.

ACKNOWLEDGMENTS

The authors are grateful to Dr. J. Crawford, Dr. D. Gordon, Dr. J. Houpt, Dr. A. Pratt, Dr. R. Renaud, Dr. P. Rosen, and the staff of the University of Toronto Rheumatic Diseases Unit for their assistance in providing us with clinical material.

REFERENCES

1. McCluskey, R. T., Benacerraf, B., Potter, J. L., and Miller, F. The pathologic effects of intravenously administered soluble antigen–antibody complexes. I. Passive serum sickness in mice. J. Exper. Med. *111*: 181 (1960).
2. Benacerraf, B., Potter, J. L., McCluskey, R. T., and Miller, F. The pathologic effects of intravenously administered soluble antigen–antibody complexes. II. Acute glomerulonephritis in rats. J. Exper. Med. *111*: 195 (1960).
3. Dixon, F. J., Vazquez, J. J., Weigle, W. O., and Cochrane, C. G. Pathogenesis of serum sickness. Arch. Path. *65*: 18 (1958).
4. Weigle, W. O. Fate and biological action of antigen–antibody complexes. Advances Immunol. *1*: 283 (1961).
5. Dixon, F. J., Feldman, J. D., and Vazquez, J. J. Experimental glomerulonephritis. The pathogenesis of a laboratory model resembling the spectrum of human glomerulonephritis. J. Exper. Med. *113*: 899 (1961).
6. Dixon, F. J. The role of antigen–antibody complexes in disease. Harvey Lect. *58*: 21 (1962–63).
7. Venters, H. D., Jr., and Good, R. A. Current concepts of the pathogenesis of the so-called collagen diseases. Paed. Clin. North Am. *10*: 1017 (1963).
8. Germuth, F. G., and McKinnon, G. E. Anaphylactic shock induced by soluble antigen–antibody complexes in unsensitized normal guinea pigs. Bull. Johns Hopkins Hosp. *101*: 13 (1957).
9. Ishizaka, K., and Campbell, D. H. Biological activity of soluble antigen–antibody complexes. I. Skin reactive properties. Proc. Soc. Exper. Biol. & Med. 97: 635 (1958).
10. Tokuda, S., and Weiser, R. S. Anaphylaxis in the mouse produced with soluble complexes of antigen and antibody. Proc. Soc. Exper. Biol. & Med. 98: 557 (1958).
11. Weigle, W. O., Cochrane, C. G., and Dixon, F. J. Anaphylactogenic properties of soluble antigen–antibody complexes in the guinea pig and rabbit. J. Immunol. 85: 469 (1960).
12. Treadwell, R. E., Wistar, R., and Rasmussen, A. F., Jr. Passive anaphylaxis in mice with homologous antiserum. I. Some quantitative aspects. J. Immunol. *84*: 539 (1960).

13. BRODER, I., and SCHILD, H. O.   The action of soluble antigen–antibody complexes in perfused guinea pig lung. Immunol. 8: 300 (1965).
14. HARTLEY, R. W., JR., PETERSON, E. A., and SOBER, H. A.   The relation of free sulfhydryl groups to chromatographic heterogeneity and polymerization of bovine plasma albumin. Biochemistry, 1: 60 (1962).
15. RINDERKNECHT, H.   Ultra-rapid fluorescent labelling of proteins. Nature, 193: 167 (1962).
16. FLODIN, P., and KILLANDER, J.   Fractionation of human serum proteins by gel filtration. Biochim. et biophys. acta, 63: 403 (1962).
17. BOURA, A., MONGAR, J. L., and SCHILD, H. O.   Improved automatic apparatus for pharmacological assays on isolated preparations. Brit. J. Pharmacol. 9: 24 (1954).
18. KABAT, E. A., and MAYER, M. M.   Experimental Immunochemistry (Charles C. Thomas, Springfield, Ill., 1961), pp. 72, 476.
19. OUCHTERLONY, O.   Diffusion-in-gel methods for immunological analysis. Progr. Allergy, 5: 1 (1958).
20. FARR, R. S.   A quantitative immuno-chemical measure of the primary interaction between I* BSA and antibody. J. Infec. Dis. 103: 239 (1958).
21. KUNKEL, H. G., MULLER-EBERHARD, H. J., FUDENBERG, H. H., and TOMASI, T. B.   Gamma globulin complexes in rheumatoid arthritis and certain other conditions. J. Clin. Invest. 40: 117 (1961).
22. CHODIRKER, W. B., and TOMASI, T. B., JR.   Low-molecular-weight rheumatoid factor. J. Clin. Invest. 42: 876 (1963).
23. BUTLER, V. P., JR., and VAUGHAN, J. H.   The reaction of rheumatoid factor with animal gamma-globulins: Quantitative considerations. Immunol. 8: 144 (1965).

PART III

Lysosomes and Inflammation

Chairman: Dean John Hamilton, Toronto

The Lysosomal Concept:
Role in Connective Tissue Disease*

W. B. CHODIRKER, M.D., F.R.C.P.(C)

IN 1955 Christian deDuve of Louvain University identified in the liver cells of the rat a series of cytoplasmic enzymes exhibiting certain common characteristics (1). All were hydrolases with acidic pH optima and all exhibited the property of latency. By latency is meant that the maximal enzyme activities are manifest only after treatment of the enzyme-rich fractions of cellular homogenates with agents capable of interfering with the integrity of membrane-bound structures. On the basis of these observations deDuve suggested that these enzymes, which are capable of digesting their own cellular constituents, are ordinarily prevented from doing so by virtue of their presence within limiting membranes. Thus he perceived of membrane-bound enzyme-containing cytoplasmic particles or organelles which he termed lysosomes.

Morphologic confirmation of the existence of a new kind of cytoplasmic organelle in cellular homogenates rich in lysosomal enzyme activity was made electron microscopically in 1956 by Novikoff and associates (2). Lysosomes or lysosome-like particles are now known to exist in virtually all cell types at one stage or another of their development and in all animal species, including man.

The enzymes that are currently recognized as belonging to the lysosomal class are given in Table I. Noteworthy is the wide range of substrate specificities, which includes proteins, nucleic acids, carbohydrates, phosphates, and sulphates.

Physiologically, lysosomes appear to act primarily as intracellular digestive systems capable of enzymically degrading a wide variety of substances of exogenous or endogenous origin. The complex sequence of intracellular events following phagocytosis or pinocytosis has recently been reviewed by deDuve (3).

The acid hydrolases, synthesized on the ribosomes, are believed to be packaged by the Golgi apparatus from which they are released in the form of small vacuoles, the lysosomes. This process occurs either spontaneously or

*From the Department of Medicine, University of Rochester School of Medicine and Dentistry, Rochester, New York.

TABLE I

LYSOSOMAL ENZYMES AND THEIR SUBSTRATE SPECIFICITIES

Enzyme	Substrate specificity
Cathepsins	Proteins
Collagenase	Proteins
Acid ribonuclease	Ribonucleic acids
Acid deoxyribonuclease	Deoxyribonucleic acids
Alpha glucosidase	Alpha glucosides
Beta-N-acetylglucosaminidase	Beta-N-acetylglucosaminidases
Beta glucuronidase	Beta glucuronides
Beta galactosidase	Beta galactosides
Alpha mannosidase	Alpha mannosides
Phosphoprotein phosphatase	Phosphoproteins, pyrophosphates
Acid phosphatase	Phosphate esters
Aryl sulphatase	Sulphate esters

in response to appropriate stimuli (phagocytosis) in most cell types. Polymorphonuclear (PMN) leucocytes are unique in this respect in that their lysosomes, the cytoplasmic inclusion granules, appear at an early stage of cell development in the bone marrow and thereafter are not inducible. Ingested materials become enclosed within a membrane derived from the cell wall forming a phagocytic vacuole or phagosome. Phagosomes and lysosomes then fuse, forming digestive vacuoles or phagolysosomes. Solubilization of the ingested material ensues, presumably owing to the presence of lysosomal enzymes. The end stage of this process is represented by residual bodies which appear to contain indigestible elements of phagocytosed materials. In some cell types the indigestible wastes may actually be excreted from the cell. Occasionally vacuoles are seen which contain mitochondria, ribosomes, or other of the cell's own organelles. The formation of these autophagic vacuoles or lysolysosomes is postulated to be a physiologic process whereby the cell consumes its own substance in a controlled manner in order to meet its metabolic needs at times when exogenously derived materials are unavailable, such as during starvation.

Knowledge is rapidly accumulating implicating lysosomes in a variety of physiologic and pathologic processes. This presentation will be restricted to a discusssion of the role or possible roles of lysosomes in the inflammatory and immunological manifestations of the rheumatic diseases.

LYSOSOMES AND INFLAMMATION

In experiments reported in 1956 and 1960 Thomas and co-workers (4, 5), extending the earlier *in vitro* observations of Fell and Mellanby (6), demonstrated the destruction of cartilage matrix in rabbits following the parenteral administration of either the hydrolytic plant enzyme papain or large doses of vitamin A. The subsequent investigations of Dingle (7) and of Weissman and

Thomas (8) strongly suggested that vitamin A produces chondromalacia by disrupting lysosomal membranes thereby exposing the cartilage matrix to the destructive effects of lysosomal enzymes. The *in vitro* breakdown of extracted chondromucoprotein by cell-free homogenates of normal blood PMN leucocytes was reported in 1960 by Ziff and associates (9). These investigators also demonstrated that homogenates of rheumatoid synovial tissue which were actively inflammatory with marked cellular infiltration had a similar effect while non-inflammatory, non-infiltrated rheumatoid synovial extracts were totally inactive in this system. Clinically, several studies (10–12) have demonstrated elevated levels of lysosomal enzymes in synovial tissue extracts and in synovial fluids obtained from patients with rheumatoid arthritis.

Observations such as these have suggested the hypothesis that hydrolytic enzymes released from lysosomes may be responsible in whole or in part for the chondromalacia and inflammation characteristic of the rheumatoid joint. In support of this concept are the 1964 experiments of Thomas (13), which demonstrated the absolute requirement of PMN leucocytes for the production of both the classical Shwartzman and Arthus reactions. Furthermore, Halpern (14) in 1964 demonstrated the inhibition of the inflammatory tissue response of the Shwartzman reaction by a protease inhibitor. Also pertinent to this discussion is the 1964 report by Janoff and Zweifach (15) of the inflammatory inducing capacity of acid-extractable fractions of isolated PMN leucocyte lysosomes on exteriorized rabbit and rat mesenteries. These investigators isolated from lysosomes a cationic protein devoid of lysosomal enzyme activity yet capable of inducing an acute inflammatory response. Enzyme-rich fractions isolated from the same lysosomes were, however, completely non-inflammatory.

The experiments cited demonstrate the capacity of lysosomal products to destroy cartilage and to induce acute inflammation under certain experimental conditions. However, the chemical nature of the lysosomal products responsible for these effects remains uncertain. Further investigations, shedding new light on these problems, will lead to a keener appreciation of the clinical significance of these phenomena.

LYSOSOMES AND IMMUNOLOGIC PHENOMENA

Much of the research currently conducted into the aetiology of the rheumatic diseases is directed towards the elucidation of the apparent disturbances in immunological processes which are so clearly manifest in rheumatoid arthritis and systemic lupus erythematosus (SLE). Several observations have suggested that lysosomes may be involved in immunologic processes. Of great interest is the finding by Miescher and associates (16) of antilysosomal antibodies in the serums of patients with SLE as well as in those of patients with infectious hepatitis. Whether these antibodies are auto-aggressive, auto-protective, or merely indifferent by-products of the disease process is at present unclear. These investigators did, however, demonstrate the ability of antilysosomal antibodies to protect lysosomes *in vitro* from disrupting influences, suggesting an autoprotective role for these antibodies. Investigations conducted by Franzl (17) have suggested that antigen degradation by macrophage lysosomal enzymes is somehow involved in the sequence of events whereby antigenic information is transmitted to the antibody-synthesizing cells, the lymphocytes and plasma cells. Furthermore, Uhr and co-workers (18) have demonstrated the inhibition of tissue immunological responses such as delayed hypersensitivity, the Arthus reaction, and passive cutaneous anaphylaxis by pretreatment of guinea pigs with agents capable of depleting cells of their lysosomal enzyme content. These observations would suggest that future investigations along similar lines may reveal an important role for lysosomes in the immunological phenomena of the rheumatic diseases.

LYSOSOMES AND EXPERIMENTAL ARTHRITIS

Another approach to the elucidation of the role of lysosomes in the rheumatic diseases was suggested by Weissman (19) in 1963 in a report which demonstrated the striking capacity of streptolysins O and S extracted from B-haemolytic streptococci to disrupt lysosomal membranes *in vivo* and *in vitro*. In 1965 Weissman and collaborators (20) reported the induction of an acute and chronic arthritis in 100 per cent of rabbits receiving as few as five intra-articular injections of small doses of streptolysin S. Pathologically, the arthritis was remarkably similar to that seen in rheumatoid arthritis and was characterized by PMN followed by lymphocytic and plasma cell infiltration of the synovial membrane with the formation of lymphoid follicles, hyperplasia, and vacuolization of the synovial lining cells, fibrinoid degeneration, vasculitis, and pannus formation with destruction of the underlying cartilage. Arthritis could not be induced in control animals receiving injections of other streptococcal toxins.

Of particular interest in these experiments was the failure of the affected animals to produce an immune response in the form of either humoral antibody or delayed hypersensitivity to the inducing agent streptolysin S. The animals did, however, produce complement-fixing antibodies to lysosomes and to a lesser extent to mitochondria. *In vitro* experiments indicated that the antilysosomal antibodies protected isolated liver lysosomes from the effects of agents capable of disrupting lysosomal membranes.

On the basis of these experiments it was hypothesized that streptolysin S disrupted lysosomes present in the synovial membrane releasing tissue-damaging substances and that the secondary auto-antibody response was autoprotective and not auto-aggressive. The relative importance of lysosomal products derived from synovial membrane on the one hand and from infiltrating PMN leucocytes and macrophages on the other in the production of this inflammatory response is at present unclear. The resolution of this conceptually important problem must await further investigations.

In view of these experiments and the current interest in pleuropneumonia-like organisms (PPLO) and L forms of bacteria as possible aetiological agents in the rheumatic diseases (21) it is of interest to note that L forms of streptococci are potent producers of streptolysins.

LYSOSOMES AND RHEUMATOID ARTHRITIS

The recent demonstration by Hollander and co-workers (22) of inclusion bodies within the cytoplasm of PMN leucocytes obtained from rheumatoid synovial fluids has stimulated a new wave of investigations into the pathogenesis of rheumatoid arthritis. The available evidence suggests that the inclusions contain immune globulins such as rheumatoid factor probably in the form of immune complexes. The phagocytosis of rheumatoid factor–gamma G globulin complexes by PMN leucocytes *in vitro* has been reported by Astorga and Bollet (23) to result in the activation of lysosomal enzymes in these cells. This phenomenon, if it occurred *in vivo*, and in the light of evidence presented earlier in this paper, may be postulated to induce the inflammatory and destructive lesions of the rheumatoid joint. In this fashion the infiltrating leucocytes may represent a pathogenetic link between the immunologic and inflammatory manifestations of rheumatoid arthritis.

LYSOSOMAL LABILIZERS AND STABILIZERS

A wide variety of chemical and physical agents are capable of disrupting lysosomal membranes (labilizers) while other agents (stabilizers) protect lysosomal membranes from disrupting influences (24). Labilizing and stabilizing agents are listed in Table II.

Ultraviolet radiation is a labilizer of particular interest. When applied to the skin of the foetal rat an acute inflammatory reaction is produced which, as pointed out by Weissman and Thomas (25), closely resembles the cutaneous photosensitivity eruptions commonly experienced by patients with SLE. Extending these findings, Weissman (26) demonstrated the production of an acute inflammatory response in the skin of patients with SLE following the local injection of vitamin A, a potent lysosomal labilizer. A much milder reaction was noted in the skin of non-SLE control subjects following the same dose of vitamin A. These observations suggest the hypothesis that an important abnormality in SLE may be an increased susceptibility of lysosomal membranes to labilizing agents.

Pharmacologic agents in general use in the treatment of the rheumatic

TABLE II

LABILIZERS AND STABILIZERS OF LYSOSOMAL MEMBRANES

Agents that labilize the membranes of lysosomes
    Physical agents
        Ultraviolet radiation
        Sonic vibrations
        Freezing and thawing
        Hypo and hyper osmolarity
        High temperature
        Waring blendor
    Chemical agents
        Endotoxins
        Streptolysins O and S

Vitamin A	Vitamin E
Progesterone	Testosterone
Deoxycorticosterone	5-Beta-H(pyrogenic) steroids
Lysolecithin	Lecithinase
Proteases	
Digitonin	
Non-ionic detergents	Bile salts
Hepatotoxins (CCl_4, P)	
Cations	Acidity

Agents that stabilize the membranes of lysosomes
    Glucocorticoids
    Chloroquine
    Antihistamines
    Cholesterol

diseases, such as adrenal corticosteroids and chloroquine, share the property of stabilizing lysosomal membranes from the disruptive effects of ultraviolet radiation and other labilizing agents. The significance, if any, of this observation with respect to the mode of action of these drugs in the rheumatic diseases is unknown at present, but this may prove to be a fruitful area for future investigation.

REFERENCES

1. DEDUVE, C. In Subcellular Particles, edited by T. Hayashi (Ronald Press, New York, 1959), p. 128.
2. NOVIKOFF, A. B., BEAUFAY, H., and DEDUVE, C. J. Biophys. & Biochem. Cytol. Supp. 2: 179 (1956).
3. DEDUVE, C. In Ciba Symposium on Lysosomes, edited by A. V. S. deReuk and M. P. Cameron (Little Brown & Co., Boston, 1963), p. 1.
4. THOMAS, L. J. Exper. Med. 104: 245 (1956).
5. THOMAS, L., McCLUSKEY, R. T., POTTER, J. L., and WEISSMAN, G. J. Exper. Med. 111: 705 (1960).
6. FELL, H. B., and MELLANBY, E. J. Physiol. 116: 320 (1952).
7. DINGLE, J. T. Biochem. J. 79: 509 (1961).
8. WEISSMAN, G., and THOMAS, L. J. Clin. Invest. 42: 661 (1963).
9. ZIFF, M., GRIBETS, H. J., and LOSPALLUTO, J. J. Clin. Invest. 39: 405 (1960).
10. LUSCOMBE, M. Nature, 197: 1010 (1963).
11. SMITH, C., and HAMERMAN, D. Arth. & Rheum. 5: 411 (1962).
12. JACOX, R. F., and FELDMAHN, A. J. Clin. Invest. 34: 263 (1955).
13. THOMAS, L. Proc. Soc. Exper. Biol. & Med. 115: 235 (1964).
14. HALPERN, B. N. Proc. Soc. Exper. Biol. & Med. 115: 273 (1963).

15. JANOFF, A., and ZWEIFACH, B. W. J. Exper. Med. *120*: 747 (1964).
16. MIESCHER, P. A., BARKER, L., VAINIO, I., and WIEDERMANN, G. *In* Injury, Inflammation and Immunity, *edited by* L. Thomas, J. W. Uhr, and L. Grant (Williams and Wilkins, Baltimore, 1964), p. 346.
17. FRANZL, R. E. Nature, *195*: 457 (1962).
18. UHR, J. W., WEISSMAN, G., and THOMAS, L. Proc. Soc. Exper. Biol. & Med. *112*: 287 (1963).
19. WEISSMAN, G., KEISER, H., and BERNHEIMER, A. W.: J. Exper. Med. *118*: 205 (1963).
20. WEISSMAN, G., BECHER, B., WIEDERMANN, G., and BERNHEIMER, A. W. Am. J. Path. *46*: 129 (1965).
21. CHRISTIAN, C. L. Arth. & Rheum. 7: 455 (1964).
22. HOLLANDER, J. L., McCARTY, D. J., JR., ASTORGA, G., and CASTRO-MURILLO, E. Ann. Int. Med. 62: 271 (1965).
23. ASTORGA, G., and BOLLET, A. J. Proc. Annual Meeting of the American Rheumatism Association, San Francisco, June 18–19, 1964, abstracted in Arth. & Rheum. 7: 288 (1964).
24. WEISSMAN, G. Fed. Proc. *23*: 1038 (1964).
25. WEISSMAN, G., and THOMAS, L. Bull. New York Acad. Med. *38*: 779 (1962).
26. WEISSMAN, G. Lancet, 2: 1373 (1964).

In Vivo and In Vitro
Studies on the Role of
PMN Leucocyte Granules in
Immediate Hypersensitivity*

H. Z. MOVAT, T. URIUHARA,†
R. K. MURRAY,
D. R. L. MACMORINE, S. WASI,
N. S. TAICHMAN,‡ and A. E. FRANKLIN

IN VIVO OBSERVATIONS ON THE ROLE OF PMN LEUCOCYTES

IN THE REVERSED ARTHUS REACTION, antigen (Ag) and antibody (Ab) combine in the walls of blood vessels; the resulting immune precipitates bind complement and are chemotactic for polymorphonuclear (PMN) leucocytes (31), which phagocytose the Ag–Ab precipitates (5). The infiltration of PMN leucocytes at the site of antigen-antibody (Ag–Ab) precipitation is associated with the production of oedema, hyperaemia, haemorrhage, and necrosis. On the other hand if an animal is made leucopenic, the Arthus reaction cannot be demonstrated (12, 25) in spite of the interaction and precipitation of immune precipitates at the same anatomical sites (4). It is obvious, then, that PMN leucocytes in some manner play a crucial role in the pathogenesis of the Arthus reaction. However, the mechanisms by which these cells mediate tissue injury (e.g. increase in vascular permeability, haemorrhage, and necrosis) remain to be elucidated.

While studying the effect of antigen–antibody interaction on the collagen fibrils of the cornea, we observed that the PMN leucocytes infiltrated the cornea at the site of the AG–Ab precipitation (16). These cells then phagocytosed the precipitates, and in this process the PMN leucocyte granules entered the phagocytic vacuoles containing the immune precipitates (Figs. 1a and 1b). Subsequent studies showed that a similar process occurred when PMN leuco-

*From the Departments of Pathology, Biochemistry, and Bacteriology, University of Toronto, Toronto. Aided by a grant from the Canadian Arthritis and Rheumatism Society.
†Research Fellow of the Medical Research Council of Canada.
‡Research Fellow of the J. P. Bickell Foundation.

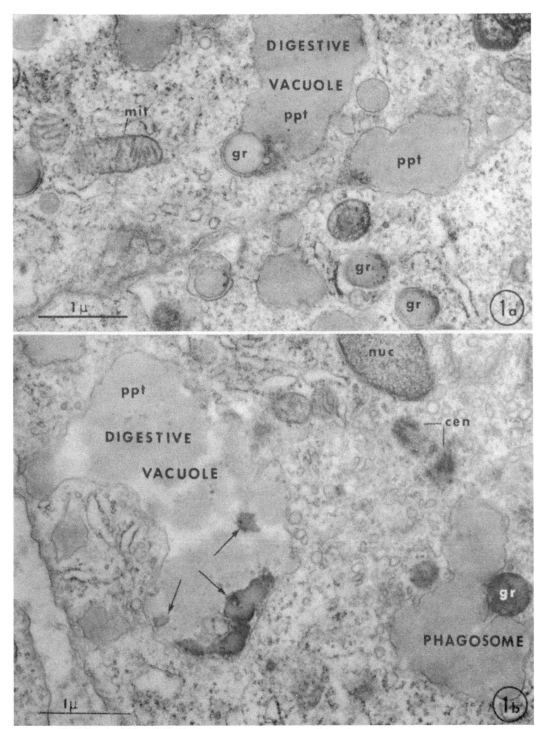

FIG. 1. Portions of two PMN leucocytes in an Arthus reaction. Fig. 1a shows an intact granule (gr) together with BSA–anti BSA precipitate (ppt) in a digestive vacuole. In Fig. 1b there are granular fragments (arrows) in the digestive vacuole. mit = mitochondrion; nuc = nucleus; cen = centriole. Fig. 1a, ×24,000; Fig. 1b, ×25,000.

cytes infiltrated the blood vessels in Arthus lesions (15, 27, 28) or during *in vitro* phagocytosis of preformed Ag–Ab complexes (17, 26). In these latter studies it was observed that within the phagocytic vacuole the PMN leucocyte granule becomes fragmented and lysed and presumably fuses with the phagocytosed material. In this process the PMN leucocytes become completely degranulated. Since PMN leucocyte granules are known to be lysosomes (6), it was postulated that the tissue injury in the Arthus reaction is due to release of hydrolytic enzymes derived from the PMN leucocyte granules (17, 28).

IN VITRO STUDIES

EXPERIMENTS WITH INTACT PMN LEUCOCYTES

Preliminary *in vitro* studies showed that when preformed Ag–Ab precipitates of bovine serum albumin (BSA)–anti BSA or horse ferritin–antiferritin were incubated with rabbit PMN leucocytes obtained from the peritoneal cavity, the phagocytic cells engulfed the Ag–Ab precipitates and became degranulated, as described above (Fig. 2). When the ambient fluid obtained from these reacting mixtures was administered intradermally in rabbits, the local injection site showed signs of increased vascular permeability, as visualized by the leakage of circulating Evans blue dye (17) (Table I); haemorrhage was commonly observed several hours after the injection, especially when higher concentrations of the fluid were employed. It was proposed that the material released from the PMN leucocytes during phagocytosis contained either (1) hydrolytic enzymes derived from the granules or (2) a degradation product of the phagocytosed material, or (3) both. Using protease inhibitors, a partial inhibition of the bluing reaction could be obtained. The permeability factor was referred to as "Pf/Phag" (permeability factor released during phagocytosis) (2).

TABLE I

Pf/Phag Induced Increase of Vascular Permeability in Rabbit Skin (Evans blue; HSA-I^{131})

(1-HOUR-OLD LESIONS)

Material injected (0.2 ml.)	Diam. bluing (cm.)	Intensity	% Trans. 620 mμ*	Radioactivity† (c.p.m.)
Sup. PMNL + Ag–Ab	1.6×1.7	++	86.0	3726
Sup. PMNL + Tyrode	1.0×1.0	+/−	95.0	1372
Sup. Tyrode + Ag–Ab	Diffuse	+/−	93.4	1520
Tyrode + Tyrode	—	—	98.2	640
Norm. skin			100.0	26

1 ml. (2 × 10⁸) PMN leucocytes incubated for 1 hr. at 37° C. with 0.8 ml. BSA–anti BSA ppt. (0.5 mg. Ab–N) and 0.2 ml. fresh rabbit serum and centrifuged at 10,400g for 20 min.

*Evans blue was extracted for 4 days at room temperature with formamide and the resulting colour read in a colorimeter at 620 mμ.

†35 μc. of I^{131}-labelled human serum albumin was injected i.v. and the radioactivity of the excised skin was determined in a Nuclear Chicago Gamma Detector.

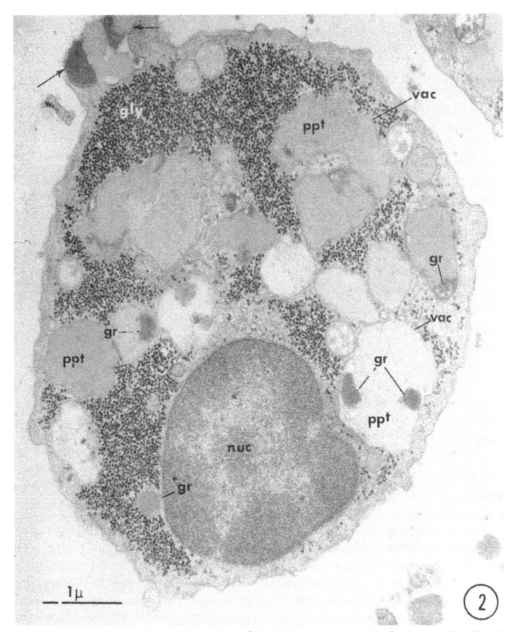

FIG. 2. Ultrastructure of a rabbit peritoneal PMN leucocyte which had been incubated with precipitates of BSA–anti BSA in a test tube for one hour. The phagocytosed immune precipitates (ppt) are seen in vacuoles (vac), occasionally in association with granules (gr) or remnants of granules. The arrows at the upper left corner of the cell point to material probably derived from a disintegrating PMN leucocyte and representing immune precipitates and fragmented granules; two pseudopods of the PMN leucocyte surround this material. nuc = nucleus; gly = glycogen. ×20,700 (from Movat *et al.*, ref. 17).

Subsequent investigations in our laboratory showed that the Pf/Phag released into the ambient fluid was heat labile and most of it was non-dialysable (Table II), indicating that Pf/Phag was predominantly enzymatic in nature. That Pf/Phag contains a protease became evident when proteolysis was demonstrated when it was incubated with various protein substrates. Peak proteolytic activity occurred at low pH values, indicating that the protease was an acid cathepsin.

TABLE II

EFFECT OF HEATING AND DIALYSIS ON PF/PHAG (INCREASED VASCULAR PERMEABILITY)

Material injected (0.2 ml.)	Visual estimation		% Trans.* 620 mμ
	30 min.	2 hr.	
Pf/Phag	1.0×0.9 −/+	1.6×1.8 ++	75.2
Pf/Phag: 50° C., 15 min.	1.2×1.2 +	1.7×1.4 ++	80.0
Pf/Phag: 60° C., 15 min.	1.2×1.0 +/−	1.5×1.4 +	87.2
Pf/Phag: 70° C., 15 min.	1.2×1.2 +/−	1.5×1.4 +/−	90.8
Pf/Phag: 80° C., 15 min.	Nil −	Nil −	93.5
Pf/Phag, dialysed	1.2×1.2 +	2.0×1.7 +++	73.1
Tyrode–gelatine	Nil −	Nil −	99.7
Normal skin			100.0

*See Table I.

EXPERIMENTS WITH ISOLATED PMN LEUCOCYTE LYSOSOMES

Ultrastructural observations and *in vitro* studies with whole PMN leucocytes indicated that during phagocytosis the granules of these cells were lysed followed by the release of lysosomal enzymes which could produce tissue injury. PMN leucocyte granules, when isolated by the method of Cohn and Hirsch (6) and lysed by freeze-thawing or ultrasonic disintegration, likewise caused an increase in vascular permeability ("bluing") when injected intradermally (17). When lysed PMN leucocyte granules were incubated with various substrates (denatured haemoglobin, BSA, BSA–anti BSA), proteolysis could be demonstrated (20). The pH optima for the enzymatic reaction varied slightly with the substrate used. When haemoglobin or BSA–anti BSA was used as substrate, maximum proteolytic activity was demonstrable at pH 2–3 (Fig. 3), while BSA gave peak activity at pH 4. More recently a second, smaller peak was obtained at pH 7–8. The significance of the two peaks of proteolytic activity is as yet uncertain, but it is possible that two or more cathepsins are present in PMN leucocyte lysosomes. It is conceivable that the acid cathepsin can act only intracellularly, as suggested by de Duve (7). When liberated, such a proteolytic enzyme would be most effective if it were released at sites where the buffering capacity of the serum and other buffers could have no effect, e.g. in aggregates of PMN leucocytes, in thrombi, or in vessels obstructed by Ag–Ab precipitates, as in the Arthus reaction (27) or in

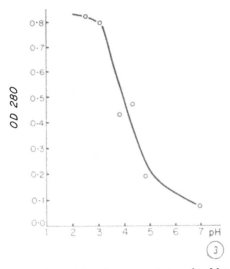

FIG. 3. Acid cathepsin activity of rabbit PMN leucocyte lysosomes on 2 per cent denatured haemoglobin. Equal volumes of lysed PMN leucocyte granules (300 mg.% protein), 2 per cent denatured haemoglobin, and buffers of various pH values were incubated at 37° C. for 24 hours, the reaction stopped with 10 per cent TCA, and the filtrate read at 280 mμ.

systemic anaphylaxis of the rabbit (18). On the other hand, the enzyme or enzymes most active at neutral or slightly alkaline pH could act, for instance, on kininogens present in the plasma and release kinins, or could have a direct proteolytic effect, as trypsin and other proteolytic enzymes may do in acute pancreatitis.

Using Ag–Ab complexes or BSA as substrate, proteolytic activity could be demonstrated also with starch gels, where partial or complete degradation of the substrate and the formation of faster-moving bands could be demonstrated (Fig. 4).

Experiments in progress are concerned with the inhibition of the proteolytic activity demonstrable in PMN leucocyte granules and with the use of synthetic substrates. Purification of the proteases will also be attempted.

TISSUE CULTURE STUDIES

From the foregoing evidence it would seem that phagocytosing PMN leucocytes release various hydrolases whose biological properties are akin to those seen following lysis of isolated PMN leucocyte granules. It would be most

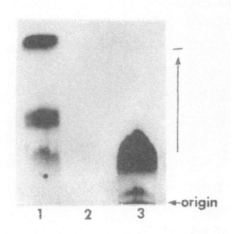

FIG. 4. Urea-starch gel electrophoresis (0.05M formate, final pH 4.0). Slot 1: BSA—anti BSA complex incubated with PMN lysosomes at pH 4.0 for 24 hours. Slot 2: PMN lysosomes incubated at pH 4.0 for 24 hours. Slot 3: BSA–anti BSA complex incubated at pH 4.0 for 24 hours. Electrophoresis was performed at room temperature (approximately 23° C.) for 20 hours with 5 volts/cm. passing through the gel (25 ma.). The gel was then stained with Amido Black B. Note breakdown of BSA–anti BSA complex with formation of faster-moving fragments (Slot 1).

interesting to study the effects of these granule-derived substances on tissue culture cells, since an *in vitro* system would eliminate any secondary alterations.

Ph/Phag, intact, or lysed PMN leucocyte granules were added to human amnion cells and to rabbit endothelial cells grown in tissue culture. At various times after the addition of these substances, fixative (osmium tetroxide) was poured on to the culture and after short fixation the monolayer was scraped off and fixed in free suspension for an additional period of time. Preliminary observations indicate that both Pf/Phag and lysed granules induce changes consisting of "granularity," rounding-up, and detachment of the cells from the tubes. At the ultrastructural level, phagocytosis of lysed PMN leucocyte granules is followed by lytic changes within the cells. The formation of autophagic vacuoles (7) and lytic changes were also observed with Pf/Phag (Figs. 5–7). With severe injury necrosis was encountered. The endothelial cells were more sensitive to injury than the epithelial cells. More recent studies using human synovial cells showed similar changes.

THE ROLE OF PMN LEUCOCYTES AND PLATELETS IN ANAPHYLAXIS

Anaphylaxis in the rabbit has been attributed in turn to spasm of the pulmonary vessels and right heart failure (3), to the release of histamine (24) or serotonin (29), and to obstruction of the pulmonary vessels by Ag–Ab complexes (8, 14). The last mechanism is generally accepted today (1).

In view of the evidence implicating PMN leucocyte granules in the mediation of allergic tissue injury, it seemed pertinent to investigate the possible role that hydrolytic enzymes, particularly proteases, may play in anaphylaxis. Although it has never been clearly demonstrated, many investigators believed that during anaphylaxis of the rabbit aggregates of leucocytes and platelets impact in the pulmonary vessel (24). During this process histamine and serotonin are released from the platelets and leucocytes into the plasma (9, 13, 29, 30). However, neither serotonin depletion (10) nor antihistamines (23) ameliorate anaphylaxis in the rabbit. We postulated that the aggregates of platelets and PMN leucocytes, if they indeed occurred, should be associated with phagocytosis of the Ag–Ab complexes and increased proteolytic activity should be demonstrable in the plasma. It should be noted that phagocytosis of latex particles (11) and of Ag–Ab complexes (19, 21) by platelets has been observed *in vitro*.

When actively immunized rabbits were challenged intravenously with the antigen used for immunization (BSA or ferritin), a fall in circulating PMN leucocytes (neutrophils) and platelets was observed (Fig. 8). This occurred concomitantly with formation of Ag–Ab precipitates in the pulmonary circulation (Figs. 9a and 9b) and the aggregation of PMN leucocytes and platelets in the pulmonary vessels (Fig. 10). At the ultrastructural level, phagocytosis of the Ag–Ab precipitates by the PMN leucocytes and degranulation of these could be demonstrated in the pulmonary blood vessels (Fig. 11). Platelets likewise phagocytosed Ag–Ab complexes (Fig. 12). We have previously presented evidence that phagocytosis of Ag–Ab complexes by platelets *in vitro* leads to platelet aggregation, which is associated with release of ADP, histamine, and serotonin (19). More recent *in vitro* experiments with platelets indicate that platelet lysosomal (granular) enzymes are also released during aggregation of platelets (22).

That proteolytic enzymes were in fact released into the plasma during anaphylaxis from PMN leucocytes and possibly from platelets was demonstrated (Fig. 13). The released protease seems to be primarily a cathepsin. In addition to the ultrastructural evidence, other findings indicate that the protease demonstrable in the plasma derived from the leucocytes and platelets. When anaphylaxis was induced in leucothrombopenic rabbits, no such proteolytic activity could be demonstrated (Table III). If rabbits with approximately

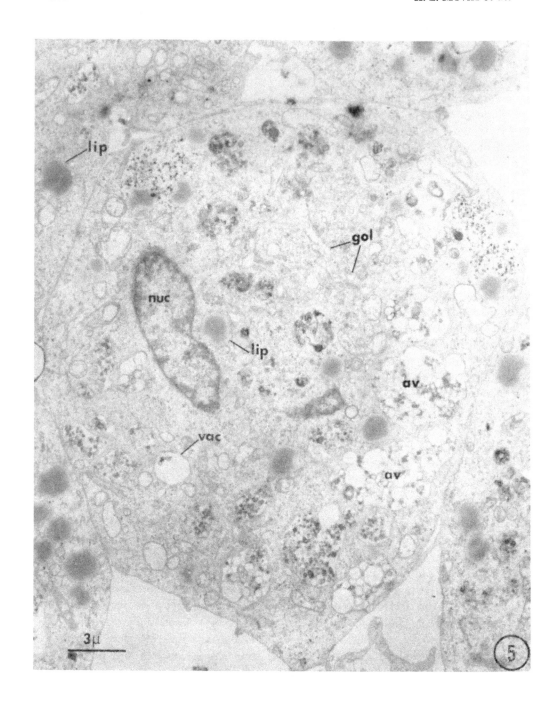

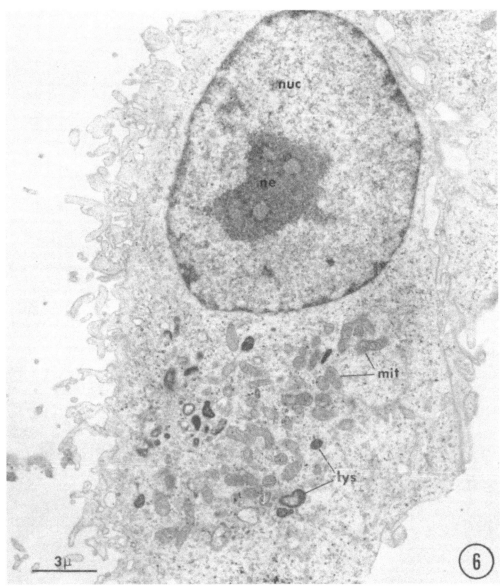

FIGS. 5 AND 6. Fig. 5 shows a human amnion cell grown in tissue culture and incubated for 4 hours with Pf/Phag. Compare with a control cell incubated with Tyrode–gelatine (Fig. 6). The control cell formed a continuous sheet with other cells and numerous microvilli. The altered cells became rounded up and often detached. Note the well-formed mitochondria (mit) and lysosomes of the control cell. The altered cells have numerous vacuoles (vac), autophagic vacuoles (av), and lipid bodies (lip). nuc = nucleus; ne = nucleolus; gol = Golgi region. Fig. 5, ×5250; Fig. 6, ×5625.

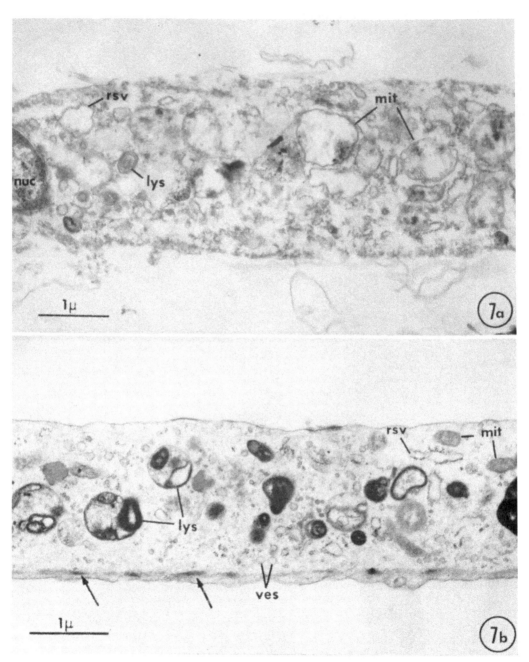

FIG. 7. Rabbit endothelial cell incubated with lysed PMN leucocyte lysosomes for 16 hours (7a) and control (7b). The control cell has numerous lysosomes (lys), a few small mitochondria (mit), rough-surfaced vesicles (rsv) and small, smooth-surfaced vesicles (ves). The treated cell appears "digested," with blurred membranes, swollen mitochondria, and few lysosomes. The arrows point to densities at the cell border, reminiscent of the attachment bodies of smooth muscle cells. Fig. 7a, ×19,300; Fig. 7b, ×21,000.

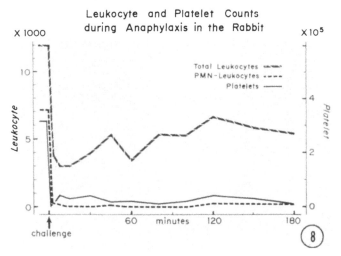

FIG. 8. The effect of challenge with antigen on the leucocyte and platelet count of a hyperimmunized rabbit. Note that the fall in WBC is due mainly to a fall in PMN leucocytes (granulocytes).

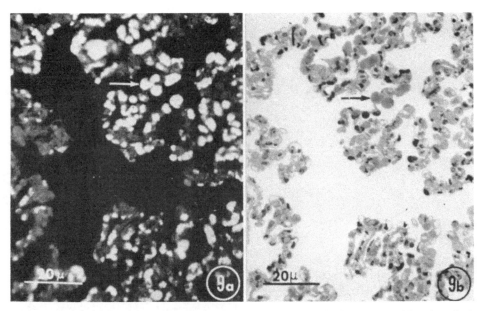

FIG. 9. Fluorescent and corresponding light micrograph of the lung of a rabbit that died of systemic anaphylaxis. The animal had circulating anti-BSA and was injected i.v. with fluorescent-labelled BSA. Many vessels are occluded by a homogeneous acidophilic material and in ultraviolet-light-fluorescent antigen-containing precipitates (arrow). ×750.

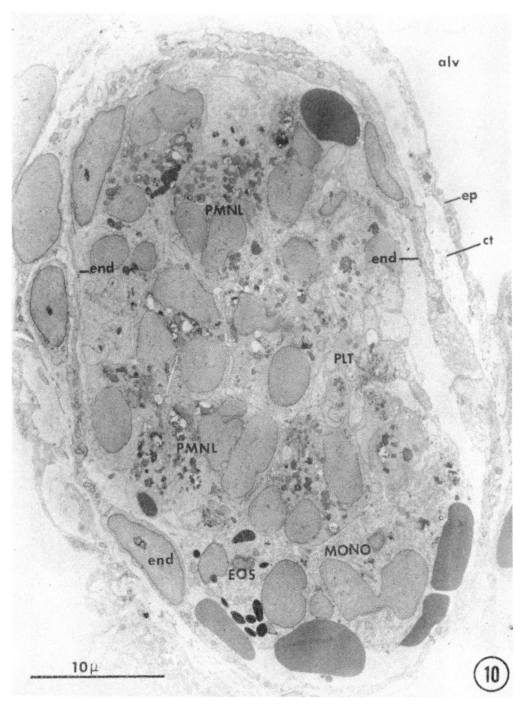

Fig. 10. Low-power electron micrograph of small pulmonary vein completely occluded by aggregated PMN leucocytes (PMNL) and platelets (PLT). An eosinophil (EOS) and monocyte (MONO) are also seen. end = endothelial lining; alv = alveolar space; ep = alveolar epithelium; et = connective tissue. ×3500.

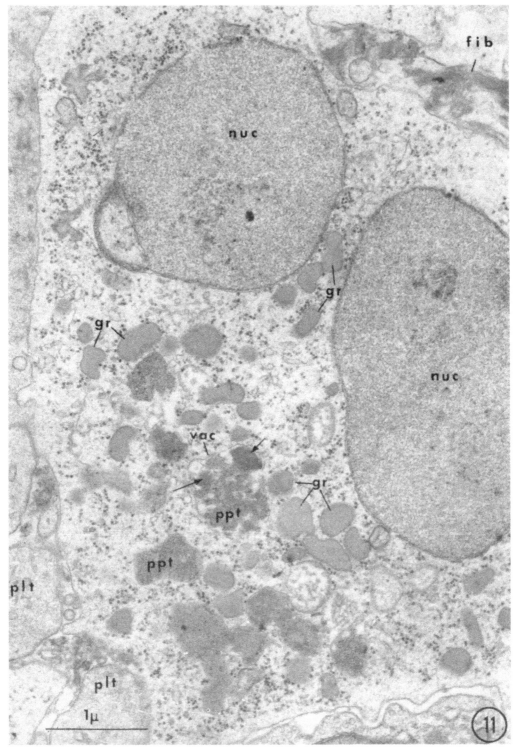

Fig. 11. PMN leucocyte in pulmonary vessel. Fragments of granules (arrows) are seen with precipitates (ppt) of ferritin–antiferritin in digestive vacuoles (vac). nuc = nucleus; gr = granule; plt = platelet; fib = fibrin. ×22,000.

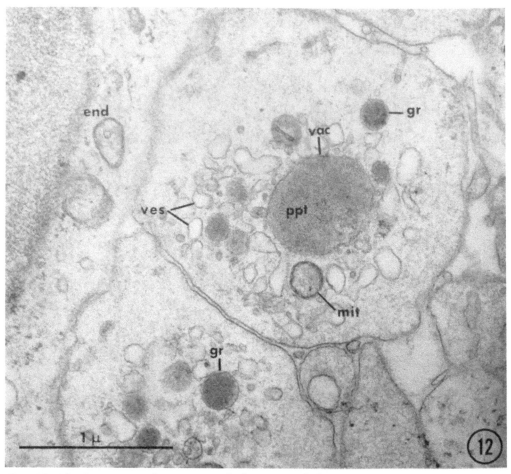

Fig. 12. Platelets in a pulmonary vessel during anaphylaxis. Ferritin–antiferritin precipitates (ppt) are present in a vacuole (vac) together with a homogeneous substance, probably lysed granules. gr = granule; mit = mitochondrion; ves = vesicle; end = endothelial cell. ×40,000.

the same levels of circulating antibody N were paired and then challenged with antigen, anaphylaxis in leucopenic animals was milder. In the animals that survived anaphylaxis the blood pressure dropped by about 25–30 per cent in leucopenic animals, as compared to about 50 per cent in those with a normal white cell count. Leucopenic animals soon recovered, whereas those without leucopenia developed protracted anaphylaxis. Finally, the lungs of leucopenics looked grossly normal, whereas animals with a normal white cell count had multiple focal and confluent areas of haemorrhage indicating that, as in the Arthus reaction, lyosomal proteases are capable of eroding vessels.

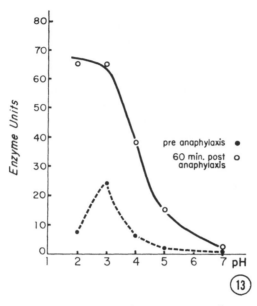

FIG. 13. Serum cathepsin activity during anaphylaxis. Effect on 2 per cent denatured haemoglobin at various pH values.

TABLE III

SERUM CATHEPSIN LEVELS DURING ANAPHYLAXIS IN RABBITS

	Enzyme units*		
Rabbits	Pre-anaph.	60-min. post-anaph.	% Increase
Normal (6)	12.10	56.0	373
Leucopenic (3)	6.71	9.10	36

*One enzyme unit produces an optical density (at 280 mμ) of 1 $\times$ 10^{-3} per hour per ml. of serum at 37° C. Equal volumes of serum, 2 per cent denatured haemoglobin, and buffer (citric acid–Na citrate pH 4.0) were incubated at 37° C. for 24 hours, the reaction stopped with 10 per cent TCA, and the filtrate read at 280 mμ. The results are average values for the number of rabbits shown in the table.

SUMMARY AND CONCLUSIONS

Ultrastructural evidence was presented that *in vivo* (Arthus reaction, anaphylaxis) when PMN leucocytes phagocytose antigen–antibody complexes, their granules (lysosomes) fuse with the phagocytosed material to form "digestive vacuoles" (7). In this process the granules become lysed and are presumably released into the tissues or into the blood.

Using *in vitro* techniques, a similar process could be demonstrated. During *in vitro* phagocytosis release of a substance(s) which probably represents lysed lysosomal enzymes occurs into the ambient fluid.

Isolated and lysed PMN granules exhibit proteolytic activity towards several substrates, including antigen–antibody complexes.

The material released from the phagocytosing PMN leucocytes and the lysed granules causes an increase in vascular permeability and haemorrhage when injected into the dermis of rabbits and degenerative changes and necrosis when added to cells grown in tissue culture.

Since antigen–antibody complexes per se cause little tissue injury, it seems reasonable to assume that severe injury leading to haemorrhage and necrosis is mediated by the PMN leucocyte lysosomal enzymes, primarily the proteases, released from these cells when they phagocytose antigen–antibody complexes.

REFERENCES

1. Austen, K. F., and Humphrey, J. H.   Advances Immunol. 3: 1 (1963).
2. Burke, J. S., Uriuhara, T., Macmorine, D. R. L., and Movat, H. Z.   Life Sci. 3: 1505 (1964).
3. Coca, A. F.   J. Immunol. 4: 219 (1919).
4. Cochrane, C. G., and Weigle, W. O.   J. Exper. Med. 108: 591 (1958).
5. Cochrane, C. G., Weigle, W. O., and Dixon, F. J.   J. Exper. Med. 110: 481 (1959).
6. Cohn, Z. A., and Hirsch, J. G.   J. Exper. Med. 116: 827 (1962).
7. de Duve, C.   The lysosome concept. Ciba Foundation Symposium on Lysosomes (J. & A. Churchill, London, 1963), pp. 1–35.
8. Dixon, F. J.   J. Allergy, 24: 547 (1953).
9. Dragstedt, C. A., Arellano, M. R., and Lawton, A. H.   Science, 91: 617 (1940).
10. Fischer, D., and Lecomte, J.   Compt. rend. Soc. Biol. 150: 1026 (1956).
11. Glynn, M. F., Movat, H. Z., Murphy, E. A., and Mustard, J. F.   J. Lab. & Clin. Med. 65: 179 (1965).
12. Humphrey, J. H.   Brit. J. Exper. Path. 36: 368 (1955).
13. Katz, G.   Science, 91: 221 (1940).
14. McKinnon, G. E., Andrews, E. C., Heptinstall, R. H., and Germuth, F. G.   Bull. Johns Hopkins Hosp. 101: 258 (1957).
15. Movat, H. Z.   The vascular changes in acute normergic (non-allergic) and allergic inflammation. *In* Methods and Achievements in Experimental Pathology, *edited by* E. Bajusz and G. Jasmin (S. Karger, A.G., Basel and New York, 1965).
16. Movat, H. Z., Fernando, N. V. P., Uriuhara, T., and Weiser, W. J.   J. Exper. Med. 118: 557 (1963).
17. Movat, H. Z., Uriuhara, T., Macmorine, D. R. L., and Burke, J. S.   Life Sci. 3: 1025 (1964).
18. Movat, H. Z., Taichman, N. S., and Uriuhara, T.   Fed. Proc. 24: 369 (1965).
19. Movat, H. Z., Mustard, J. F., Taichman, N. S., and Uriuhara, T.   Proc. Soc. Exper. Biol. & Med. 120: 232 (1965).
20. Murray, R. K., Wasi, S., and Macmorine, D. R. L.   Fed. Proc. 24: 368 (1965).
21. Mustard, J. F., and Movat, H. Z.   In preparation.
22. Mustard, J. F., Movat, H. Z., Macmorine, D. R. L., and Senyi, A.   Proc. Soc. Exper. Biol. & Med. 119: 988 (1965).
23. Reuse, J. J.   Antihistamine drugs and histamine release, especially in anaphylaxis. Ciba Foundation Symposium on Histamine (J. & A. Churchill, London, 1956), pp. 150–4.
24. Rocha e Silva, M.   Histamine, Its Role in Anaphylaxis and Allergy (C. C. Thomas, Springfield, Ill., 1955).

25. STETSON, C. A., Jr.   J. Exper. Med. *94*: 347 (1951).
26. URIUHARA, T.   Fed. Proc. *23*: 390 (1964).
27. URIUHARA, T., and MOVAT, H. Z.   Lab. Invest. *13*: 1057 (1964).
28. ——— Exper. & Molec. Path. (in press).
29. WAALKES, T. P., WEISSBACH, H., BOZICEVICH, J., and UDENFRIEND, S.   J. Clin. Invest. *36*: 1115 (1957).
30. WAALKES, T. P., and COBURN, H.   J. Allergy, *30*: 394 (1959).
31. WARD, P. A., and COCHRANE, C. G.   J. Exper. Med. *121*: 215 (1965).
32. WASI, S., URIUHARA, T., TAICHMAN, N. S., MURRAY, R. K., and MOVAT, H. Z.   In preparation.

Platelet Aggregation, Phagocytosis, and Vessel Permeability[*]

M. F. GLYNN,[†] J. F. MUSTARD,
H. A. SMYTHE, and H. Z. MOVAT

AGGREGATED PLATELETS are found in many intravascular reactions associated with inflammation. For example, they are present in the Arthus reaction, anaphylaxus, and the Schwartzmann reaction. Recent evidence indicates that the platelet, like the leucocyte, is capable of phagocytosis (1–4) and that it also undergoes degranulation (4, 5). Furthermore, the platelet granules have been identified as being in part composed of lysosomes (6). In view of this evidence we have examined the changes produced in the platelet by a variety of stimuli including some of those associated with inflammatory reactions.

The factors that induce platelet aggregation, swelling, and degranulation can be classified into two groups: enzymes such as thrombin, trypsin, pronase, and chymotrypsin and surfaces such as collagen, heat-aggregated protein antigen–antibody (AG/AB) complexes, and protein-coated polystyrene particles (3–5, 7–9). As can be seen in Fig. 1, when AG/AB complexes, aggregated protein, or protein-coated particles of polystyrene of a size that can be ingested come in contact with the platelet membrane, the particles are taken up by the platelet (3, 4, 8, 10). In Fig. 2, it can be seen that platelets exposed to polystyrene for 60 minutes at 37° C. show considerable change in their ultrastructure, which includes swelling and loss of glycogen, granules, and mitochondria. The unit membranes of the platelets, however, appear to remain intact. We have found that a similar series of morphological changes occur in the platelet when it is exposed to thrombin, AG/AB complexes, aggregated protein, or uric acid crystals.

[*]From the Blood and Vascular Disease Research Unit, Departments of Medicine and Pathology, University of Toronto, and Sunnybrook Hospital, Department of Veterans Affairs, Toronto.

This work was supported in part by grants from the Department of Veterans Affairs, Ontario Heart Foundation, Medical Research Council MT 1309, and the Department of National Health and Welfare.

[†]Fellow, National Heart Institute, National Institutes of Health, Bethesda, Maryland.

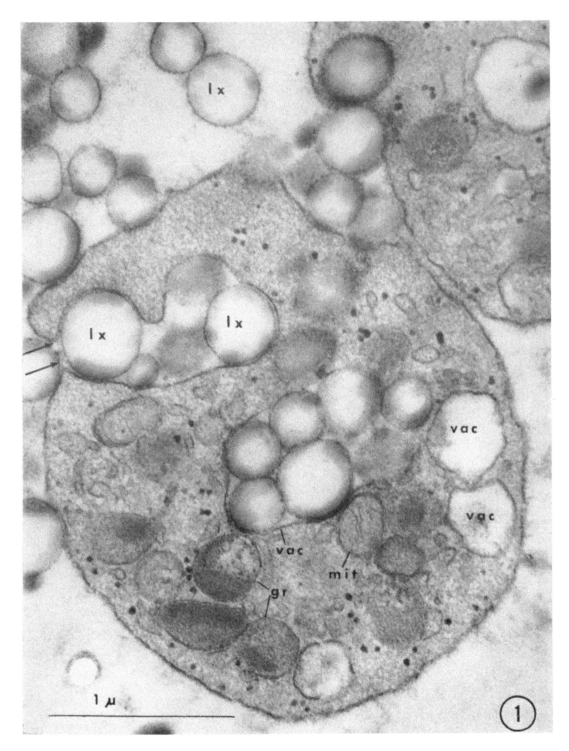

Fig. 1.

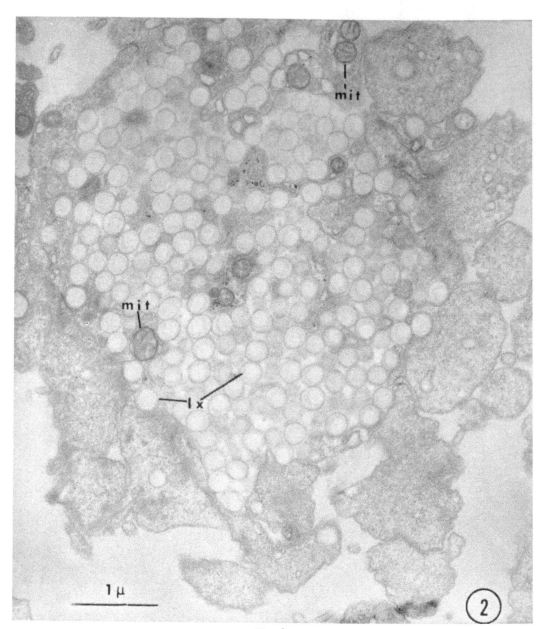

Fig. 2.

In our initial studies with polystyrene particles and platelets it was demonstrated that the platelet aggregation induced by latex was probably mediated through release of platelet adenosine diphosphate (ADP) (3). This release of ADP was associated with a fall in the platelet adenosine triphosphate (ATP) level. Studies with the other compounds that have been found to induce these changes have revealed that they too produce a fall in platelet ATP and increased amounts of ADP in the ambient fluid (Table I). Further proof that ADP is the key factor in inducing aggregation in these experiments is the observation that prior exposure of a platelet to adenosine monophosphate (AMP) or adenosine, compounds known to inhibit the aggregating effect of ADP (11), prevents platelet aggregation induced by the various stimuli. In Table II the effect of AMP on latex-induced aggregation is shown. These compounds, however, do not prevent platelet phagocytosis (4).

TABLE I

PLATELET NUCLEOTIDE RELEASE

Platelet suspension* plus	Platelet ATP (μg./ml. platelet suspension)	Supernatant	
		ADP	AMP
		(μg./ml. supernatant)	
Tyrode	47.8	44.6	1.0
Collagen suspension	20.5	73.2	65.8
AG/AB complex	4.0	139.8	95.4
Thrombin 10 μ/ml.	3.6	171.8	41.2
Uric acid crystals	10.4	96.3	70.0
Latex	—	60.5	52.0

*10 part platelet suspension plus 1 part of the solutions or suspensions listed. Agitation at 37° C. for 10 minutes.

TABLE II

AMP- AND LATEX-INDUCED PLATELET AGGREGATION*

Platelet-rich plasma plus	Counts per unit volume	
	Threshold 7	Threshold 30
	67,400	1900
Saline + latex	24,500	4100
AMP + saline	68,500	1900
AMP + latex	48,900	2900
Saline + saline	67,400	1900

*The methods used have been described.

The chelation of divalent cations by disodium ethylenediamine tetra-acetate (EDTA) also blocks ADP-induced platelet aggregation. In Table III it can be seen that although EDTA does not prevent the release of nucleotide into the ambient fluid when platelets are exposed to most of these stimuli, such as latex, aggregation nevertheless does not take place. The aggregation in these

TABLE III

THE EFFECT OF LATEX ON PLATELET AGGREGATION IN EDTA PLATELET-RICH
PLASMA*

	Counts per unit volume			
	Threshold 7		Threshold 50	
Sample	Pre-latex	Post-latex	Pre-latex	Post-latex
1	40,400	40,400	2600	2700
2	48,300	46,000	3200	3400
3	58,500	57,300	2500	2500
4	52,600	48,900	3100	2800
5	48,300	39,200	4500	3500

*Details of the methods used have been published (3).

studies was assessed using the Coulter counter, details of which have been described elsewhere (3). Furthermore, our observations have indicated, as can be seen in Fig. 3, that very little, if any, phagocytosis of polystyrene occurs in the presence of EDTA (3, 4). However, we have found that adherence of polystyrene to the membrane of the platelet still occurs (12). This is analogous to what has been reported for platelet adherence to collagen fibres (13).

There are changes in platelet serotonin and histamine associated with these stimuli. The release of radioactive serotonin and histamine from prelabelled platelets in a suspension exposed to these various agents is shown in Table IV.

TABLE IV

C^{14}-SEROTONIN AND H^3-HISTAMINE RELEASE*

Platelet-rich plasma (citrate) plus	Counts per minute/ml. supernatant	
	C^{14}-serotonin	H^3-histamine
Tyrode	48.7	368.0
Thrombin (10 μ/ml.)	3149.6	782.0
Trypsin (1 mg./ml.)	3367.0	734.0
Latex (1:10)	2808.9	1360.0
AG/AB complex	3086.4	921.0
Collagen	3210.3	—

*The methods used have been described (3, 8).

Although far from conclusive, there is evidence that at least some of the factors producing these effects also lead to metabolic changes. The addition to the platelet suspension of an appropriate amount of iodoacetate prevents the release of ADP (Table V). This evidence may indicate that some sulphydryl groups are involved in this process and that perhaps glycolysis itself plays a part. Further evidence that platelet metabolism may be involved comes from the demonstration that thrombin causes increased oxygen consumption by platelets (14).

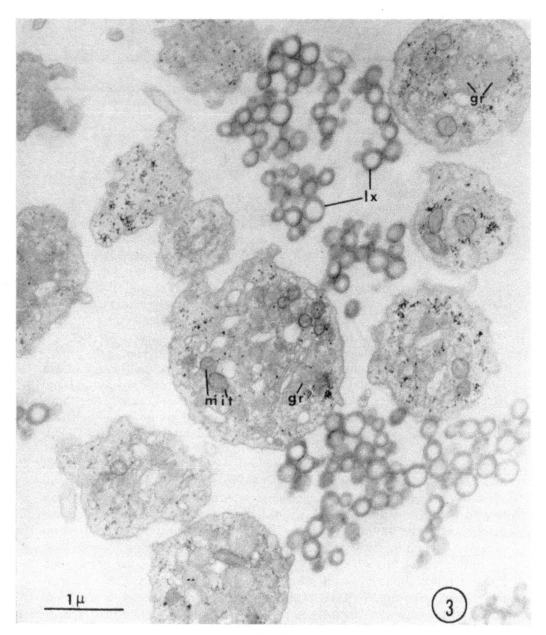

FIG. 3.

TABLE V

IODOACETATE AND PLATELET NUCLEOTIDE RELEASE

Platelet suspension* plus	Platelet ATP (μg./ml. suspension)	Nucleotide ADP (μg./ml.)	Supernatant AMP (μg./ml.)
Collagen + buffered saline	2.05	7.32	—
Collagen + iodoacetate†	3.84	3.82	—
AG/SB complex + buffered saline	0.40	13.98	9.54
AG/AB complex + iodoacetate†	3.60	2.84	4.12
Tyrode + buffered saline	4.78	4.46	2.10
Tyrode + iodoacetate†	3.50	1.60	2.32

*10 parts platelet suspension plus 1 part collagen or other material and 1 part saline or iodoacetate.

†Concentration 10 mM. (Final concentration 0.83 mM.)

The results from these and other investigations suggest that some proteolytic enzymes and protein surfaces when in contact with the platelet membrane cause changes in the platelet which lead to: a fall in platelet ATP, increased ADP in the ambient fluid, platelet aggregation, release of platelet serotonin and histamine, and loss of platelet granules. We have found that platelet degranulation is associated with increased acid phosphatase in the ambient fluid. When the particle is of appropriate size these changes are associated with the uptake by the platelet.

The effect of these platelet aggregates on the vessel wall may be complex. There is good evidence that serotonin, histamine, and lysosomal enzymes can influence vessel permeability (15, 16, 17). Preliminary experiments indicate that platelet granules, like the granules of polymorphonuclear cells, have proteolytic properties with peak activities at low pH values, suggesting that they contain acid cathepsins as well as enzymes such as acid phosphates (18). We have examined the effects of the various stimuli on the release of factors from the platelet which influence vessel permeability (19). In Table VI it can be seen that the supernatant from platelet suspensions exposed to these stimuli caused increased bluing when injected intradermally into rabbits previously treated with Evans blue (1.0 ml./kg. of 0.5 per cent solution). In the experiment shown here the rabbit had also been injected with I[131]-labelled serum albumin. The radioactivity of the injection sites is also shown. There is little doubt that all the factors, including ADP, which produce platelet aggregation induced release of factors which increase vessel permeability (19). Furthermore, even exposure to AMP, which does not cause platelet aggregation, appeared to cause some increase in the ambient fluid of factors that increase vessel permeability. Pretreatment of rabbits with antihistamine prior to injection of the supernatant material diminished the response but did not completely suppress it (20). Furthermore, granules isolated from platelets and exposed to immune complexes released factors which increased vessel per-

TABLE VI

PLATELETS AND VESSEL PERMEABILITY

Supernatant from platelet suspension* plus	Injection site		
	Evans blue bluing		I^{131} albumin (c.p.m.)
	Area, cm.	Intensity	
Tyrode	Nil	Nil	1.223
AG/AB complex	1.0×1.0	++	6.493
Thrombin 100 u/ml.	1.0×1.1	++	3.311
Collagen	1.1×1.1	+	3.302
Uric acid crystals	0.8×0.9	+/−	1.692
Latex (undiluted)	Diffuse†	+/−	2.000
Control*—Supernatant from Tyrode solution plus			
AG/AB complex	Nil	Nil	1.100
Thrombin	Nil	Nil	1.024
Collagen	Nil	Nil	940
Uric acid crystals	Nil	Nil	1.200
Latex	Nil	Nil	976

*10 parts of the platelet suspension or Tyrode solution (control) were incubated with 1 part of the solution or suspension indicated for 10 minutes at 37 °C. The mixtures were then centrifuged at 7000 r.p.m. and the supernatant injected intradermally into a rabbit previously given Evans blue and I^{131} albumin.
†Outer margin not clearly defined.

meability which were not blocked by antihistamines. Platelets depleted of serotonin by reserpine treatment still have a considerable activity, which increases vessel permeability when exposed to factors such as AG/AB complexes (20). These observations suggest that serotonin, histamine, and probably platelet lysosomal enzymes could be important in inducing increased vessel permeability in areas of platelet aggregation.

A variety of factors appear to induce metabolic changes within the platelet leading to a fall in platelet ATP and increased amounts of ADP in the ambient fluid, which induces aggregation. These changes are associated with swelling and loss of platelet granules and the release of factors which increase vessel permeability. Although not generally recognized, the platelet may play an important part in the inflammatory response seen in areas of vessel and tissue injury and may be of importance in the body's defence against foreign particles and micro-organisms in the blood.

REFERENCES

1. DAVID-FERREIRA, J. F. Demonstration du pouvoir phagocytaire des plaquettes sanguines chez le lapin. Proc. European Regional Conf. Elect. Micr. (Delft) 2: 917–20 (1960).
2. SCHULZ, H. Ueber die Phagozytose von kolloidalem Siliziumdioxyd durch Thrombocyten mit Bemerkungen zur submikroskopischen Struktur der Thrombozytenmembran. Folia Haemat. (N.F.), 5: 195–205 (1961).

3. GLYNN, M. F., MOVAT, H. Z., MURPHY, E. A., and MUSTARD, J. F. Study of platelet adhesiveness and aggregation with latex particles. J. Lab. Clin. Med. *65*: 179–201 (1965).

4. MOVAT, H. Z., WEISER, W. J., GLYNN, M. F., and MUSTARD, J. F. J. Cell Biol. (to be published).

5. FRENCH, J. E., and POOLE, J. C. F. Proc. Roy. Soc. B, *157*: 170 (1963).

6. MARCUS, A. J., and ZUCKER-FRANKLIN, D. Enzyme and coagulation activity of sub-cellular platelet fractions (Abstract). J. Clin. Invest. *43*: 1241 (1964).

7. HOVIG, T. Release of a platelet-aggregating substance (adenosine diphosphate) from rabbit platelets induced by saline "extract" of tendons. Thromb. et Diath. Haem. *9*: 264–78 (1963).

8. MOVAT, H. Z., MUSTARD, J. F., TAICHMAN, N. S., and URIUHARA, T. Proc. Soc. Exper. Biol. & Med. (to be published).

9. RODMAN, N. F., MASON, R. G., McDEVITT, N. B., and BRINKHOUS, K. M. Am. J. Path. *40*: 27 (1962).

10. DAVID-FERREIRA, J. F. *In* International Review of Cytology, Vol. 17 (Academic Press, New York, 1964), p. 99.

11. BORN, G. V. R. Nature, *194*: 927 (1962).

12. GLYNN, M. F., HERREN, R., and MUSTARD, J. F. To be published.

13. HOVIG, T. Thromb. et. Diath. Haemorrh. *9*: 264 (1963).

14. HUSSAIN, Q. Z., and NEWCOMB, T. T. J. Appl. Physiol. *19*: 297 (1964).

15. MAJNO, G., and PALADE, G. E. Studies on inflammation I. The effect of histamine and serotonin on vascular permeability: and electron mucroscopic study. J. Biophys. & Biochem. Cytol. *11*: 571–605 (1961).

16. GOLUB, E. S., and SNITZNAGEL, J. K. Fed. Proc. *25*: 509 (1964).

17. MOVAT, H. Z., TAICHMAN, N. S., URIUHARA, T., and WASI, S. Rabbit anaphylaxis—The role of PMN-leukocytes and platelet pysosomes. Fed. Proc. *24*: 369 (1965).

18. WASI, S., MUSTARD, J. F., and MOVAT, H. Z. Unpublished observations.

19. MUSTARD, J. F., MOVAT, H. Z., MACMORINE, D. R. L., and SENYI, A. Proc. Soc. Exper. Biol. & Med. (to be published).

20. MUSTARD, J. F., MACMORINE, D. R. L., and SENYI, A. Fed. Proc. *24*: 154 (1965).

Skin Window Studies in
Rheumatoid Arthritis*

R. D. WILKINSON,† S. KIM,‡ and A. SARGENT§

THE SKIN WINDOW TECHNIQUE has been applied to the investigation of specific immunologic systems in an effort to relate antigen-antibody interaction with cellular events (1, 2). Cell populations available for evaluation on skin window slides may be divided into four groups: polymorphonuclear basophils, eosinophils, and neutrophils, and the heterogeneous mononuclear group consisting of monocytes, lymphocytes, macrophages, and plasma cells. The several characteristic cellular reaction profiles which have emerged with the use of this technique are depicted in Fig. 1 as the average percentage of cells counted at 3, 8, 24, and 27 hours in 10 or more subjects.

The cellular response to simple abrasion of the skin is the basic control in these profiles. The effect of a test substance is measured by injecting it intradermally and abrading the resultant injection wheal for skin window testing.

The response to simple skin abrasion in normal and rheumatoid subjects consists of an early neutrophilia, which is overshadowed by an influx of mononuclears at 6 and 24 hours, but which recurs at 27 hours. Basophils and eosinophils are not seen.

Local histamine challenge of normal subjects induces the same non-specific response, whereas in pollen-allergic subjects histamine evokes trace basophilia and weak, sustained eosinophilia. Allergen challenge of pollen-allergic subjects induces basophilia and prominent sustained eosinophilia, superimposed on the usual neutrophil–mononuclear swing.

A contrasting profile is encountered in subjects sensitive to poison ivy who are challenged with *Rhus oleo* resin. The basophil response is relatively dominant at 24 and 27 hours, eosinophilia is weak and sustained, and the mononuclear response tends to persist through the later hours.

Additional characteristic patterns have been described in chronic ulcerative

*From the Royal Victoria Hospital, Montreal.
†Research Fellow, Department of Immunochemistry and Allergy, and Clinical Assistant, Division of Dermatology.
‡Fellow, Department of Medicine.
§Research Fellow.

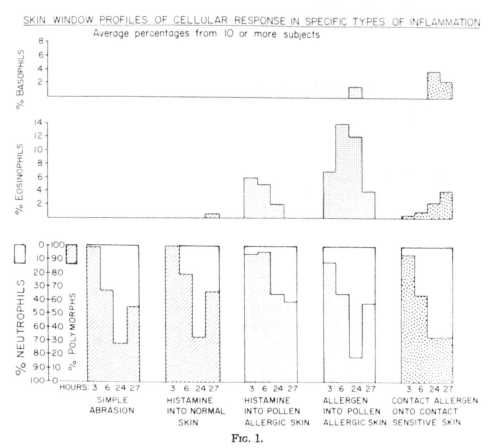

SKIN WINDOW PROFILES OF CELLULAR RESPONSE IN SPECIFIC TYPES OF INFLAMMATION
Average percentages from 10 or more subjects

FIG. 1.

colitis (3), interstitial cystitis (4), Hurler's syndrome (5), and bacterial hypersensitivity (6).

The present study was designed to establish profiles of cellular response in rheumatoid arthritis. Since rheumatoid factor has an antibody-like affinity for human gamma globulin, particularly aggregated gamma globulin (7), cellular responses to these reactants and to native and polymerized DNA, and finally to nucleoprotein-coated latex particles, were evaluated in 10 patients with rheumatoid-factor-positive rheumatoid arthritis, and in 6 healthy student volunteers.

MATERIALS AND METHODS

Testing materials were prepared as follows:

1. Commercial immune gamma globulin was prepared as a 1 per cent solution in saline.*

*Immune serum globulin (human), Connaught Laboratories.

2. A portion was aggregated by heating it at 63° C. for 30 minutes (8).

3. High-purity native calf thymus DNA was prepared in a 0.1 per cent solution, rendered bacteria-free by millipore filtration.*

4. Polymerized DNA was derived from the above by heating as described by Stollar and Levine (9).

5. Commercial nucleoprotein-coated and uncoated latex particles were prepared as 1 per cent suspensions sterilized by ultraviolet irradiation.†

The skin window technique used in these experiments incorporated fixed time intervals of 3, 6, 24, and 27 hours for slide changes, and adapted a motorized grinding burr for abrading the test sites. Initially 500 consecutive cells were differentially counted, but because of inaccuracy when cell distribution on slides was uneven, this procedure was dropped in favour of scan estimation of group percentages of the total number of intact cells on each slide. This procedure tended to correct for uneven cell distributions and, in our hands, was efficient and reliable.

RESULTS AND DISCUSSION

Intradermal skin tests were read at 15 minutes and at 24 hours (Table I). All the positive reactions were weak, and consisted of persisting induration and erythema of the injection wheal. Neither halo erythema nor pseudopods were seen. There was no significant difference in the skin test reactivity between the rheumatoid and control groups.

TABLE I

PER CENT POSITIVE INTRADERMAL SKIN TESTS

	15 min.		24 hr.	
	Rheumatoid*	Normal*	Rheumatoid	Normal
Aggregated gamma globulin	90	87	0	0
Native gamma globulin	90	75	0	0
Polymerized D.N.A.	20	12	0	0
Native D.N.A.	0	12	0	0
Nucleoprotein–latex	20	0	10	0
Latex	20	0	20	0

*10 rheumatoid arthritics and 6 normal subjects.

For each challenge material 40 test and control skin window slides were evaluated. Neither eosinophilia nor basophilia occurred in response to the reactants tested, nor were there significant variations in the mononuclear cell reactions between the test subjects and controls. Finally all slides were evaluated for changes in cellular morphology which might be considered

*Calf thymus DNA Lot 400 302, California Corporation for Biochemical Research.
†Hyland Laboratories, Latex-Nucleoprotein Reagent.

specific, such as the LE cell phenomenon, Russell-body formation, or unusual granulation, but none was found.

CONCLUSIONS

It is concluded that under the conditions of these experiments, native and aggregated gamma globulin failed to induce specific cellular reaction patterns in rheumatoid patients with circulating rheumatoid factor. The nucleic acid and nucleoprotein reactants were also inactive. It is suggested that the interaction between rheumatoid factor and gamma globulin evokes a cellular response in the skin window which cannot be differentiated from reaction to simple injury. Efforts to evaluate the cellular responses to these reactants in systemic lupus erythematosus are under way.

SUMMARY

A comparison was made between 10 rheumatoid arthritic and 6 normal volunteers by means of skin test reaction and skin window cell responses to a group of auto-antigenic reactants. A simple irritant type of response was obtained in each instance. Significant differences between test and control subjects were not observed.

This work was supported by the Canadian Arthritis and Rheumatism Society and the Medical Research Council of Canada.

REFERENCES

1. REBUCK, J. W., and CROWLEY, J. H. Ann. New York Acad. Sci. 59: 757 (1955).
2. EIDINGER, D., WILKINSON, R. D., and ROSE, B. J. Allergy, 35: 77 (1964).
3. PRIEST, R. J., REBUCK, J. W., and HARVEY, G. T. Gastroenterology, 38: 715 (1960).
4. BOHNE, A. W., HODSON, J. M., REBUCK, J. W., and REINHARD, R. E. J. Urol. 88: 387 (1962).
5. CARLISLE, J. W., and GOOD, R. A. A.M.A. J. Dis. Child. 99: 193 (1960).
6. HU, F., FOSNAUGH, R. P., and LIVINGOOD, C. C. J. Invest. Dermat. 41: 325 (1963).
7. CHRISTIAN, C. L. J. Chron. Dis. 16: 875 (1963).
8. ——— J. Exper. Med. 108: 139 (1958).
9. STOLLAR, D., and LEVINE, L. J. Immunol. 87: 477 (1961).

Gamma-Globulin-Induced Synovitis: Studies on the Pathogenesis of Rheumatoid Joint Inflammation*

ANDRE LUSSIER, M.D.

ROPES AND BAUER (1) in their classical work noted the possibility of cytoplasmic vacuolization of the leucocytes found in the synovial fluid. Hollander and his group (2) showed the presence of leucocytes containing cytoplasmic inclusion granulas in synovial fluids from rheumatoid patients, so he called them R.A. cells. Delbarre and his group (3) confirmed this finding, and because of their morphology—these inclusion-body cells have the appearance of grapes —he named them synovial ragocytes (from the Greek name ραγος meaning "grape").

Then emerged the possibility that the intracytoplasmic granules were phagocytized complexes of altered gamma globulin with rheumatoid factor and the hypothesis (4) that the inflamed joint results from the phagocytosis of intra-articular complexes of rheumatoid factor and 7S gamma globulin by leucocytes. This mechanism could be somewhat analogous to crystal-induced synovitis.

Supporting such a concept are (1) the release of rheumatoid factor from washed rheumatoid synovial cells fractured by ultra-sound (5), (2) the demonstration by immunofluorescent staining of intracytoplasmic particulate 7S and 19S gamma globulins in rheumatoid synovial fluid leucocytes, (3) the *in vitro* phagocytosis of complexes of rheumatoid factor and aggregated 7S gamma globulin by normal leucocytes (6).

To test *in vivo* this hypothesis, on the suggestion of Dr. Ronald Restifo, it was decided to perform intra-articular injections of 7S gamma globulins. If definite inflammation resulted and the cells showed the specific phagocytized granules and intracytoplasmic 7S and 19S gamma globulins stained by immunofluorescence, and finally proper controls were negative, we could feel surer that the rheumatoid joint inflammation was specifically the leucocytic reaction to rheumatoid factor and gamma$_{ss}$ globulin.

*Work done during the tenure of a fellowship of the Canadian Arthritis and Rheumatism Association, at the Hospital of the University of Pennsylvania, under the direction of Dr. Joseph Hollander, Chief of the Arthritis Section, and in collaboration with Drs. Ronald A. Restifo and Arnold J. Rawson.

Comparisons were made between native and isolated gamma globulins, aggregated and non-aggregated gamma globulins, gamma globulins from rheumatoid and non-rheumatoid individuals, and autologous and homologous gamma globulins.

Preparations of purified 7S gamma globulins were obtained on DEAE cellulose columns, then controlled by immunoelectrophoresis and cultured before being injected. Proper concentrations were determined by the modified method of Folin–Ciocalteau (7, 8) employing a standard curve constructed with human FII.

Aggregation of gamma globulin was performed by heating in a water bath at 63° C. for 10 minutes.

Protein-free buffer, which had been passed through DEAE cellulose, and in all respects treated in the same manner as the protein, served as a control solution.

Patients were volunteers from the Arthritis Clinic of the Hospital of the University of Pennsylvania. The rheumatoid patients, except one, had a serum latex fixation titre of 1:160 or more. Gamma globulin solution was injected into one knee, and an equal volume of control buffer was injected into the other knee.

Criteria used for grading experimental arthritis were clinical (symptoms and signs), synovianalysis, and the presence of R.A. cells. Also in use was the technique of immunofluorescence, which consists of fixation of washed joint fluid cells in cold acetone with subsequent exposure of the cells to rabbit anti-human 7S gamma globulin serum or to rabbit anti-human 19S gamma globulin serum. Fluorescence was developed by subsequent exposure of the cells to fluorescein-tagged sheep anti-rabbit globulin serum.

The results of various experimental combinations are summarized in Table I. It will be noted that, in general, acute arthritis was produced in rheumatoid patients only and, in these, only by the injection of autologous gamma globulin which had been separated from their own serum. Five of the six trials of autologous, rheumatoid 7S gamma globulin elicited an acute reaction. In the one for which there was no reaction, it was later found that the patient had a negative serum latex fixation test. When purified rheumatoid 7S gamma globulin was injected into osteo-arthritic knees, there was no inflammatory response in five such trials. In five of six instances, the injection of non-rheumatoid, purified 7S gamma globulin into the knees of patients with rheumatoid arthritis provided no response, but one patient of this group did exhibit a mild response. In this case, synovianalysis did not reveal any leucocyte with cytoplasmic inclusion granule. There were three trials with homologous rheumatoid 7S gamma globulin, none of which produced an inflammatory response. The result of the use of autologous 7S gamma globulin in a uraemic patient was likewise negative.

The injection of 2 to 4 c.c. of autologous whole serum into the knees of

TABLE I

RESULTS FROM INTRA-ARTICULAR INJECTION OF PURIFIED 7S

	Donor of 7S	Recipient	Number of patients	Number of trials	Inflammatory response (0 to ++++)
Autologous	1. Rheumatoid arthritic	Self	5	6	+(1), ++(3), +++(1), ++++(1)
	2. Uraemic	Self	1	2	0 (2)
Homologous	3. Rheumatoid arthritic	Rheumatoid arthritic	2	3	0 (3)
Heterologous	4. Rheumatoid arthritic	Osteo-arthritic	4	5	0 (5)
	5. Normal	Rheumatoid arthritic	5	7	0 (6), + (1)

seven rheumatoid patients produced no evident reaction. In three instances the serum was heated to 63° C. for 10 minutes, and in the remainder the serum was untreated. FII has also been injected without any subsequent flare-up (9).

In Table II is seen the detailed summary of the results for rheumatoid patients who received autologous isolated gamma globulin. This patient received 3 mg. of aggregated purified 7S gamma globulin in the left knee. A marked effusion developed in that knee after a 45-minute interval. Within 24 hours 50 c.c. of a highly inflammatory fluid was aspirated, and again on the second day. The patient was later given an injection of normal 7S gamma globulin in the same knee and did not show any inflammatory response whatsoever.

TABLE II

DETAILS FROM INTRA-ARTICULAR INJECTION OF AUTOLOGOUS RHEUMATOID 7S GAMMA GLOBULIN IN A KNEE JOINT

Quantity of 7S gamma glob.: 3 mg.	Synovial fluid aspirated:
Time of response: 45 min.	Quantity: 50 c.c.
Inflammatory response: acute (+++)	R.A. cells: present†
Duration of inflammation: 3 days*	Cell count: 62,000
	Latex fixation: positive
	7S and 19S fluorescence: positive‡

*The induced articular inflammation had to be stopped by the intra-articular injection of steroid.

†R.A. cells were seen in fluid aspirated 24 hours after the installation of gamma globulin, but only once in fluid aspirated earlier.

‡Similarly, 7S and 19S fluorescence was positive only in fluid aspirated 24 hours after the globulin injection.

N.B. It is of importance to remember that both aggregated and non-aggregated gamma globulins were injected; they both provoked inflammation.

Since the discovery by Cecil (10) in 1931 that rheumatoid sera possess a peculiar agglutinating activity, an army of researchers have come out with different publications about the rheumatoid factor (thus making it rheumatoid factors). But two schools still persist: one considering R.F. as an aetiological agent and the other, simply as a witness of the disease. In support of the latter view is the study of Harris and Vaughan: plasma or plasma containing peripheral leucocytes from high-titred rheumatoid arthritic patients was transfused repeatedly to non-rheumatoid individuals and did not provoke any disease (11). Similarly, in our experience, the autologous whole serum in six trials failed to produce arthritis following intra-articular instillation in rheumatoid patients. Physiological buffer or "inhibitors" (globulin β_2 ?) present in the serum might explain the absence of flare-up. Another possibility would be that rheumatoid factor is an antibody to determinants which are exposed on gamma globulin previously altered by the process of separation but which are not exposed on native gamma globulin present in whole serum (12).

In the present study, five of six trials of the injection of autologous isolated 7S globulin into the knee joints of rheumatoid patients resulted in unequivocal severe arthritis with exudates simulating those found in spontaneous rheumatoid arthritis. By contrast, isolated 7S gamma globulin from rheumatoid patients produced no reaction when injected into joints of osteo-arthritics; nor did arthritis follow the injection of autologous isolated 7S gamma globulin into a patient with uraemia.

Though preliminary, this study lends some support to the view that the rheumatoid factor may be, at least indirectly, of aetiologic significance in so far as the genesis of the arthritis of rheumatoid disease is concerned, and more importantly it might suggest that different antigenic determinants of 7S gamma globulin may be active in different individuals and that particular rheumatoid factors may be specific for these groupings (13). The specific direction of some rheumatoid factors to buried determinants of 7S gamma globulin has been demonstrated by Osterland *et al.* (14). The relationship of such specificity to Gm group or to H chains of 7S gamma globulin (15–17) is a possibility. Further studies along this line might be of great value. If this study about gamma-globulin-induced synovitis brings more questions than answers to our mind, it still fulfils its aim in the search for truth.

REFERENCES

1. Ropes, M. W., and Bauer, W. Synovial Fluid Changes in Joint Disease (Harvard University Press, Cambridge, Mass., 1953).
2. Hollander, J. L., Rawson, A. J., Restifo, R. A., and Lussier, A. J. Studies of the pathogenesis of rheumatoid joint inflammation. Arth. & Rheum. 7: 314 (1964).
3. Delbarre, F., Kahan, A., Amor, A., and Krassinine, C. Le ragocyte synovial, son intérêt pour le diagnostic des maladies rhumatismales. Presse méd. 72 (no. 37): 2129–32 (1964).
4. Hollander, J. L. Personal communication (1964).
5. Astorga, G., and Bollet, A. J. Diagnostic specificity and possible pathogenetic significance of inclusion-body cells in synovial fluid. Arth. & Rheum.
6. Parke, R. L., and Schmid, F. R. Phagocytosis of particulate complexes of gamma globulin and rheumatoid factor. J. Immunol. 88: 519 (1962).
7. Lowry, O. H., and Bessey, O. H. The adaptation of the Beckman spectrophotometer to measurements in minute quantities of biological materials. J. Biol. Chem. 163: 633 (1946).
8. Scheidegger, J. J. Unc. micro-methode de l'immuno-électrophorèse. Intern. Arch. Allergy, 7: 103 (1955).
9. Restifo, R. Personal communication (Feb. 1965).
10. Cecil, R. L., Nichols, E. E., and Stainsby, W. J. The etiology of rheumatoid arthritis. Am. J. M. Sci. 181: 12 (1931).
11. Harris, J., and Vaughan, J. R. Transfusion studies in rheumatoid arthritis. Arth. & Rheum. 4: 47 (1961).
12. James, K., Henney, C. S., and Stanworth, D. R. Structural changes occurring in 7S gamma globulin. Nature, 202: 563 (1964).
13. Osterland, C. K., Harboe, M., and Kunkel, H. G. Rheumatoid factor (7S and 19S types) reacting with different portions of the gamma globulin molecule. Arth. & Rheum. 5: 312 (1962).
14. Williams, R. C., Jr. Reaction of human and rabbit anti-gamma-globulin factors with heavy and light chains of gamma globulin. Arth. & Rheum. 7: 368 (1964).
15. Franklin, E. C., Fudenberg, H., Martensson, L., Maltzer, M., and Stanworth, D. Genetic control of gamma globulins in man; its structural basis and biologic significance. Third International Symposium of Immunopathology, *edited by* Miescher and Graber (B. Schwabe, Basel, 1963).
16. Alepa, F. P. Personal communication (1964).

PART IV

Other Studies in Aetiology

Chairman: Professor K. J. R. Wightman, Toronto

Searches for an Infective Agent in Human Arthritis*

DENYS K. FORD, M.D.

THE PATHOLOGY of rheumatoid arthritis is characterized by the cellular reaction of a persistent antigenic stimulation. Table I lists the most frequently discussed aetiological processes that might give rise to such an immunopathological lesion, and it is readily seen that in three of the five possibilities a microbiological agent might be involved. In rheumatoid arthritis there is no clinical evidence to suggest an infective origin but in two closely allied forms of arthritis, Reiter's syndrome and ankylosing spondylitis, there is circumstantial evidence suggesting that genito-urinary infection is a precipitating factor in a proportion of cases. Over the past five years a search has been made at the University of British Columbia to obtain direct or indirect evidence that microbiological agents might be implicated in the aetiology of some forms of human non-suppurative arthritis.

TABLE I

RHEUMATOID ARTHRITIS

An immunologically produced lesion due to:
1. Aberrant lymphoid clones reacting against synovium
2. Loss of natural tolerance to synovial antigens
3. Altered synovial antigens (chemicals, viruses)
4. Foreign antigens in joints
5. Common antigenicity between infecting organisms and synovium

In recent years polyarthritis has been seen in British Columbia in association with three "viral" epidemics. In 1957, an outbreak of rubella was complicated by transient polyarthritis in affected young adult women. In 1963, acute polyarthritis was seen in four members of a Haida Indian family who had complained of "flu" immediately prior to the onset of their arthritis; a further four members of the family had severe arthralgia. In 1964 a widespread epidemic of erythema infectiosum occurred in the Greater Vancouver area and 16

*From the Department of Medicine, University of British Columbia, Vancouver.

individuals were seen in whom transient polyarthritis arose as a sequel to the erythema infectiosum. Unfortunately in none of these situations was it possible to obtain the causative agent of the primary epidemic, and therefore no laboratory studies could be performed to illuminate the pathogenesis of the accompanying arthritis.

Over the past 10 years urethral, conjunctival, and synovial exudate from patients with Reiter's syndrome has been inoculated into a variety of cell lines to attempt the demonstration of viral cytopathogenic agents. Hela, Chang conjunctival, amnion, synovial, and embryonic lung cultures have been the cells of human origin employed for these studies and both Rhesus and African monkey kidney cultures have also been used. To the present time no cytopathogenic agent has been recovered.

The yolk sacs of embryonated eggs have been inoculated with similar exudate but the claim of Siboulet and Galistin (1) has not been confirmed, and no agent which would give rise to inclusion bodies or malformation of the embryos has been isolated.

On the assumptions that synovial cells from rheumatoid subjects might contain a latent virus, and that this hypothetical latent virus might interfere with the multiplication of a second virus, synovial cell cultures from rheumatoid and non-rheumatoid individuals were infected with Newcastle disease virus. The multiplication of the virus in the two types of cultures was compared, but it was not possible to demonstrate a reduced multiplication in the rheumatoid cultures.

TABLE II

HUMAN MYCOPLASMAL STRAINS

Mouth and resp. tract.	Genital tract
M. pneumoniae	M. hominis Type 1
M. salivarum	M. fermentans
M. orale (Pharyngis)	"T-strain" mycoplasma

During the past five years, the genital strains of mycoplasmas have been studied and attempts made to relate them to non-gonococcal urethritis and Reiter's syndrome. Table II shows the seven distinct strains of mycoplasmas isolated from humans; it is to be anticipated that additional strains will be discovered in the near future.

The mycoplasmas are characterized by their small size, the 0.2 μ diameter of their smallest granules being about that of the vaccinia virus. They are also characterized by having no rigid cell wall so that they may exist as granules, larger bodies, or filaments. Because they have no rigid cell wall, they are resistant to penicillin; on the other hand, they are sensitive to the tetracyclines. They are cultivated on specially supplemented bacteriological agars and broths and are handled in the laboratory by usual bacteriological techniques.

At least three serologically distinct strains have been isolated from the human genital tract. Morphologically these strains fall into two groups, large-colony strains and strains characterized by their very small colony size and named T-strains by Shepard (2). Data on the isolation of mycoplasmas from the human genital tract are summarized in Table III. It is evident from these findings that both morphological types are found in "control" subjects with no genito-urinary symptoms. They are likewise also found frequently in asymptomatic women. However, the incidence of T-strains in men with non-gonococcal urethritis is higher than in all the other groups studied. This fact coupled with the response of abacterial non-gonococcal urethritis to tetracycline suggests, but does not prove, that these organisms are one and possibly the major cause of non-gonococcal urethritis.

TABLE III

INCIDENCE OF GENITAL MYCOPLASMAS

	Males			Females
	Services recruits	Gaol inmates	Cases of N.G.U.	"Private" gynaecology patients
No. of cases studied	100	100	100	100
No. of mycoplasmas isolated				
T-strains only	14⎫21	18⎫47	57⎫79	34⎫40
Both strains	7⎭	29⎭	22⎭	6⎭
Large-colony strains only	3⎭10	8⎭37	5⎭27	7⎭13
Total mycoplasmas	24	55	84	47

Table IV shows the frequency of isolation of mycoplasmas from the genital tract of those patients having Reiter's syndrome. It can be seen that the incidence of the organisms is not significantly different from that in patients with uncomplicated non-gonococcal urethritis. Moreover, the organisms have never been isolated from synovial fluid. Clearly there is no evidence from these data to indicate that these genital strains of mycoplasmas are related to Reiter's syndrome, and there is a strong suggestion that, if an aetiological relationship does exist, it will have to be an indirect one, perhaps analogous to the relationship of streptococci to rheumatic fever.

TABLE IV

INCIDENCE OF T-STRAIN MYCOPLASMA FROM THE GENITO-URINARY TRACT OF PATIENTS WITH REITER'S SYNDROME

25 episodes of arthritis following urethritis in 23 patients
18 occasions adequate urethral specimens obtained for mycoplasmal culture
10 occasions T-strain mycoplasma cultured from urethra

In June 1964, it was claimed (3) that mycoplasmas could be isolated from the synovial fluid of patients with rheumatoid arthritis, Reiter's syndrome, and systemic lupus erythematosus by means of blind passage through African monkey kidney or human embryonic lung cultures. To examine this question further, synovial fluid from 20 patients with rheumatoid arthritis, 2 patients with Reiter's syndrome, and 1 patient with systemic lupus erythematosus was inoculated into the two already mentioned cell cultures and also human amnion cells. Culture fluid was tested for mycoplasmas at weekly intervals until five to seven blind passes had been made at 3-week intervals. No mycoplasmas were isolated by these techniques in Vancouver.

SUMMARY

Circumstantial evidence suggests that some forms of "rheumatoid-like" arthritis may be related to infection with microbiological agents. No direct evidence favouring such a hypothesis has been obtained up to the present and various unsuccessful experimental approaches have been described in this paper. Current knowledge of both viruses and mycoplasmas is so limited, however, that further attempts to search for relationships between these microbiological agents and "rheumatoid-like" arthritis are fully justified.

REFERENCES

1. SIBOULET, A., and GALISTIN, P.   Arguments in favor of a virus etiology of non-gonococcal urethritis. Brit. J. Ven. Dis. 38: 209 (1962).
2. SHEPARD, M. C.   T-form colonies of pleuropneumonia-like organisms. J. Bact. 71: 362 (1956).
3. BARTHOLOMEW, L. E., and HIMES, J.   Isolation of mycoplasma (PPLO) from patients with rheumatoid arthritis, systemic lupus erythematosus and Reiter's syndrome. Arth. & Rheum. 7: 291 (1964).

Tryptophan Metabolism and Rheumatoid Arthritis*

J. B. HOUPT, M. A. OGRYZLO, M. A. HUNT, and
A. A. FLETCHER†

IN 1958, Nishimura and co-workers (6) demonstrated the presence of an abnormal metabolite of tyrosine (2,5-dihydroxyphenylpyruvic acid) in the urine of patients with "collagen disease." In repeating this work, McMillan (4) was unable to confirm this finding but noted instead an increased excretion of 3-hydroxyanthranilic acid (3-HAA) in patients with rheumatoid arthritis. This was confirmed by Bett in 1962 (1), who reported as well an increase in excretion of kynurenine (KYN). Following a tryptophan load, there was an abnormally large increase in KYN excretion, which was blocked if pyridoxine was given prior to the tryptophan load. A functional deficiency of pyridoxine in patients with rheumatoid arthritis was suggested. Here we shall review the studies that have implicated an abnormality of tryptophan metabolism in this disease and discuss our attempts at affecting the activity of the disease with low tryptophan diets.

Tryptophan is an essential amino acid, which is an important constituent of plasma proteins, haemoglobin, thyroglobulin, Nissl substance, and many other body proteins. Experimental deficiency in animals leads to a disturbance in growth, loss of hair, cataracts, anaemia, reduction in total plasma proteins, and fatty infiltration of liver. The minimal requirements in man are reported to be 100–250 mg. per day (Fig. 1). Its degradation may take three pathways:

(1) A small amount is broken down via 5-hydroxytryptophan to 5-hydroxy-tryptamine (serotonin) and excreted as 5-hydroxyindoleacetic acid. Patients with *carcinoid* syndrome divert their tryptophan breakdown via the serotonin pathway (and are susceptible to pellagra from the resultant nicotinic acid deficiency).

*From the Department of Medicine, University of Toronto, the Clinical Investigation Unit, Sunnybrook Hospital, and the Rheumatic Disease Unit, Wellesley Hospital, Toronto. This study was supported by grants-in-aid from the Canadian Arthritis and Rheumatism Society and the Canadian Life Insurance Officers Association.
†Deceased.

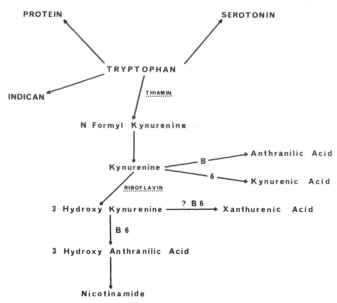

FIG. 1. An outline of the pathway from tryptophan to nicotinamide showing the suggested sites of action of the vitamins:
thiamin, riboflavin, and pyridoxine (B6).

(2) Tryptophan in the gastro-intestinal tract may be degraded to indolic
substances such as indican. *Hartnup disease,* a rare hereditary affliction presenting clinically with a combination of pellagra and attacks of cerebellar
ataxia, is characterized biochemically by defective renal tubular reabsorption
of a large number of amino acids, and defective absorption of tryptophan in
the jejunum. Patients with this disease excrete large amounts of indolic
substances in their urine, presumably because ingested tryptophan is degraded
by gastro-intestinal bacteria to its indolic compounds, which are then absorbed
and excreted by the kidney.

(3) The major pathway of breakdown, however, is via kynurenine. In this
scheme, the indole ring of tryptophan is broken by tryptophan pyrrolase to
form N-formyl kynurenine. This is then degraded to *kynurenine* (KYN)
(affected by thiamin) to 3-hydroxykynurenine (affected by riboflavin) to 3-
hydroxyanthranilic acid (affected by pyridoxine) to *nicotinic acid.* Pyridoxine
also influences the breakdown of kynurenine to kynurenic acid and anthranilic
acid, and may be effective in the breakdown of 3-hydroxykynurenine to
xanthurenic acid.

The excretion of 3-HAA was studied by Spiera (7) in a group of patients
with rheumatoid arthritis and other connective tissue disorders. He found that
10 of 26 patients with rheumatoid arthritis and 3 of 8 patients with "collagen
disease" excreted excessive quantities of this compound in the urine. The
quantity excreted did not-correlate well with any other clinical or laboratory

parameter studied. Over the past two years there have been several further papers documenting the excretion of various other metabolites of tryptophan by patients with rheumatoid arthritis. Several authors have documented abnormalities in urinary metabolite excretion only after a tryptophan load, as Bett (1) suggested in 1962. In her study, 11 patients with rheumatoid arthritis excreted significantly more KYN following a tryptophan load in 24 hours than did 12 controls. This elevated excretion of KYN was blocked by pretreatment with pyridoxine suggesting a functional deficiency of pyridoxine. Flinn *et al.* (2) reported significantly elevated levels of hydrokynurenine and kynurenine in patients with rheumatoid arthritis following such a tryptophan load. McKusick *et al.* (3) reported that patients with active rheumatoid arthritis excrete significantly less pyridoxine in the urine than controls. In Flinn's study, basal pyridoxine (pyridoxic acid) was within normal limits; however, administration of pyridoxine restored tryptophan metabolism towards normal. Pinals (5) reported an excessive excretion of kynurenine and 3-hydroxykynurenine as a common but non-specific occurrence in patients with rheumatoid arthritis. These metabolites were also found to be elevated in patients with scleroderma, systemic lupus erythematosis, recent myocardial infarction, carcinoma of bladder, megaloblastic anaemia, and tuberculosis.

SUNNYBROOK EXPERIENCE

Over the past two years we have been attempting to document the urinary excretion products of tryptophan metabolism in patients with rheumatoid arthritis. The main difficulty has been methodologic since the early investigators estimated their results from visual analysis of chromatograms. Miss M. Hunt has now perfected techniques for the quantitative spectrophotometric analysis of five of the main excretion products: (1) KYN, (2) 3-HAA, (3) xanthurenic acid (X.A.), (4) kynurenic acid (K.A.), and (5) nicotinamide (NIC) (Table I).

TABLE I

Tryptophan Metabolites in Urine (MG./24 HR.)

	KYN	K.A.	X.A.	3-HKN	3-HAA	NIC
Normal	2.56	4.26	0.20	5.95	2.71	3.90
Rheumatoid	5.93	5.10	0.12	7.98	4.39	4.31

The normal range for these has been determined by an analysis of the 24-hour urine collections of 10 ambulatory healthy persons. Ten patients with rheumatoid arthritis have been studied as well as two patients with vasculitis and one patient with carcinoid syndrome. Four of the rheumatoid patients had excretion products within the normal range; the other six showed elevations of one or more of the excretion products. It is seen in this table that although an elevated excretion of KYN and 3-HAA seems apparent in patients with rheumatoid arthritis, the overlap is too great to make this observation significant.

Pursuing his contention that abnormal handling of foodstuffs contributes to some diseases, Dr. Fletcher treated five patients with rheumatoid arthritis with diets low in tryptophan with protein derived from gelatin powder with a subsequent impressive lowering of erythrocyte sedimentation rate and moderate fall in plasma fibrinogen level. Two patients with active rheumatoid arthritis have been studied for prolonged periods of time while being treated with a low tryptophan diet in the Clinical Investigation Unit (C.I.U.). While they were on this low tryptophan diet their ESR and plasma fibrinogen level fell impressively; although the patients claimed to feel better subjectively, clinical improvement (as, for instance, in the disappearance of effusions) was not apparent. When the patients were placed back on normal diet, the values of these quantities rose to previous control levels.

PATIENT 1 (J.C.S.; SEE FIG. 2)

This latex-positive, nodular, severely erosive rheumatoid arthritic was leading a bed-chair existence when he was admitted to the C.I.U. on January 10, 1964, with an ESR of 75 mm. hour and a fibrinogen level of 600 mg./100 c.c. He was on prednisone 13 mg./day and aspirin 75 grains/day and these drugs

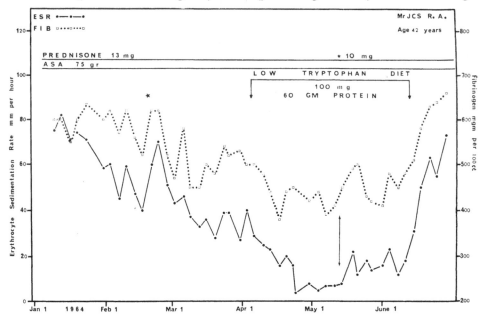

FIG. 2. The effect of a low tryptophan, 60-gm. protein diet on plasma fibrinogen and erythrocyte sedimentation rate. Note the spontaneous fall during the first two months of observation.

were continued. Of interest is the fact that the ESR and fibrinogen level fell steadily over the next three months while he was on a normal ward diet, and receiving physiotherapy and a continuation of the same dose of salicylates and steroid. This observation points up the difficulties in evaluating therapeutic measures in this disease, and emphasizes the fact that adequate control should be obtained prior to any of these studies. During the third week in February, the ESR and fibrinogen level rose; at this time, which is indicated by the star in Fig. 2, the patient complained of a "head cold." On April 3, with the ESR at 40 mm./hour and the plasma fibrinogen level at 500 mg./100 c.c., he was started on a low tryptophan (100 mg. approximately) diet containing 60 gm. of protein, mainly in the form of powdered gelatin. The ESR and plasma fibrinogen level fell over the next 30 days to a low of 5 mm./hour and 380 mg.%. On May 11, the dose of prednisone was dropped from 13 to 10 mg., the ESR settled out at approximately 20 mm./hour, and the plasma fibrinogen level at 450 mg.%. On June 12, having been on the low tryptophan diet for 69 days, the patient was started on a normal diet once again. The ESR and fibrinogen level climbed to previous control levels of 73 mm./hour and 660 mg.% at the time of discharge on June 29, 1964. (During 43 control days, while on a diet containing 13.0 gm. nitrogen, this patient excreted a mean of 10.53 gm. of nitrogen in the urine daily. During the first 30 days on the low tryptophan diet containing 11.9 gm. of nitrogen he excreted a mean of 10.11 gm. of nitrogen in the urine daily indicating no significant negative nitrogen balance.) At the time of discharge, the patient was ambulatory with two canes only. He attributed his rehabilitation to the low tryptophan "rice" diet; however, we must not lose sight of the fact that he was receiving intensive physiotherapy during this period.

This patient was readmitted on August 10, 1964, with an ESR of 48 mm./hour and a fibrinogen level of 500 mg./100 c.c. plasma (Fig. 3). He was kept on prednisone 10 mg./day and aspirin 75 grains/day. On September 15 he was started on a low tryptophan diet consisting of 25 gm. of protein made up of jelly instead of the objectionable gelatin powder. On this regimen the ESR and fibrinogen level once again fell to 6 mm./hour and 450 mg.%. On September 28 he had severe symptoms of an exacerbation of a chronic duodenal ulcer. Aspirin administration was stopped on October 3 but was started again on October 12 at the request of the patient at a dose of 40 grains per day. During this period the ESR rose to 36 mm./hour. On October 21, one litre of milk daily was added (giving him 34 gm. protein and 470 mg. tryptophan). The ESR climbed to 45 mm./hour by November 9, when the diet was changed to an uncontrolled gastric 3. The ESR and fibrinogen level climbed during this period to 60 mm./hour and 600 mg.%. At the request of the patient he was once again started on the low tryptophan diet on November 24, with the addition of 40 ounces of milk to this regimen. The ESR fell to 40 mm./hour and the fibrinogen level to 450 mg./100 c.c. over the next three weeks. The

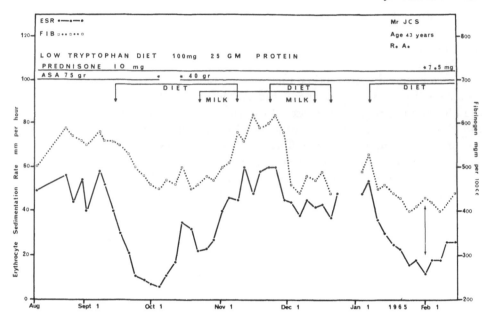

Fig. 3. The effect of a low tryptophan, 0.25-gm. protein diet on erythrocite sedimentation rate and plasma fibrinogen. Note fall with institution of "diet" and rise at time of exacerbation of peptic ulcer "milk."

patient went home for Christmas and after returning he requested that we try the low tryptophan rice diet again without milk. Once again the ESR fell over the next 4 weeks to 15 mm./hour and fibrinogen to 400 mg.%. On February 2, 1965, the dose of prednisone was dropped from 10 to 7.5 mg./day. The study is continuing.

PATIENT 2

Mr. A. C. is a 67-year-old latex-positive patient with non-deforming rheumatoid arthritis of two years' duration (Fig. 4). On admission to the Unit in August 1964, his ESR was 115–120 mm./hour and his plasma fibrinogen level 600–640 mg./100 c.c. Through the course of the study he was kept on 60 grains of aspirin daily. On September 14, he was started on a diet containing 29 gm. of protein (jelly) and approximately 100 mg. tryptophan. The ESR and fibrinogen level fell dramatically over the next 3 weeks to 66 mm./hour and 460 mg.%. When he was put back on a normal diet, the ESR and fibrinogen level both rose to 112 mm./hour and 560 mg.%. On October 29, he was started once again on the low tryptophan diet, and again one can see a dramatic fall in ESR and fibrinogen level to approximately 65 mm./hour and 450 mg.%. When he was taken off the diet, the ESR and plasma fibrinogen level climbed to previous control values.

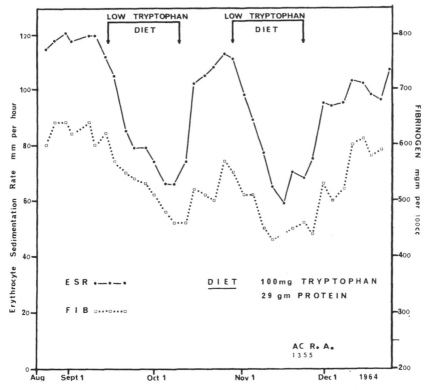

Fig. 4. The effect of a low tryptophan, 29-gm. protein diet on erythrocyte sedimentation rate and plasma fibrinogen.

CONCLUSIONS

The increased excretion of tryptophan metabolites in a large percentage of patients with rheumatic diseases seems to be well established. It is not clear whether this abnormality is due to (1) a shunting of tryptophan via the kynurenine pathway secondary to increased tryptophan pyrrolase activity or (2) the inhibition of pyridoxal-dependent hepatic enzymes or functional deficiency of pyridoxine. The pattern of urinary metabolites differs from that seen in pyridoxine deficiency since xanthurenic acid is usually elevated in this situation and is not significantly so in rheumatoid arthritis. No data on the output of 3-HAA after pyridoxine administration are available.

Abnormalities of the serotonin pathway have been suggested but not substantiated since excretion of 5-hydroxyindoleacetic acid has been reported to be normal in rheumatoid arthritics.

The significance of the abnormality is uncertain; since identical defects are present in many diseases, it suggests that the phenomenon is secondary and not of aetiologic significance. However, in view of the complexity of tryptophan metabolism and our present lack of knowledge, this conclusion is probably not warranted, and further study of these abnormalities especially in relation to pyridoxine reversal seems justified.

As well, the observed phenomena of a fall in ESR and plasma fibrinogen level coincident with a low tryptophan diet require clarification. To date, only two other therapeutic manoeuvres achieve comparable results: fasting or protein deprivation and steroid administration.

Our original studies were conducted with isocaloric 60–70 gm. protein diets using gelatin as the protein source. During two such studies negative nitrogen balance did not occur and so protein deprivation as such cannot be implicated in these phenomena.

It has been suggested that the observed fall in sedimentation rate is due to a deficiency of fibrinogen secondary to the dietary deficiency of tryptophan. This may be so; however it is unlikely, as we do not really achieve complete tryptophan deficiency and normal plasma fibrinogen contains only 3.29 per cent tryptophan (Documenta Geigy Tables).

Whether or not the basic abnormality in rheumatoid arthritis is linked with the abnormal metabolism of the essential amino acids, and whether the relative deficiency of tryptophan affects disease activity or not, remain to be clarified.

We gratefully acknowledge the nursing and dietary assistance of Miss I. Rowland, R.N., and Miss B. Robertson, B.SC., and the technical assistance of Miss M. Hunt.

REFERENCES

1. BETT, I. M.   Ann. Rheum. Dis. *21*: 63 (1962).
2. FLINN, J. H., *et al.* Arth. & Rheum. 7 (3): 201 (1964).
3. McKusick, A. B., *et al.*   Arth. & Rheum. 7 (6): 636 (1964).
4. McMILLAN, M.   J. Clin. Path. *13*: 140 (1960).
5. PINALS, R. S.   Arth. & Rheum. 7 (6): 662 (1964).
6. NISHIMURA, N., *et al.*   A.M.A. Arch. Dermat. 77: 255 (1958).
7. SPIERA, H.   Arth. & Rheum. 6 (4): 364 (1963).

DISCUSSION

DR.   M. A. OGRYZLO (Toronto): We are currently taught that diet plays no significant role in rheumatoid arthritis, yet the belief that nutritional factors may be important is probably as old as medicine itself. The older members of this group will recall that the programmes of the old, original American Association for the Control of Rheumatic Diseases, the fore-runner of the present A.R.A., contained many papers on nutritional aspects of this disease. The late Dr. A. A. Fletcher, Dr. Ralph Pemberton, and many others believed that there might be an underlying metabolic fault in rheumatoid arthritis, and looked largely to the digestive tract for the answer to these questions. It was then customary to treat rheumatoid patients with suspected colonic dysfunction with diets consisting largely of carbohydrates and fats, which would be, presumably, very comparable to what has been used here, and which seemed to help some patients. They were encouraged by their results in rheumatoid patients, and certainly carried them on for long periods of time.

Fasting would often do the same thing and produce the same type of improvement. I have here, just to interject a lighter vein to this discussion today, a letter from a patient who wrote: "Dear Sir: I have suffered from rheumatoid arthritis for twenty years, diagnosed by a specialist. For fifteen years I have known it was caused by my diet. If I went on a drastic diet, eating almost nothing, I could nearly cure my swollen joints, but I could not keep on such a diet. As soon as I began to eat even moderately normally, my pains and swollen joints returned." This type of letter or comments by patients who have made the observations themselves is not uncommon.

During the past fifteen years, together with Dr. Fletcher, we have become interested in a variety of dietary measures, and these preliminary results given by Dr. Houpt today may be of some significance particularly when others have reported abnormalities in tryptophan metabolism in this disease. One must admit that any relationship between the abnormalities demonstrated and the activity of rheumatoid arthritis is very tenuous. However, the study is important in that it does demonstrate that diet can, in fact, alter disease activity.

The introduction of ACTH and steroids about 15 years ago gave us probably the most potent suppressive anti-inflammatory agents we have ever had. Perhaps the best indices of activity of an inflammatory process are the erythrocyte sedimentation rate and plasma fibrinogen. With pharmacologic doses of ACTH or corticosteroids, disease activity can be suppressed, with a dramatic fall in the E.S.R. and plasma fibrinogen (Fig. 1).

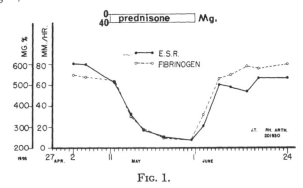

Fig. 1.

Very few measures other than ACTH and the corticosteroids will produce such dramatic changes, although a comparable effect on plasma fibrinogen level and sedimentation rate has been demonstrated by Dr. Houpt in the present study. It seems probable that tryptophan may not be the whole answer. We have done other studies in the past on patients using diets that are simply low-protein diets. In one study, for example, the protein content of the diet was changed from 68 gm. to 14.5 gm. and then back to 68 gm. (Fig. 2). The effect here on the sedimentation rate and plasma fibrinogen level was comparable to what was shown. It, in effect, would be a low tryptophan diet as well, but it would also be deficient in other essential amino acids.

In another patient the diet was changed from 74 gm. of protein to 16 gm. and back to 74 gm. (Fig. 3). There was a drop in the plasma fibrinogen level and sedimentation rate, with a rebound much the same as you see with corticosteroids, when the high protein diet was resumed, another drop with the resumption of the low protein diet, and an even sharper rebound after reverting to the high protein diet.

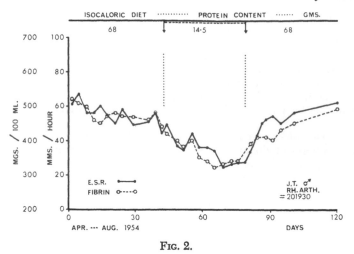

FIG. 2.

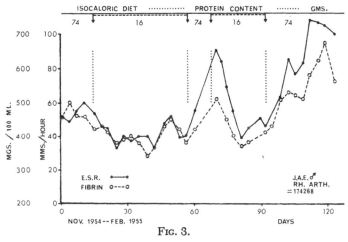

FIG. 3.

What these observations mean, we are not certain, but we know that steroids do interfere with protein synthesis and induce a negative nitrogen balance. Also, that fasting, low protein diets, and deprivation of essential amino acids can produce comparable effects. The possibility that a tryptophan-containing kinin peptide may be involved merits further consideration.

DR. MELLORS: As I understand fibrinogen levels, they have a close correlation with the erythrocyte sedimentation rate. ESR and fibrinogen then are related to each other. My question is this: Is fibrinogen unusually rich in the amino acid tryptophan, and what is known about tryptophan and its influence on fibrinogen synthesis itself?

DR. HOUPT: Fibrinogen contains approximately 3.6 per cent tryptophan. It certainly is not rich in tryptophan. This figure is taken from the Geigy Handbook, and there are many other amino acids that are present in much higher percentages in fibrinogen.

PART V

Immune Mechanisms

Chairman: Dr. M. A. Ogryzlo, Toronto

An Electron Microscopic Study of
the Skin Lesions of
Experimental Delayed Hypersensitivity*

JOHN C. WYLLIE, M.D.

DELAYED HYPERSENSITIVITY is a potentially tissue-damaging abnormal immuno-logical response, apparently mediated by "sensitized" mononuclear cells. Prior exposure of the organism to the antigen has resulted in the development of a population of specifically sensitized mononuclear cells capable of reacting with that antigen. This reaction is damaging to cells and possibly also to inter-cellular components in its vicinity. The pathogenesis and nature of the cell injury are unknown.

Delayed hypersensitivity to a purified protein, ovalbumin, can be readily induced in the guinea pig. Typical delayed hypersensitivity reactions, charac-terized by an increased vascular permeability, oedema of the epidermis and dermis, and infiltrations of mononuclear cells, can be elicited thereafter. The light-microscopic observations of Waksman (1), based on a similar lesion (the tuberculin reaction), indicated that specific injury to epidermal cells occurred. This injury was due apparently to the presence of a sensitized histiocyte.

It was of interest to us to study this reaction with the electron microscope in an attempt to define (1) the nature of the epidermal lesion and (2) its relationship to the infiltrating mononuclear cells.

Guinea pigs were sensitized with ovalbumin by the method of Salvin (2). Six days following sensitization, delayed hypersensitivity reactions were induced in flank skin by the intradermal injection of a minute dose of oval-bumin. The guinea pigs were killed at intervals of 4, 8, 12, 18, 24, and 48 hours thereafter. The skin lesions produced were excised, fixed in osmic acid, and processed for electron microscopy by techniques described in detail else-where (3). Thin sections were examined in an RCA EMU-3D electron microscope.

*From the Department of Pathology, Kingston General Hospital and Queen's University, Kingston, Ontario.

Supported by a grant-in-aid of research from the Canadian Arthritis and Rheumatism Society, Toronto, Ontario.

A delayed hypersensitivity reaction is a slowly evolving indolent process that reaches its maximum development 18–24 hours after induction. It appears on the skin surface as a well circumscribed slightly elevated indurated erythematous lesion. It is characterized, on microscopic examination, by the appearance of oedema in dermis and epidermis and the slow infiltration of mononuclear cells, both lymphocytes and macrophages (monocytes and histiocytes). We have paid particular attention to the lesion in the epidermis.

Oedema fluid appears in the intercellular space of the epidermis. Normally, the epidermal cells are closely approximated, bound together by attachment bodies, or desmosomes (Fig. 1). As the oedema fluid accumulates around

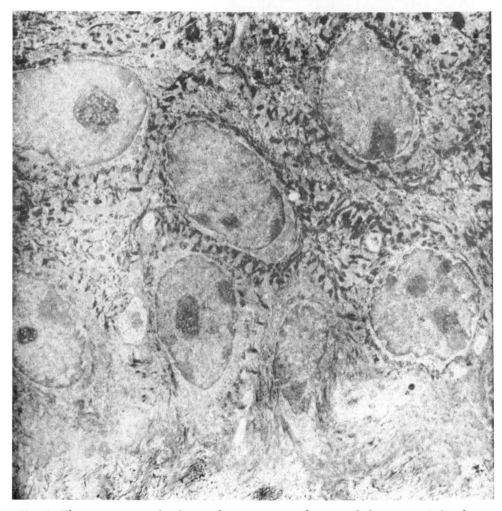

Fig. 1. Electron micrograph of normal guinea-pig epidermis including part of the dermis (bottom). The epidermal eclls are closely approximated and contain bundles of electron-dense tonofibrils. Uranyl acetate stain. About 6000×.

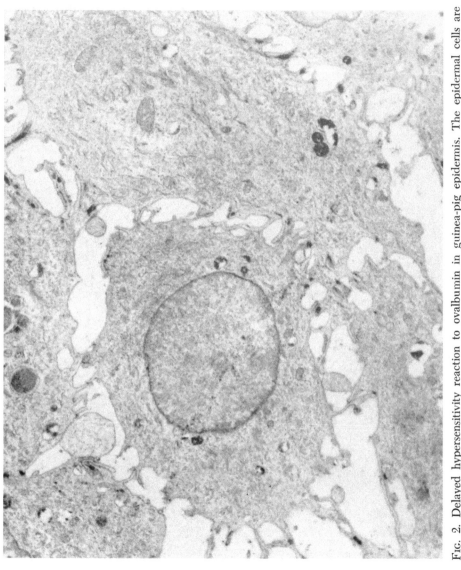

FIG. 2. Delayed hypersensitivity reaction to ovalbumin in guinea-pig epidermis. The epidermal cells are separated by moderate amounts of oedema fluid. The attachment regions are stretched. Note the loss of tonofibrils and the appearance of electron-dense round bodies in these cells. Electron micrograph; uranyl stain. About 12,000×.

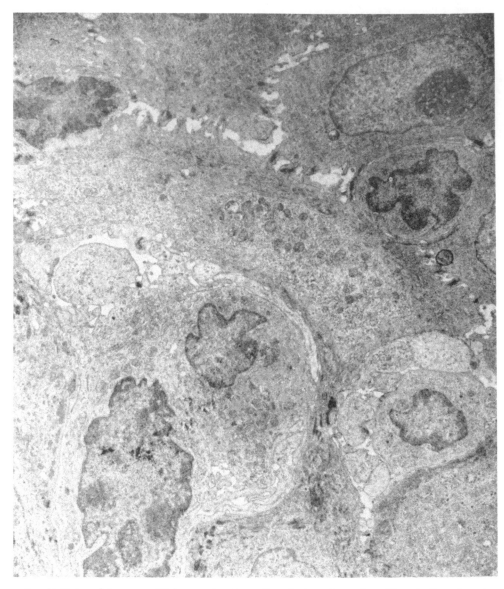

FIG. 3. Delayed hypersensitivity reaction to ovalbumin in guinea-pig epidermis. Lymphocytes and macrophages are infiltrating the epidermis. Electron micrograph; uranyl acetate stain. About 7850×.

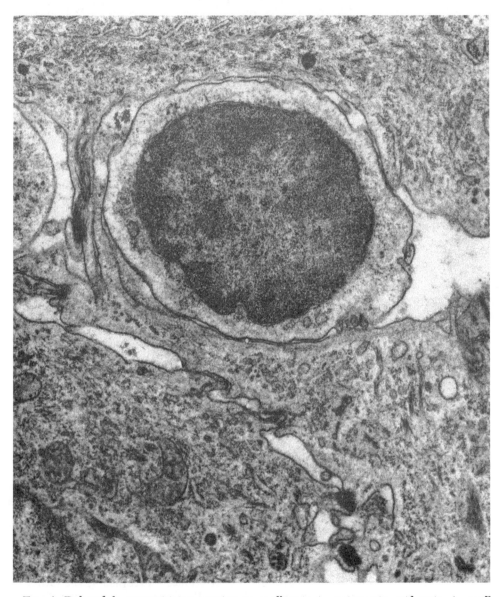

Fig. 4. Delayed hypersensitivity reaction to ovalbumin in guinea-pig epidermis. A small lymphocyte is seen within the epidermis. The epidermal cells in contact with it show no evidence of injury apart from a reduction in the number of their tonofibrils. Electron micrograph; uranyl acetate stain. About 17,000×.

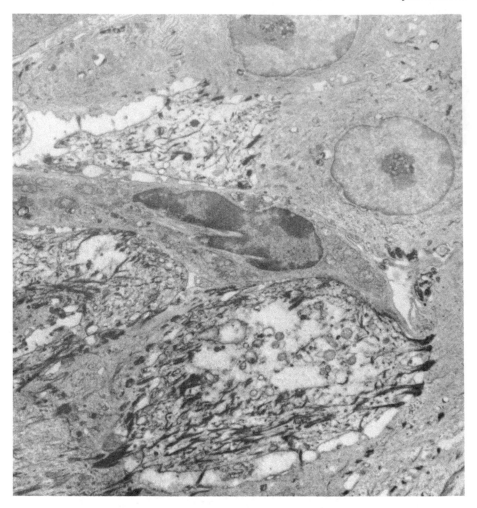

FIG. 5. Delayed hypersensitivity reaction to ovalbumin in guinea-pig epidermis. A macrophage lies in close contact with a group of severely oedematous epidermal cells. Electron micrograph; uranyl acetate stain. About 6000×.

these cells, it pushes them apart, stretching and finally rupturing their attachment zones (Fig. 2). The breaks do not occur through desmosomes, which are very stable structures, but through the attenuated cytoplasm, on either side. The epidermal cells in the regions of intercellular oedema show a striking loss of tonofibrils (Fig. 2). In addition, dense, round bodies appear in their cytoplasm (Fig. 2), some of which contain remnants of mitochondria. This cellular injury could not be correlated with the infiltrating mononuclear cells.

Mononuclear cells, both lymphocytes and macrophages (monocytes and histiocytes), infiltrate the epidermis during the course of a delayed hypersensitivity reaction (Fig. 3). For the most part, we could not attribute specific epidermal cellular injury to the presence of these cells. They did cause displacement of epidermal cells and breaks in their attachment zones, but these injuries were mechanical in origin. The contact zones between an invading mononuclear cell and adjacent epidermal cells were carefully scrutinized. No damage to the cell membrane or to cytoplasmic organelles could be detected in the epidermal cells (Fig. 4). Very rarely, however, a severely damaged and oedematous epidermal cell was observed in close contact with an infiltrating macrophage (Fig. 5).

The mode of production of cellular injury by sensitized mononuclear cells is not known. Waksman (1) felt that he could correlate epidermal cell damage with the immediate presence of an invading histiocyte. Our observations show that epidermal cell injury does occur during the course of a delayed hypersensitivity reaction. Usually this injury consisted of loss of tonofibrils and changes in mitochondria. It was observed in the foci of epidermal intercellular oedema and could not be correlated with invading mononuclear cells. In fact, the majority of the invading mononuclear cells did not specifically injure epidermal cells, apart from mechanical disruptions. Only rarely were severely injured epidermal cells encountered in close contact with macrophages. Although this lesion, owing to its infrequency, could not be evaluated, it may represent a damaging interaction between a sensitized macrophage and an antigen-containing epidermal cell.

REFERENCES

1. WAKSMAN, B. H. A comparative histopathological study of delayed hypersensitivity reactions. *In* Ciba Foundation Symposium on Cellular Aspects of Immunity, *edited by* G. E. W. Wolstenholme and M. O'Connor (Little, Brown and Co., Boston, 1960), p. 280.
2 SALVIN, S. B. Occurrence of delayed hypersensitivity during the development of Arthus type hypersensitivity. J. Exper. Med. *107*: 109 (1958).
3. WYLLIE, J. C., MORE, R. H., and HAUST, M. D. Electron microscopy of epidermal lesions elicited during delayed hypersensitivity. Lab. Invest. *13*: 137 (1964).

The Organ and Species
Distribution of the Hepatocellular
Antigens of the Rabbit*

A. U. SARGENT, M. RICHTER,
and J. MYERS

IN THE COURSE of an investigation of the immunological aspects of chronic liver disease, we had cause to investigate the organ and species specificity of hepatocellular antigens (1). For this purpose rabbit anti-rat liver, rat anti-rabbit liver, and rabbit anti-rabbit liver sera were employed as reagents to demonstrate the organ specificity of the hepatic antigens.

MATERIALS AND METHODS

A. PREPARATION OF ANTIGENS

The livers as well as the other required organs were obtained from exsanguinated Wistar rats and albino New Zealand rabbits. The individual livers were minced with scissors and passed through a tissue press to remove the connective tissue and vascular components. When examined by light microscopy the resultant liver preparation consisted almost entirely of parenchymal cells. The liver preparation was then lyophilized and stored in a desiccator until required. Rat or rabbit heart, kidney, and lung were prepared in a similar fashion.

B. IMMUNIZATION PROCEDURES

For purposes of immunization, the lyophilized liver was homogenized in saline and then emulsified in complete Freund's adjuvant and injected into the footpads of the rabbits and rats. A total of five injections was given, at 10-day intervals. Ten days after the final injection the animals were bled and their sera tested for the presence of anti-liver antibodies.

*From the Division of Immunochemistry and Allergy Research, McGill University Clinic, Royal Victoria Hospital, Montreal.

C. HAEMAGGLUTINATION STUDIES

Boyden's method for the indirect or passive haemagglutination technique was followed throughout (2). Sensitization of the tanned cells was accomplished by mixing them thoroughly with a saline extract obtained from a suspension of lyophilized heart, kidney, or liver, previously determined to be optimal for the sensitization of tanned red cells.

D. ABSORPTION OF ANTI-SERA FOR USE IN HAEMAGGLUTINATION EXPERIMENTS AND FLUORESCENT MICROSCOPY

The following procedures were undertaken to establish the specificity of the anti-liver sera for hepatocellular antigens.

1. Citrated rat or rabbit blood was added to an equal volume of anti-liver sera diluted tenfold in phosphate-buffered saline. After incubation at room temperature for two hours, the suspension was centrifuged and the supernatant removed and stored at −20° C. until required.

2. Lyophilized rat or rabbit heart, kidney, or lung was added to 10-fold dilutions of anti-liver serum previously absorbed with citrated rat or rabbit blood. The antisera and the lyophilized organ were carefully homogenized with a Potter homogenizer and allowed to incubate with constant shaking at room temperature for two hours. The suspension was then centrifuged and the supernatant removed and employed to demonstrate the organ specificity of the hepatocellular antigens.

E. IMMUNOFLUORESCENT STUDIES

Immunofluorescent studies were performed utilizing a modification of the indirect method of Weller and Coons (3). The sections of tissue to be studied were processed according to the method of Sainte-Marie (4).

RESULTS

A. THE SPECIFICITY OF ANTI-LIVER SERA FOR HEPATOCELLULAR ANTIGENS

Rabbit anti-rat liver serum absorbed with citrated rat blood was capable of agglutinating cells sensitized with rat heart, kidney, lung, and liver. After absorption of the immune serum with lyophilized rat heart or lung, only cells sensitized with rat kidney and liver were agglutinated. Antiserum absorbed with rat kidney, however, was found to react specifically with cells sensitized with the immunizing liver preparation.

When these studies were repeated with indirect fluorescent microscopy, an identical series of results was obtained.

A somewhat more restricted pattern of organ reactivity was obtained with rat anti-rabbit liver sera. These sera consistently agglutinated cells sensitized with rabbit kidney and liver, but failed to agglutinate cells sensitized with rabbit heart or lung. Absorption of these sera with rabbit kidney rendered them specific for rabbit liver. When rabbit anti-rabbit liver serum was exposed to a similar panel of sensitized cells, only those cells sensitized with rabbit liver were agglutinated.

B. SPECIES SPECIFICITY OF HEPATOCELLULAR ANTIGENS

Rabbit anti-rat liver sera rendered specific for liver antigens by absorption with rat kidney and citrated blood were used in conjunction with rat anti-rabbit liver sera absorbed with rabbit blood and kidney to determine the species distribution of the organ-specific hepatocellular antigens. For this purpose, cells sensitized with rat, dog, cat, human, and rabbit liver were prepared. When aliquots of either immune sera were added to the various sensitized cells, agglutination was observed to occur. Maximal antibody activity was recorded when the antisera were added to cells sensitized with the specific liver preparation used for immunization. When the sensitized cells were tested against rabbit anti-rabbit liver serum, a similar pattern of reactivity was observed, with the exception that cells sensitized with human liver were not agglutinated by the immune serum.

C. ATTEMPTS TO BREAK TOLERANCE TO THE HEPATOCELLULAR ANTIGENS OF THE RABBIT BY IMMUNIZATION WITH RAT OR RABBIT LIVER

A group of albino New Zealand rabbits were immunized with lyophilized rabbit or rat liver emulsified in complete Freund's adjuvant. A total of 8 to 10 injections were given at intervals of two to four weeks. Upon completion of the immunizing schedule the sera were collected and assessed for their capacity to agglutinate cells sensitized with rabbit liver. Serum obtained from both groups of rabbits was able to agglutinate cells sensitized with homologous rabbit liver.

DISCUSSION

The experiments in Section A demonstrate the extreme heterogeneity of the antigens comprising the immunizing emulsion of rat or rabbit liver. The relative distribution of those antigens, which are shared with rat or rabbit heart, lung, and kidney, was established by the absorption experiments. It would appear in the case of the rat that heart and lung share a common group of antigens with liver and kidney, while the kidney contains antigens common to the liver which are not present in either heart or lung. Similarly our results suggest that rabbit liver shares certain antigens with rabbit kidney, in addition to which it possesses antigens unique to itself. The specific reaction with rat or rabbit liver resisted all absorption save that with rat or rabbit liver respectively.

The study of the species distribution of the organ-specific hepatocellular antigens suggests that each animal species tested contained at least certain antigens in common with those present in rat and rabbit liver. The species distribution of the organ-specific hepatocellular antigens of the rat is the subject of a further report (5).

Immunization of rabbits with either rabbit or rat liver resulted in the production of antibodies that react with homologous rabbit liver. The antibody manifested strict organ specificity, while cells sensitized with rabbit kidney were not agglutinated by the immune serum. It is significant that rat anti-rabbit liver sera were capable of agglutinating cells sensitized with rabbit kidney, in a manner analogous to that observed with rabbit anti-rat liver sera.

Our data suggest, therefore, that immunization of rabbits with either rat or rabbit liver resulted in the production of antibodies that react with homologous rabbit liver. The antibody appears to be specific for the organ-specific hepatocellular antigens of the rabbit. The more widely distributed antigens which rabbit liver shares with kidney do not appear to be involved in the process. These findings would, therefore, tend to confirm the experiments which demonstrated the presence of such liver-specific antigens. A more detailed presentation of this work as it applies to the rat is to be published shortly (5, 6, 7).

REFERENCES

1. SARGENT, A. U., and RICHTER, M.   Fed. Proc. *21*: 20 (1962).
2. BOYDEN, S.   J. Exper. Med. *93*: 107 (1951).
3. WELLER, T. H., and COONS, A. H.   Proc. Soc. Exper. Biol. & Med. *86*: 789 (1954).
4. SAINTE-MARIE, G.   J. Histochem. *10*: 250 (1962).
5. SARGENT, A. U., RICHTER, M., and MYERS, J.   Immunology, *10*: 199 (1966).
6. RICHTER, M., SARGENT, A. U., MYERS, J., and ROSE, B.   Immunology, *10*: 211 (1966).
7. SARGENT, A. U., MYERS, J., and RICHTER, M.   J. Immunol. *96*: 268 (1966).

Studies on the Pathogenesis of the Liver Lesions in Runt Disease*

K. ARAKAWA and J. W. STEINER

THE PATHOGENESIS of lesions which are said to be of the delayed hypersensitivity type has interested us, as it has Dr. Wyllie. For the purpose of elucidating the mechanisms involved, we have selected a study of runt disease, a disease produced by the injection of homologous, i.e. isogenic, spleen cells, that is to say, spleen cells of one member of a strain of mice into a member of a different strain of mice.

Theoretically, one would anticipate that, when cells that are, presumably, reacting with histocompatibility antigens are transplanted, lesions would develop in every organ in the body, since histocompatibility antigens are thought to be distributed evenly throughout the organism. However, it has been well established in the literature that this is not true. Lesions occur predominantly in lymphoid tissue, liver, and lung, but they do not affect any other organs.

We have selected the liver for study. Other investigators have mentioned in passing that lesions occur in the liver, but most of them have concentrated on the spleen and lymph nodes, arguing that these are the target organs of the transplanted cells. We find that in spleen and lymph nodes we cannot discover what is going on because the cells that are allegedly attacking the tissue and the cells that are allegedly being destroyed are identical. In the liver this problem does not exist, in that the cells that are being destroyed, namely parenchymal liver cells, are fundamentally different from the cells that are supposedly attacking the lymphoid cells of the donor.

We have used the classical model for producing runt disease. We injected spleen cells of a donor strain into new-born mice of a different strain, and observed them over a period of 21 days. The splenic cells transferred consisted of lymphocytes (almost 99 per cent), with a very small sprinkling of plasma cells, polymorphonuclear leucocytes, and some endothelial cells. Some of the animals developed runt disease, but others remained normal, and these were found to be tolerant thereafter to the splenic cells of the donors.

*From the Department of Pathology, University of Toronto, Toronto, Ontario.

In our particular strain combination—and one must emphasize this because the criteria of the disease vary from author to author and one must set up one's own criteria in order to achieve reproducibility of results—the main criterion for runting was an arrest of growth within 10 days of birth. We discounted all animals that died before the third day of life, because we assumed that they may have died as a result of some conditions associated with the handling or the trauma of injection. If there was a sudden arrest of weight gain between the third and tenth day, we considered this the main criterion of the transplantation or runting disease. Additional criteria were loss of weight and subsequent death. In every animal that was clearly runting, depletion or disappearance of lymphocytes from lymphoid tissues occurred. In the majority of the animals there were no circulating lymphocytes to be found, nor were any lymphocytes found in the tissues. Thirdly, there was a marked hyperplasia of reticulo-endothelial cells, i.e. Kupffer cells, in the liver. Fourthly, coagulative necrosis of hepatic cells was very characteristic; and fifthly, there was perivascular mononuclear cell proliferation in the liver and lung. In many instances we killed the animals before all of the criteria outlined had developed.

We have examined 289 normal animals together and have compared these with two groups. In experiment 1 we injected animals intravenously with spleen cells, and in experiment 2 we injected our animals intraperitoneally. The mortality in the intravenously injected group was high (about 29 of the 195 died), whereas in the intraperitoneal injection group none died. The incidence of runt disease was about 60 per cent in intravenously injected cases, and about 33 per cent in intraperitoneally injected cases; so we can conclude from this that runting disease is more readily produced by the intravenous introduction of the cells than by the introduction of the cells intraperitoneally. In our particular strain this finding is not the same as that described by other authors.

Now the question always arises: Is this a so-called graft-versus-host reaction or transplantation disease; is it truly an immunological disease? We think it is, and one of the pieces of evidence, which we feel suggests fairly conclusively that an immunological event is involved, is that if one uses spleen cells of unpresensitized donors, that is to say, one strain of spleen cells injected into another recipient, the incidence is about 62.1 per cent if the injection is intravenous. If about two to three weeks prior to the transplantation of the spleen cells, the donor is brought into contact with either liver or spleen tissue of the prospective recipient, then the incidence rises to 87 per cent and, in some instances, we have been able to get an incidence of 100 per cent. In other words, presensitization does aggravate and increase the incidence of the disease, and this in itself would suggest that an immunological process is involved.

The weight-gain chart of mice injected intravenously showed a characteristic pattern. The animals were all injected with an identical dose of spleen cells, and for the first five days they all gained weight at a steady rate. Thereafter, the control mice continued to gain weight at a steady rate while the mice that had been injected and showed no criteria of runting, either grossly, clinically, or microscopically, also continued to gain weight at the same rate. The runted mice stopped gaining weight at this point, and there was quite an abrupt loss of weight from then on.

In the intraperitoneally injected group, the same thing happened, but the mice continued to gain weight for a somewhat longer period of time. However, the injected mice began to lose weight steadily about the seventh or eighth day. It is clear then that after intraperitoneal injection the loss of weight produced by the transplanting of spleen cells was not as abrupt as it was in the intravenously injected animals.

A comparison on the ninth day following injection of spleen cells of a normal mouse and a runting mouse revealed characteristic findings. The runted mice usually showed a lack of fur, and they had a peculiar wobbly gait, which was partly due to the fact that their hind legs were somewhat deformed as a result of muscle atrophy. In addition, they developed a very marked exfoliative dermatitis, with scaly skin which became extremely excoriated and rather thick. This was characteristic, but in our strain combination it was not an invariable phenomenon.

When the abdomen of these animals was opened there were two striking features: first there was marked splenomegaly; and, secondly, hepatic necrosis had developed. It is a mystery to us why many authors have ignored this lesion in the liver, which is surely extremely striking. In many instances the entire liver is necrotic.

It is important to note that in the cases in which the necrosis was mild it was invariably present near the free border of the liver, and rarely did it involve the upper border or the right lobe. The specific reasons for this are not clear at the present time.

Under the light microscope there were certain paramount features. First, the necrosis usually began near the free margin of the liver and extended into the parenchyma. No matter how widespread the necrosis, in a given liver it was more or less of the same age. The necrosis apparently occurred on one day, and thereafter there was no further progression, at least not in the animals that were killed before the 21st day of the experiment.

In some of the animals, liver parenchyma remained intact in the midst of this holocaust. In the progression with time there was, first of all, coagulative necrosis. Gradually the parenchymal cells disappeared, but the Kupffer cells often survived in the midst of this destruction. There was very often a dilatation of sinusoids, and we interpreted this as being secondary to the necrosis. The necrosis was subcapsular, and we assume that this dilatation of sinusoids was simply due to the fact that sinusoidal flow was obstructed at this point. In the liver itself aggregates of cells were found. Some of these were haematopoietic cells, which were markedly increased in number, owing to the fact that all of these animals had a Coombs-positive haemolytic anaemia. There were other cells, present, which were usually large reticulum cells, and a very large complement of plasma cells. However, even in serial sections, one did not necessarily find areas of necrosis with the immunologically competent cells in the immediate vicinity. In fact, it was much more frequent to find areas of necrosis with no immunologically competent cells adjacent to them.

In portal tracts there was a proliferation of cells, which were mostly reticulum cells and macrophages. I wish to stress the fact that in these areas there were no lymphocytes whatsoever, and this was so in all organs, including the lymph nodes and spleen. Occasionally a thrombus was found in one of the hepatic arteries, but this was a rather unusual finding in these animals.

In some areas intact liver cells were found, and in between there were scattered cells, with extremely eosinophilic cytoplasms. Now it has been suggested that this eosinophilic phenomenon was in some way related to the presence of immunologically competent cells, but, as can be shown in the electromicrograph, this point cannot be supported. All of the cells seen were haematopoietic cells, and there was no particular relationship between this kind of degeneration and the presence of immunologically competent cells in the liver.

Occasionally large aggregates of lymphoid cells, many of them reticulum cells, were found in the liver, and there was no evidence of any kind of necrosis or degeneration in the vicinity of such aggregates.

A striking feature in the livers was a hypertrophy and hyperplasia of Kupffer cells. It is very difficult to say, at present, whether the hyperplasia of Kupffer cells was secondary to the necrosis, or whether it was a primary event. At any rate, no antibody has been identified in these Kupffer cells in such areas, and at present we interpret the Kupffer-cell hyperplasia as being secondary to the destruction of liver cells.

At a later stage in the process of necrosis there were occasional polymorphs, and even the Kupffer cells underwent degeneration and necrosis, with the ultimate complete disappearance of the liver cells. Thus, even if the Kupffer cells were primarily involved in the necrosis, they certainly disappeared thereafter, and consequently can no longer be invoked as causative.

The ultimate fate of these lesions was remarkable, in that the majority of them became calcified, and often there were found giant cells and a granulomatous kind of inflammation which ultimately led to fibrosis of the lesion. This is very unusual in the liver, even in inflammations known to be allergic.

We have been searching, by means of the electron microscope, for any possible evidence bearing on the pathogenesis of these lesions. First, in some areas sinusoids were found to be occluded. In them there were clumps of platelets and even polymorphonuclear leucocytes. Such sinusoids were found very frequently in these livers and the question arises: Were these sinusoids occluded as a primary phenomenon, i.e., did thrombosis lead to necrosis, or is this thrombosis secondary to the necrosis due to spaces in the sinusoids? This question we cannot answer at present.

There was evidence of some immunological activity in the liver in that aggregates of a fibrillar material which has no periodicity and which we interpret as amyloid "deposition" were found between Kupffer cells and liver cells. The quantities of amyloid present were so small that we have been unable to demonstrate it by light microscopy. However, other workers have found amyloid in the spleen and other organs.

Lastly, we found large numbers of plasma cells in the livers of the animals, between the fifth and seventh day. Plasma cells are not normally found in the livers of neonatal mice on the fifth or seventh day, but in mice that were runting plasma cells were extremely numerous. We do not know whether these cells were of donor or recipient origin, and opinions on this point are divided. What I wish to stress here is that these cells proliferated directly adjacent to liver cells, and yet we find no evidence of injury to these cells.

In conclusion, we have been studying a model in which we hoped to demonstrate that immunologically competent cells, with a known immunological commitment against cells of the recipient, would indeed attack the recipients and destroy the recipient cells. We have been unable to find any evidence of this, either by light microscopy or by electron microscopy. Therefore we feel that the lesions are probably non-immunological.

We postulate that the graft-versus-host reaction, that is to say the reaction of the transplanted cells against the host tissue, is immunological; the fact that presensitization will accentuate the lesions provides the evidence. However, not all the lesions in the recipient animals are immunological. In the liver, for example, the lesions are probably vascular and not related to the direct immunological activity of the transplanted spleen cells.

We consider the graft-versus-host reaction as being an immunological event which leads to the loss of weight and to the various clinical features shown by these animals. We also consider that this reaction is associated with hypertrophy of Kupffer cells, an increase in immature haematopoietic cells, and a perivascular mononuclear cell proliferation. These three features produce an increase in liver volume, which, in turn, produces a disturbance of the circulation, because the liver enlarges at a rate that is greater than the capsular enlargement. The disturbance of circulation leads to anoxia and degeneration and necrosis under the capsule, so that an immunological event has secondary effects and produces an essentially ischaemic injury.

DISCUSSION

CHAIRMAN: Thank you. Dr. Steiner's paper is open for discussion.

DR. M. D. HAUST: I have one question of Dr. Steiner, and one suggestion to make. Would it be possible, Dr. Steiner, that the accumulation of haematopoietic foci in these new-born animals is due to their new-born nature, because in human neonatal subjects we see foci of haematopoiesis regularly in the livers and the spleen. The suggestion to utilize a female animal as a donor might be helpful; with sex chromosome being present in the nuclei one might be able to distinguish, on injection into the male recipient, whether or not these are his own plasma cells or those of the donor.

DR. STEINER: The new-born mice have haematopoiesis up to about the tenth day. the haematopoiesis is gradually reduced, whereas in runted animals it increases, and this is directly related to the development of the Coombs-positive haematopoietic anaemia. We know that there is an increase in haematopoiesis, but we do not think that the haematopoiesis is in any way related to the destruction of the liver which occurs.

Secondly, regarding the use of different sexes of animals for donor and recipient, this has been done by a number of investigators, and opinions are completely divided as to the identity of the cells that appear in the liver. Some say that they are of donor origin because they find, for example, that, if female recipients are used, "X" chromosome bearing cells are found in the liver; other investigators deny this, and it is at present not at all clear which cells are proliferating in the liver. We are saying that it doesn't matter two hoots to us what the cells are or from whom they originate. All we say is that the necrosis is not due to the cells or to the direct activity of these cells.

DR. D. FORD (*Vancouver*): What is the present status of runting disease, both in this situation and in thymectomy runting, in germ-free animals?

DR. STEINER: Runt disease is known today to be a highly non-specific phenomenon. It can be produced by a variety of methods, for example, thymectomy; injections of sterile vaccine will produce runt disease, viral infections will produce runt disease, and all of these have one thing in common—lymphoid depletion. It is quite likely that the over-all clinical picture of the disease is due to the lymphoid depletion, rather than to any specific destructive activity.

We have selected one lesion, mainly because we felt that the fact that this disease is caused by lymphoid depletion does not mean, necessarily, that each and every lesion in the animal is caused by the same mechanism. There can be all kinds of mechanisms involved.

We have been collaborating with Dr. Soloman, in Paris, who has injected germ-free animals for us. These germ-free animals, following the same procedure as used by us, also get runt disease. Now it is true that some of these germ-free animals may still harbour viruses, but the fact is that they do develop runt disease and liver lesions that are identical with those observed by us.

DR. ZIFF: I might say that thymectomized animals will not runt in the germ-free animal, but immunological runting, by contrast, does happen in the germ-free animal.

DR. BARNETT: Apparently, Dr. Steiner, these lesions are not associated with cellular infiltrate. To support your hypothesis that they are not immunologic, have you excluded the possibility that the lesion may be due to a circulating antibody? We see that the runted animal does have a circulating antibody as evidenced by a Coombs-positive anaemia: are there immunoglobulins and complement in these lesions?

DR. STEINER: We have done the immunological chemistry on these lesions and we have not been able to convince ourselves that any antibody can be demonstrated in them. Antibody can be demonstrated in any hepatic necrosis, but we have not been able to demonstrate it to any unusual extent in these animals. These are new-born animals, which are incapable, at least at this stage, of producing any large quantity of antibody.

CHAIRMAN: Are there any other questions? I think Dr. Steiner's suggestion or hypothesis that this is an anoxic thing is very interesting, but in clinical situations we see many types of diseases in which the liver is enlarged mechanically or otherwise because of various factors; yet we see very little in the way of circulatory disturbances that lead to necrosis on that basis. Do you know of any counterpart to this in clinical disease?

DR. STEINER: I think that we have become so obsessed with the concept of immunological destruction that we ignore the possibility that other factors may be involved. In liver disease a typical example is obstruction of the common bile duct. We say that obstruction of the common bile duct is due to leakage of bile, and bile is an agent that injures cells; but it has now been shown conclusively that the necrosis of the liver in biliary obstruction is due to thrombosis, to occlusion of small capillaries and sinusoids in the liver; and I think we must keep an open mind about the mechanisms of immunological destruction because such factors as vascular factors can be extremely important, and the actual destruction may be mediated by things other than antibody or antibody-bearing cells.

Evidence for Separate Control of Haemopoietic and Immunologic Functions in the Mouse[*]

E. A. McCULLOCH, J. C. KENNEDY,
L. SIMINOVITCH, and J. E. TILL

BOTH the haemopoietic and immunological systems may be considered as cell-renewal systems (1) characterized by continuous replenishment of their cellular constituents. It has long been appreciated that the cells of the blood have limited life spans and that the senescent cells are replaced through the proliferation and differentiation of precursors in haemopoietic tissue (2). More recently, it has become apparent that cellular proliferation is also a very important part of immunological responses (3). Further, in responding to antigenic stimulation, cells not only proliferate, but also acquire a new function, the production of specific antibody protein. Therefore, differentiation may also be considered as an important part of the immune response.

Cell-renewal systems depend for their integrity and continuing function on those cells within them which have extensive proliferative capacity and can renew themselves as well as differentiate. Such cells are often called stem cells and are responsible, through their proliferation and differentiation, for the replacement of the short-lived cells that carry out specific functions. Evidence is accumulating that, for the haemopoietic system, stem cells are important targets for control mechanisms (4, 5). It is, therefore, of some interest to know whether or not the haemopoietic system and the immunological system depend upon a common class of stem cells. For example, in certain clinical states it might be desirable to suppress the function of the immunological system. However, complete suppression of haemopoiesis inevitably leads to death. If both systems depend on the activity of a common stem, it would appear unlikely that the immunological system could be effectively repressed without eventually endangering the life of the patient because of haemopoietic failure. Alternatively, if each system is maintained by separate

[*]From the Department of Medical Biophysics, University of Toronto, and the Ontario Cancer Institute.

independent stem cells, it might be feasible to affect the one while leaving the other functionally intact.

A resolution of this controversial question may perhaps be achieved if both the haemopoietic and immunological systems are studied using similar methods and under similar conditions. It is especially important that each be studied at the cellular level. The purpose of this paper is to present the results of experiments in which the cellular basis for haemopoiesis and the cellular basis for haemolysin production are compared. The results indicate that the production of blood cells and the production of antibody-producing cells are independently controlled functions. The findings are compatible with the view that each function is dependent upon the activity of a separate stem cell.

MATERIALS AND METHODS

THE SPLEEN-COLONY TECHNIQUE

The spleen-colony method (6, 7) used for studying haemopoietic stem cells is shown in Fig. 1. Cells are obtained from the haemopoietic organs of normal donors, dispersed, and counted. An appropriate number is then injected into each of a group of heavily irradiated recipient animals. After 9 to 14 days the survivors are killed and their spleens fixed in Bouin's solution. These spleens are seen to contain discrete round or oval nodules that are colonies of proliferating and differentiating haemopoietic cells. These colonies have been shown to consist of the progeny of single cells by direct cytological means (8).

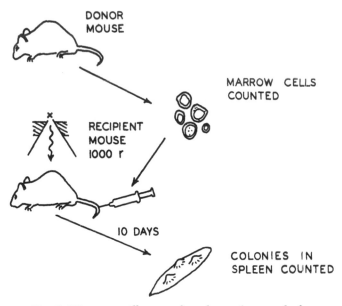

FIG. 1. Diagram to illustrate the spleen-colony method.

The cells of origin, which we have termed colony-forming cells, are considered to be examples of the stem cells of the haemopoietic system since they have the capacity for extensive proliferation, self-renewal, and differentiation (9). Spleen colonies are readily counted, and their number is linearly related to the number of haemopoietic cells injected into the recipients (6, 7). Thus, by counting spleen colonies one may obtain an estimate of the number of this class of haemopoietic stem cells.

THE JERNE PLAQUE-FORMING CELL TECHNIQUE

The method used for detecting cells engaged in the immune response is shown in Fig. 2. This is the method of Jerne and Nordin (10) for measuring quantitatively the number of haemolysin-producing cells in a cell suspension. Normal mice are immunized by receiving an intravenous injection of sheep erythrocytes. After a period of time, usually four days, their spleens are removed and a cell suspension prepared. An appropriate number of cells from this suspension is mixed with sheep red cells in agar. In this way the

JERNE ASSAY FOR PLAQUE-FORMING CELLS

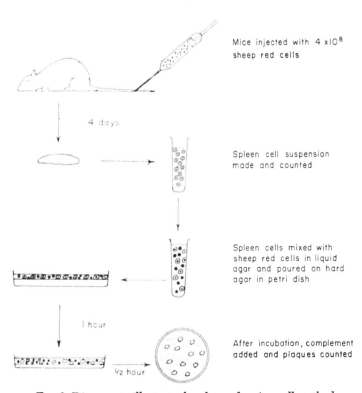

FIG. 2. Diagram to illustrate the plaque-forming-cell method.

haemolysin-producing cells in the spleen-cell suspension are immobilized in close contact with sheep red cells. The mixture is incubated for one hour and at the end of this time complement is added. This results in a zone of lysis about each cell that releases haemolysin during the incubation period. These zones of lysis, or plaques, are readily counted; their number is linearly related to the number of nucleated spleen cells added to the plate, and evidence has been presented that each plaque results from the activity of a single cell (10). Very few plaque-forming cells of this kind are present in the spleens of unimmunized animals, but following the injection of sheep red cells their number increases, until, at the height of the immune response, each spleen contains between 10^4 and 10^5 plaque-forming cells. Their number, therefore, provides a measurement of the extensive proliferation and differentiation occurring in the spleen in response to antigenic stimulation.

RESULTS

Ionizing radiation provides a useful tool for investigating tissue function at the cellular level. The dose of radiation absorbed by tissue can be measured accurately, and is free from the pharmacological considerations that affect the results obtained by the use of drugs. In addition, a large body of information exists relevant to the effects of radiation on cellular function (for example, see (11)). For these reasons, a comparison was made of the effects of gamma radiation on colony formation and plaque-cell formation, with a view to seeing if the two functions respond differently.

SENSITIVITY OF PLAQUE-CELL FORMATION AND COLONY FORMATION TO GAMMA RAYS IN VIVO

The radiation survival curves obtained when cells of mouse spleen are exposed to gamma rays and tested for colony formation and production of plaque-forming cells are shown in Fig. 3. In each case the survival of the function, expressed as a logarithm of the fraction of the value obtained for unirradiated control cells, is plotted on the vertical axis against the radiation dose in rads plotted on the horizontal axis. The survival curve for colony formation was obtained by a transplantation method (7). Cells from normal mouse spleen were injected into irradiated recipients, and after two hours these animals, containing the injected cells, received varying amounts of additional radiation. The spleen cells under test received only this second dose of radiation, and it is this dose that is plotted in the figure (12).

The survival curve for production of plaque-forming cells shown at the bottom of Fig. 3 was obtained by irradiating groups of mice with varying doses of gamma rays and within two hours administering sheep red cells intravenously (13). After four days pooled spleen-cell suspensions from each group were assayed for content of plaque-forming cells. Control experiments

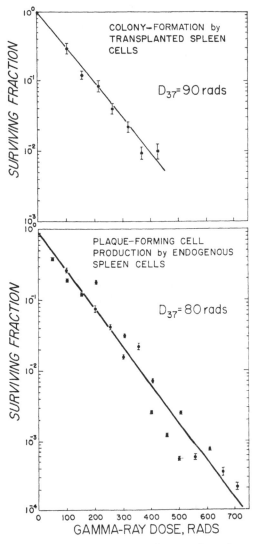

FIG. 3. Gamma-ray survival curves for colony formation (top) and the production of plaque-forming cells (bottom) by spleen cells.

indicated that the resulting radiation survival curve is not strongly dependent on the dose of antigen or the time of assay during the first four days (13).

It is evident from the figure that the two radiation survival curves are very similar. Both are simple negative exponentials. In each case the D_{37} dose (dose required to reduce survival to 0.37) is very similar. These experiments, there-fore, detect no difference between the radiation responses of colony-forming cells and the progenitors of plaque-forming cells. However, both processes, colony formation and plaque-cell formation, depend on cell proliferation, and it is known that the sensitivity of this cellular function to ionizing radiation is very similar for mammalian cells, regardless of the organ or species from which the cells are obtained (11). The similarity of the two survival curves presented in Fig. 3 cannot, for this reason, be considered as evidence of a common stem for the two functions. Rather, a sensitivity to the initial radiation injury shared with most mammalian cells is being displayed. However, there are other aspects to radiation responses of tissue than the production of the initial injury. For example, it remained possible that studies of repair of the initial injury might require specific responses from each system, and this will be considered next.

REPAIR OF RADIATION DAMAGE

A major mechanism for the repair of radiation-induced damage to cellular systems is the proliferation of surviving cells. The kinetics of this proliferation in normal tissue might be expected to be a function of control mechanisms affecting the damaged tissue. Repair of radiation injury may be studied to advantage by using a fractionated-dose technique. Representative data from a large series of experiments on the repair of damage to the colony-forming cell system in mouse spleen (14) are shown in Fig. 4. In these experiments, the

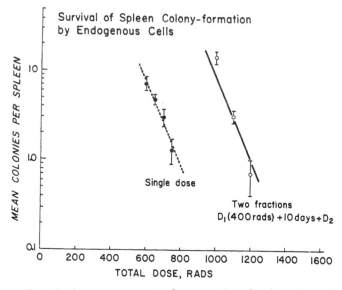

FIG. 4. Gamma-ray survival curves for the formation of spleen colonies from endogenous colony-forming cells. Left: single exposure. Right: total dose in two fractions, with 10-day time interval. First dose: 400 rads.

endogenous spleen-colony method was used. Groups of animals received varying doses of radiation, and after 11 days their spleens were examined for colonies. In the figure, the logarithm of the mean number of colonies per spleen is shown as a function of the radiation dose. The curve on the left is the result obtained when the radiation was delivered as a single dose. It is a negative exponential with a D_{37} very similar to that obtained in the experiments shown in Fig. 3, using the transplantation method. The curve at the right of the figure represents the results obtained when all of the mice received a first dose of 400 rads, and then were allowed to rest for 10 days. After that time sufficient additional radiation was given to provide the doses shown on the graph. The spleens were examined for colonies 11 days after the second radiation dose. It is evident that the slopes of the two curves are very similar, but that very much larger amounts of radiation are required for the two-dose method to achieve the same reduction in colony formation obtained by a single exposure. The extent of the separation between these two curves is indicative of the proliferation of the cells surviving the first

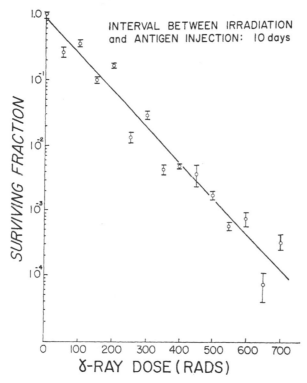

Fig. 5. Gamma-ray survival curves for production of plaque-forming cells obtained when an interval of 10 days was allowed between irradiation and antigen injection.

radiation dose. Indeed, experiments of this design, using varying intervals between the two doses, have been used to measure the doubling time of colony-forming cells (14). From the data shown in Fig. 4, it is apparent that extensive repair of radiation damage to the colony-forming system occurred within 10 days.

The results of experiments designed to measure repair of radiation-induced damage to the immunological system are shown in Fig. 5. In these experiments groups of mice received varying doses of radiation, and were then allowed a period of 10 days for repair. After this interval sheep red cells were injected, and after four days spleens were assayed for plaque-forming cells. The results are presented in the figure as a radiation survival curve. The line shown is the survival curve of Fig. 3, in which the interval between irradiation and antigen injection was two hours. The points indicate the data from experiments in which 10 days elapsed between irradiation and antigen injection. It is evident that these points yield a survival curve not different from that previously obtained. This finding is interpreted to mean that, for all doses tested, no repair of radiation-induced damage to the plaque-forming cell system had occurred. This result, indicating no repair to this part of the immune system in 10 days, is in striking contrast to the extensive repair observed in the same time interval in the colony-forming cell system. Thus, in respect to their capacity to repair radiation-induced injury, the colony-forming and plaque-cell-forming systems are very different.

DISCUSSION

Our experimental results have been presented in the form of a comparison between spleen-colony formation, and the production of haemolytic plaque-forming cells. Each system is considered as a cell-renewal system; in the case of spleen-colony formation it has been shown that single cells with the properties of stem cells give rise to large numbers of differentiated progeny and smaller numbers of new colony-forming cells (9). Evidence has also been presented which suggests that the cells in mouse spleen which respond to antigenic stimulation by sheep red cells (antigen-sensitive cells) do not themselves produce haemolysin, but respond to stimulation by proliferation and differentiation, with the production of plaque-forming cells (13). In our experiments, ionizing radiation has been used as a tool to explore the relationship between colony-forming cells and antigen-sensitive cells. The results show that a functional separation between the two is possible, since radiation-induced damage is repaired at different rates in the two systems. This separation is compatible with the view that each system is maintained by the activity of independent stem cells having no common precursor in adult life. Support for this view has been obtained in a further series of experiments in which sheep cells were given to mice during the process of colony growth. When colonies had developed, these were dissected from supporting splenic tissue, and both colonies and areas of spleen free of colonies were assayed for plaque-forming cells. No correlation was found between the presence of colonies and the presence of plaque-forming cells (15).

The spleen-colony method and the Jerne plaque-forming cell method provide model systems for experimentation. Extrapolation of the results obtained using such models to haemopoiesis or immunologic response must be made with caution. However, it is evident from the results of our experiments that, in terms of model systems, immunological responsiveness may be suppressed without suppressing haemopoiesis. Thus, if mice received repeated small doses of radiation at approximately weekly intervals, regeneration of colony-forming cells would occur between doses, and the animals would not die of marrow failure. However, regeneration of immune capacity would not occur between doses, and the cumulative effect of repeated exposure would finally lead to failure to respond to antigen. Such a regime would, of course, not be practical in man, since repeated exposures to small doses of radiation would certainly be leukaemogenic. However, the results obtained in the model systems support the hope that clinically practical methods for the suppression of immunity may be developed.

ACKNOWLEDGMENTS

These investigations were supported by the National Cancer Institute of Canada, the Defence Research Board (Grant 9350–14), the Medical Research Council of Canada (Grant Ma–1420), and the National Research Council of Canada (Grant T–1714).

REFERENCES

1. LEBLOND, C. P., and WALKER, B. E.   Physiol. Rev. *36*: 255 (1956).
2. CRONKITE, E. P., FLIEDNER, T. M., BOND, V. P., and ROBERTSON, J. S.   Anatomic and physiologic facts and hypotheses about hemopoietic proliferating systems. *In* Conference on Fundamental Problems and Technics for the Study of the Kinetics of Cellular Proliferation, Salt Lake City, 1954. The Kinetics of Cellular Proliferation, *edited by* F. Stohlman, Jr. (Grune & Stratton, New York, 1959), p. 1.
3. MAKINODAN, T., KASTENBAUM, M. A., and PETERSON, W. J.   J. Immunol. *88*: 31 (1962).
4. LAJTHA, L. G., GILBERT, C. W., PORTEOUS, D. D., and ALEXANIAN, R.   Ann. New York Acad. Sci. *113*: 742 (1964).
5. TILL, J. E., McCULLOCH, E. A., and SIMINOVITCH, L.   Proc. Nat. Acad. Sci. U.S.A. *51*: 29 (1964).
6. TILL, J. E., and McCULLOCH, E. A.   Radiat. Res. *14*: 213 (1961).
7. McCULLOCH, E. A., and TILL, J. E.   Radiat. Res. *16*: 822 (1962).
8. BECKER, A. J., McCULLOCH, E. A., and TILL, J. E.   Nature *197*: 452 (1963).
9. SIMINOVITCH, L., McCULLOCH, E. A., and TILL, J. E.   J. Cell. Comp. Physiol. *62*: 327 (1963).
10. JERNE, N. K., and NORDIN, A. A.   Science *140*: 405 (1963).
11. WHITMORE, G. F., and TILL, J. E.   Ann. Rev. Nucl. Sci. *14*: 347 (1964).
12. SIMINOVITCH, L., TILL, J. E., and McCULLOCH, E. A.   Radiat. Res. *24*: 482 (1965).
13. KENNEDY, J. C., TILL, J. E., SIMINOVITCH, L., and McCULLOCH, E. A.   J. Immunol. *94*: 715 (1965).
14. TILL, J. E., and McCULLOCH, E. A.   Ann. New York Acad. Sci. *114*: 115 (1964).
15. KENNEDY, J. C.   Unpublished experiments.

Studies on the *In Vivo*
Handling of the Third
Component of Complement*

C. KIRK OSTERLAND, M.D.,
U. NILSSON, M.D., and
H. J. MÜLLER-EBERHARD, M.D.

COMPLEMENT is a highly complex system of serum factors with the capacity to damage cell membranes. There are nine or ten components, and these are activated by antigen-antibody interaction in a sequential manner, which results finally in membrane damage and the neutralization of the complement activity itself.

There is quite good evidence now that tissue damage produced by immuno-logical mechanisms, at least in some cases, is mediated by this complement system. In the presentation of this material I shall provide a certain amount of background to complement studies. For some of you it will be a review; for others it will probably be an introduction to complement.

The experiment to be described is in its early stages, so that the results are of a preliminary nature.

First of all, as an indicator of complement fixation, sheep cells sensitized with subagglutinating quantities of anti-sheep cell haemolysin have been used extensively. This is a convenient system for demonstrating the degree of haemolysis, since the amount of haemoglobin liberated can be measured spectrophotometrically and thereby quantitated and extrapolated to have a meaning in terms of degree of haemolysis or units of complement activity.

Recently the new and powerful techniques of protein separation have been applied to the separation of this haemolytic activity into various fractions from whole serum. Using such fractions, considerable data have been accumulated on their interaction in the various steps leading to immune haemolysis. With the use of purified components, the kinetics of the reaction steps are also being defined.

Table I shows the sequence of events occurring for the complement compon-

*From Washington University School of Medicine, St. Louis, Missouri, and Scripps Research Institute, La Jolla, California.

TABLE I

(1)	E	$+A \xrightarrow[\text{Ca}^{++}]{}$	EA
(2)	EA	$+C'1q, r, s \longrightarrow$	EAC'1a
(3)	EAC'1a	$+C'4 \longrightarrow$	EAC'1a, 4
(4)	EAC'1a, 4	$+C'2 \xrightarrow[]{\text{Mg}^{++}}$	EAC'1a, 4, 2a
(4a)	↑		
(5)	EAC'1a, 4, 2a	$+C'3 \longrightarrow$	EAC'1a, 4, 2a, 3
(5a)	EAC'1a, 4, 3		
(6)	EAC'1a, 4, 2a, 3	$+C'5, 6 \longrightarrow$	EAC'1a, 4, 2a, 3, 5, 6
(7)	EAC'1a, 4, 2a, 3, 5, 6	$+C'7 \longrightarrow$	EAC'1a, 4, 2a, 3, 5, 6, 7
(8)	EAC'1a, 4, 2a, 3, 5, 6, 7	$+C'8 \longrightarrow$	E* (damaged cell)

ents during immune haemolysis. In this table E refers to erythrocyte membrane, A to antibody and C to complement—the particular component being designated by a number.

In the first step C'q, C'r, and C's are fixed and an esterase activity is generated; such an erythrocyte is then called C'a, where "a" stands for activated. As shown, calcium ions are necessary for this step.

The second component to become attached is the C'4; the esterase activity of C'1 is necessary for this reaction. The C'4 component which has been isolated by Dr. Müller-Eberhard and identified on immuno-electrophoresis patterns as β_{1E} protein, apparently combines directly with the erythrocyte membrane.

In the next step C'2 becomes fixed loosely to the complex and then is acted upon also by the esterase activity of C', with the result that an active part of C'2 becomes attached to the complex, probably on a receptor site on C'4. An inactive fragment C'2i is released in the fluid phase. This step, which requires the participation of Mg^{++} ions, generates a C'1a, 4, 2a complex.

The component that is able to combine with this complex has been defined as C'3 and is identified by immuno-electrophoresis as β_{1C} globulin in human serum. Some of the C'3 molecules are attached firmly to the complex, while the others are released into the fluid phase in a physicochemically altered form which is haemolytically inactive and shows slightly enhanced electrophoretic mobility. This product has been designated as β_{1G}.

Two factors, C'5 and C'6 react next. The former has been isolated and identified by Dr. U. Nilsson and Dr. Müller-Eberhard. With the fixation of these two factors the whole complex becomes stabilized, with the final two steps involving C'7 and C'8 leading to loss of the cell membrane integrity and actual haemolysis.

The component being studied in these experiments is the C'3 or β_{1C} component. Immuno-electrophoretically, as the name suggests, this component migrates in the β_1 region and is characterized by its lability in serum (being altered by hydrazine or ammonia treatment or even by simple aging).

The altered protein has a faster electrophoretic mobility and a smaller molecular weight. It is designated β_{1A} globulin. This must be distinguished from the β_{1G} globulin liberated from the C′3 component during actual fixation of the complement. This protein, like β_{1A}, has more rapid electrophoretic mobility, but is not of lower molecular weight than β_{1C}.

β_{1C} was isolated in pure form following the method of Nilsson and Müller-Eberhard by the steps shown in Table II. It should be noted that all steps are performed at 4° C. Using this technique, it was possible to obtain preparations of β_{1C} which were pure as judged by gel diffusion methods and ultracentrifugation.

TABLE II

1. Euglobulin preparation from fresh normal human serum, by dialysis against pH 5.4 λ/2.02 phosphate buffer
2. Centrifugation and collection of euglobulin precipitate
3. Wash precipitate, and dissolve in pH 7 λ/2.1 phosphate buffer
4. Clear lipids by ultracentrifugation
5. Dialysis and TEAE column chromatography
6. Detection of activity using haemolytic system deficient in C¹3

Purified β_{1C} was then labelled with I^{125}, using a method of Dr. F. J. Dixon which employs chloramine T and sodium metabisulphite. Hot labelling is achieved without the use of carrier iodine. This labelled protein retained full haemolytic activity. It was sterilized by passage through a Seitz filter and was deemed ready for use when a culture proved the absence of contamination.

To date, five patients have been injected with β_{1C} in order to determine the biological half-life of this protein. Approximately 35 μc. was administered, following which serial blood samples were taken for counting. Stool and urine specimens were also collected for counting, and protein-bound and non-protein-bound counts were estimated by precipitating the sample with 5 per cent TCA. Thyroidal uptake of the label was blocked during the experiment by the administration of Lugol's solution. Samples were counted in a Packard automatic well-type gamma spectrometer.

In the five patients tested the biological half-life of the protein ranged from 1.2 to 2 days. The patient with the most active "immunological" disorder did not yield the shortest half-life, but the actual recovery of label in the urine was less in his samples than in those of the other subjects. In all cases the label excreted in the urine was in the free form, while that in the serum remained protein bound. By making an immuno-electrophoresis of a patient's serum and subsequent autoradiography of a dried plate, it was possible to demonstrate that the injected material remained in the β_{1C} form *in vivo*.

To date, it has not been possible to subject to biopsy an active lesion in a patient who has been injected with the labelled β_{1C}. It may be possible to detect preferential deposition (fixation) of label in these areas. By this sort of technique it is hoped to define another parameter in the immunological defect of patients with the "collagen" or "auto-immune" type disorders.

DISCUSSION

DR. PRICE: Would you need to postulate a re-use of complement, since you said that there was no correlation between the activity of the disease and the turnover rate of complement? Would you have to postulate that it is being used over and over—one molecule?

DR. OSTERLAND: I obviously didn't make myself clear on that point. This is apparently a rapidly turned-over protein—so rapidly turned over that, at least in the five cases studied, we could not demonstrate any difference in the disappearance rate. Now there are many parameters that you can study in these experiments. There is a difference in recovery of the label that is administered; but, thus far, the disappearance curves in the actively ill patients and in the controls seem to be the same.

A Complement and Antigen Defect in Certain Inbred Strains of Mice: An Instance of Eniotypy*

B. CINADER, S. DUBISKI, and
A. C. WARDLAW

OUR INTENTION in this paper is to discuss certain aspects of molecular polymorphism in mammals, with particular reference to its effect on the specificity of the antibody response of different individuals within a species. The general discussion will be based an experimental evidence on an antigen defect (lack of MuB1) in inbred mice and on a defect in haemolytic complement which is a functional consequence of the loss of the antigen. The immunological reactivity of the complement-deficient mouse and its potential as a research tool will be considered.

1. THE ROLE OF POLYMORPHISM IN THE REGULATION OF IMMUNOLOGICAL SPECIFICITY

A number of different processes regulate the quantity and specificity of antibody production. Some of these regulatory mechanisms are under the direct control of genes (2, 22, 37), others are feed-back mechanisms (45, 54, 65), and yet others are inhibitory processes, functioning mainly in the recognition and exclusion from immunogenicity of certain antigenic determinants.

In any disease involving or affecting the regulation of the antibody response (auto-antibody formation, atopy, myeloma), the study of the regulatory mechanisms and the phenomena underlying them are of obvious importance. The regulatory mechanism that prevents auto-antibody formation is based on acquired immunological tolerance to autologous determinants. Determinants on foreign macromolecules which are thus excluded from immunogenicity are those that are identical with determinants of autologous macromolecules. Since

*From the Subdivision of Immunochemistry, Division of Biological Research, Ontario Cancer Institute; the Department of Immunology, Toronto Western Hospital; and the Department of Medical Biophysics and Pathological Chemistry, and Connaught Medical Research Laboratories, University of Toronto, Toronto.

the structure of autologous macromolecules varies from individual to individual, immunogenicity of determinants on a foreign antigen also varies in different individuals. As a consequence, the variation in the immune response of normal individuals depends on the polymorphism of individual macromolecules. We have discussed this "steering mechanism" in detail elsewhere (10, 11, 14).

2. ALLOTYPY AND ENIOTYPY

The protein composition of individuals of the same species shows many differences. This polymorphism is essentially of two types. The first type is one in which an isofunctional protein is present in all individuals and the individuals differ from one another by the amino-acid sequence in a limited region of the molecule. Most instances of molecular polymorphism so far studied are of this kind. When they have been revealed by isologous antibody, they are designated as allotypes (47). We propose to extend this term to include all kinds of polymorphism of the first type. Many instances of this type of polymorphism are now known, and Tables I and II show some examples of serum

TABLE I

ALLOTYPY OF SERUM PROTEINS OF MOUSE, MAN, AND RABBIT

Name and/or function of the molecule	Species	Locus	No. of alleles	References
Albumin	Man		2	(20, 36)
Beta-lipoprotein	Man	Ag	3	(9, 30)
		Lp	2	(6)
			2	(7)
Group-specific protein	Man	Gc	2	(16)
Haptoglobin	Man	Hp	5	(58, 44)
Immunoglobulin	Mouse	*	8	(19, 26, 29, 34, 39)
		*	3	(26)
		*	2	(27)
	Man	Gm	15	(61, 62)
		InV	3	(42)
	Rabbit	Aa	3	(18)
		Ab	3	(18)
		Ms	2	(33)
Transferrin	Mouse	Trf	2	(17)
	Man	Tf	12	(23)

*Notation under discussion.

protein and enzyme polymorphism selected from the steadily increasing amount of information.

Individuals of the same species may also differ from one another by a second type of variation which we propose to call the *eniotype** and which consists in

*Eniotype indicates "a type occurring in some," derived from ἐνίοτε (somewhere).

TABLE II

POLYMORPHISM OF ENZYMES IN MOUSE AND MAN

Enzyme	Species	Source of enzyme	Locus	No. of alleles	Differences in the allelic products detected by	References
Acid phosphatase	Man	Erythrocytes	P	3	Electrophoretic mobility	(31)
Alkaline phosphatase	Man	Serum	Pp*	2	Electrophoretic mobility	(4)
δ-Alpha-amino-levulinate dehydratase	Mouse	Liver	Lv	2	Activity	(56)
Beta-glucuronidase	Mouse	Liver	Gg	2	Activity†	(48)
Catalase	Mouse	Blood		2	Activity†	(21)
Catalase	Man	Blood		2	Activity†	(64, 1)
Catalase	Man	Erythrocytes		2	Electrophoretic mobility	(3)
Esterase	Mouse	Erythrocytes	Ee-1	2	Electrophoretic mobility	(49)
			Ee-2	2		(49)
Esterase	Mouse	Kidney	Es-3	2	Activity and electrophoretic mobility	(55)
			Es-4	2		(55)
Esterase	Mouse	Serum	Da	2	Electrophoretic mobility	(50)
Esterase	Man	Erythrocytes		2	Activity	(57)
Glucose-6-phosphate dehydrogenase	Man	Erthrocytes	G-6-PD‡	8	Activity and/or electrophoretic mobility	(35)
Lactic dehydrogenase	Man	Erythrocytes		2	Electrophoretic mobility	(43)
Phosphoglucomutase	Man	Erythrocytes	PGM	2	Electrophoretic mobility	(59)
Pseudocholinesterase	Man	Serum	Ch$_I$	4	Activity	(24, 40)

*Associated with blood groups.
†Enzyme activity has not been detected so far, for the product of one of the alleles.
‡X-linked.

the *presence* or *absence* of certain proteins. This second type of polymorphism is not as well understood or fully documented as is the first type. Nevertheless, it may occur quite frequently and may, in many instances, have detrimental consequences, as, for example, in various clotting deficiencies such as congenital afibrinogenaemia, haemophilia, Christmas disease, absence of factors 5, 7, 8, and 10 (8, 60) and in such metabolic deficiencies as total albinism (tyrosinase), Von Gierke's disease (glucose-6-phosphatase), familial goitrous cretinism (iodotyrosine deshalogenase), phenylketonuria (phenylalanine hydroxylase), and Cugler–Najjar syndrome (glucuronyl-transferase) (25, 32), and acatalasaemia (1, 64); see Table II. In none of the cases enumerated above has it been definitely established whether the deficiencies are due to total failure to synthesize the molecule (*eniotypy*) reduction in the quantity of the molecules synthesized (*plethotypy**), or loss of function resulting from amino-acid substitution of the functionally crucial portion of the molecule (*allotypy*). Rigid criteria for discrimination between these different variations are needed and we shall attempt to illustrate the application of such criteria to the identification of *eniotypy*. This type of polymorphism will have a profound effect on the tolerance exclusion of determinants from immunogenicity and is, therefore, of considerable interest in connection with the "steering mechanism," referred to in the introductory paragraphs. We shall present an instance in which it is clearly established that some individuals of a species do, and other individuals do not, synthesize a certain type of molecule. The example to be documented is the eniotypic variation of a mouse antigen which we have called MuB1 (12) and which we believe may be identical with the C′5 component of the complement system. (It is perhaps unnecessary to point out that all experimental demonstrations of the absence of a substance are limited by the sensitivity of the detection techniques available. With MuB1, the deficient animal is either totally deficient or contains an amount that has so far eluded detection and is below the threshold at which tolerance is induced (see p. 210).)

3. MuB1 AS AN ANTIGEN

MuB1 was discovered in the course of systematic investigations of the allotypy of mouse-serum proteins (12, 13, 15, 19). These investigations have involved taking the serum of some inbred mice, emulsifying it with Freund's complete adjuvant, and injecting it into other strains of inbred mice. At a later date, an Ouchterlony diffusion test in agar was set up to see whether the serum of the recipient contained antibodies directed against any factors in the donor serum. MuB1 was first detected (and shown to be distinct from other allotypic factors) in the donors of sera used for immunization and was subsequently detected in the serum of a considerable proportion of the inbred strains tested.

*Plethotypy is a type difference characterized by quantity, derived from πλῆθος (quantity).

4. MuB1 AS AN INSTANCE OF ENIOTYPIC POLYMORPHISM

(a) CRITERION BASED ON THE USE OF A HETEROLOGOUS ANTIBODY

The antigen, MuB1, is normally detected by its reaction with an isologous antibody (i.e. an antibody raised in an MuB1-negative mouse). This antibody reacts with a single antigen in the serum of 60 per cent of inbred strains of mice and fails to react with the serum of the remaining 40 per cent. The question arose whether MuB1-negative animals contained an antigen that was under the controle of a gene, allelic to the gene controlling synthesis of MuB1 in the MuB1-positive animals, or whether MuB1-negative mice lacked a product genetically and structurally related to MuB1. In other words, was the difference between MuB1-negative and -positive mice *allotypic* or *eniotypic*?

To approach this problem we elicited antibody to MuB1 in animals belonging to another species, and indeed, to another order than the mouse, i.e., the rabbit, and examined the reaction of this heterologous antibody with the serum of MuB1-negative mice. We found no evidence of interaction between this antibody to MuB1 and the serum of MuB1-negative animals. This constitutes strong evidence that MuB1-negative animals do not contain the molecule having structural similarities to MuB1, as can be seen from the following argument.

Antibody to MuB1 raised in a species other than the mouse would be expected to be directed not only against those determinants in which MuB1 differs from a hypothetical antigen in an MuB1-negative animal, but also against those structural portions of the molecules which are shared between MuB1 and the hypothetical molecule in MuB1-negative animals. The absence of any reactivity between the rabbit antibody to MuB1 and the serum of MuB1-negative animals would, therefore, exclude the presence of the hypothetical antigen in MuB1-negative animals, unless it were assumed that determinants shared between MuB1 and the hypothetical antigen were exactly the same as the autologous determinants of the rabbit, so that they would all be excluded from immunogenicity.

(b) CRITERION BASED ON THE RELATIVE SPECIFICITY OF ISOLOGOUS AND HETEROLOGOUS ANTIBODY

The most striking difference between *eniotypy* and *allotypy* would be in the specificity of the antibody raised in animals lacking allotypic or eniotypic determinants respectively. The animal in which the allotypic determinant is missing would not be tolerant to this particular determinant but would be tolerant to all the other determinants of the molecule. Thus, it would synthesize antibody only to the particular determinants which, in an allotypic variation, constitute the variable region of the molecule. The situation would be markedly different in an animal totally deficient in an antigen. Such an animal would not be tolerant to any part of the molecule, and would, therefore, be able to make antibody to all the determinants of that molecule.

In order to examine this criterion further, we shall discuss specificity differences, in terms of the structure of autologous macromolecules and immunogens. Attention will first be given to the phenomenon of "faulty perspective" (38) and subsequently to the specificity of antibody to an antigen formed in an animal that has no appreciable tolerance to any determinant of the antigen.

(i) *"Faulty Perspective"*

If antibody is raised in a species closely related to that of the donor, the resulting antibody discriminates between the antigens of the donor and the antigens of animals closely related to the donor, but shows relatively little or no reactivity with antigens of animals distantly related to the donor. On the other hand, antibody raised in animals distantly related to the donor of antigen does not discriminate between donor antigens and the antigens of animals closely related to the donor, but shows cross-reactivity not only with the antigens from animals closely related to the donor, but also with antigens from animals distantly related to the donor. This difference in specificity, depending on the relation between the donor of antigen and the donor of antibody, was recognized by Landsteiner (38), who called the phenomenon "faulty perspective." We can interpret this phenomenon in terms of the "steering mechanism" (10, 11, 14).

The proteins of the members of one species differ from the proteins of the members of another species by many amino-acid changes in configuration; proteins of different individuals of any one species differ from one another by considerably fewer amino-acid substitutions. This means, for example, that, although the proteins of different mice differ from one another in varying degrees, they all differ greatly from those of chickens. However, the proteins of mice, in general, differ from those of chickens more than they differ from animals of a species more closely related to mice (that is of the same mammalian order); for example, they resemble the proteins of rats more closely than those of chickens. Therefore, in considering the possibilities of producing antiserum, we have at least three possibilities to consider. In the case of a mouse, these could be as follows:

(*a*) A member of the same species whose proteins differ in only some respects from those of the donor of the antigen (another mouse).

(*b*) A member of a closely related species (a rat).

(*c*) A member of a distantly related species (a rabbit).

Figure 1 illustrates some of the factors involved in making antibody against one individual in another member of the same species, which differs from the donor in allotype. We shall consider this situation in mice.

The antigen molecule illustrated on the left represents that of one kind of

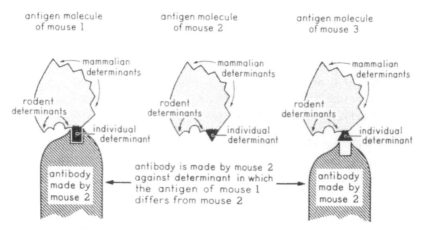

antigen molecule of mouse 1

antigen molecule of mouse 2

antigen molecule of mouse 3

mammalian determinants

mammalian determinants

mammalian determinants

rodent determinants

rodent determinants

rodent determinants

individual determinant

individual determinant

individual determinant

antibody made by mouse 2

antibody is made by mouse 2 against determinant in which the antigen of mouse 1 differs from mouse 2

antibody made by mouse 2

FIG. 1. Antibody formation when donor of antigen and donor of antibody show allotypic differences.

inbred mouse (mouse 1). It is injected into a second type of inbred mouse (mouse 2), whose corresponding antigen molecule is shown in the middle. It is seen that *all but one* of the determinants are identical in both mice; hence both mice are tolerant to these particular determinants, which consequently do not elicit antibody formation. Mouse 2, therefore, makes antibody only against the one determinant (shown in black) in which the antigen of mouse 1 and that of mouse 2 differ from one another. When this antibody is mixed with the corresponding antigen of mouse 3 (shown on the right), it does not react with the one determinant that is different in mouse 3 because this determinant is different from the determinant in mouse 1 to which antibody was made. The antibody that is made in mouse 2 is, therefore, extremely specific for one individual strain of inbred mice (mouse 1) and not for other members of the species.

We shall next consider the situation that obtains when a member of a distantly related species is used for making antibody (Fig. 2).

The antigen of the donor rodent (mouse 1) is shown on the left, while the corresponding antigen molecule of the rabbit into which the antigen of the mouse 1 is injected is shown in the middle. The antigens of the rabbit show extensive differences from those of the rodent and hence the rabbit is tolerant to only a few determinants (called "mammalian determinants" on Fig. 2). Consequently it synthesizes antibody against many of the determinants of the rodent antigen. When this antiserum is mixed with the antigens of a second mouse (shown on the right), the antibody reacts strongly with all of these determinants except the one shown in black. In this situation, virtually all of the antibody made against one type of rodent can react with another type of rodent.

Thus, "faulty immunological perspective" depends on the structural relation-

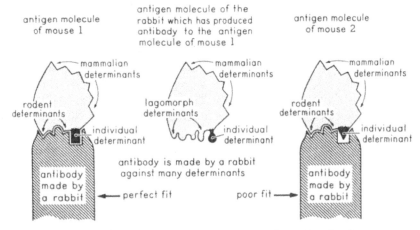

FIG. 2. Antibody formation when a member of a distantly related species is used for making antibody.

ship between the autologous macromolecules of the donor of antibody and the donor of antigen. If the donor of the antigen and the donor of the antibody have very similar determinants, antibody is made only to the few determinants that differ and that are to be found only in animals closely related to the donor of antigen. As a consequence, the antibody discriminates between the antigen donor and its closest relative, but shows little cross-reactivity with antigens of distantly related species. If, however, the macromolecules of the donor of antigen and the donor of antibody are very different from one another, antibody is made to very many determinants and this multispecific antibody will react to a very similar extent with the antigens of the donor and with those of animals closely related to the donor, but will also cross-react with antigens of distantly related species.

(ii) *Inversion of "Faulty Perspective"*

We have indicated in the foregoing that an antibody to an isologous protein, raised in the same species of animal as that of the donor of the antigen, normally shows a very narrow specificity, and reacts, as a rule, only with individuals of the same species as the donor of the antibody and antigen. The antibody to MuB1 did not show the narrow specificity that one normally finds in isologous situations, but, on the contrary, showed a very wide cross-reaction with an antigen present in the serum of many other mammals. An antigen, reacting with the murine antibody to MuB1, was found in the serum of species belonging to 13 of the 15 orders of mammals tested, and among 63 of the total of 85 mammalian species whose serum was examined. The antibody reacted equally with the sera of normal rabbits and also with the sera of rabbits deficient in complement. It reacted with the serum of all humans tested, including the serum of 30 Eskimos and 20 Amerindians from the Queen Charlotte Indian Reserve. There were a few species, such as minks, in which the serum of some individuals gave a reaction with the antibody, while that of other individuals did not. There were also a few mammalian species, such as moose and deer, which lacked an antigen that reacted with the mouse antibody, but, in general, the majority of mammals possessed the antigen that reacted with the antibody to the mouse antigen. Thus, the antibody to MuB1 reacted with the corresponding antigen in other mammals, in a very different way to that observed with allotypic antibodies (15).

The wide range of cross-reactions observed with the mouse antibody to MuB1 was in marked contrast to the activity of the antibody to MuB1 obtained in the rabbit, an animal belonging to an order (Lagomorpha) other than the Rodentia. The quantity of the antibody so obtained was 40 per cent of that elicited in mice in strain AH/J and 200 per cent of that elicited in mice of strain DBA/2J. It showed less reactivity with the serum of rodents than either of the murine antibodies and none with sera of mammals belonging to other orders. Cross-reactions occurred with rat and hamster sera only. Thus, antibody to the mouse protein, MuB1, raised in an animal of an order (Lagomorpha) other than that of the mouse, showed a narrower specificity range than antibody raised in the mouse (order, Rodentia). The unusually wide cross-reactivity of the antibody to MuB1 obtained from MuB1-negative animals is best explained by the absence of tolerance to any of the determinants of MuB1 in the MuB1-negative mouse and, hence, to the total absence of a molecule corresponding to MuB1 in such animals.

It is convenient, in this context, to consider the determinants of a protein in terms of their evolutionary stability. Accordingly, one might postulate mammalian determinants, which remain unchanged throughout all the orders of Mammalia, order determinants (say Rodentia determinants), which remain unchanged during the evolution of the order, and finally species determinants, which remain unchanged during the evolution of the species. Where two individuals of the same species differ in an allotypic determinant only, both individuals would possess general mammalian determinants in their circulation, as well as order and species determinants. When an animal is tolerant to the determinants of an autologous protein, all the determinants of this protein are excluded from immunogenicity in it. Thus, one would expect that antibody against a serum protein, raised in an animal of the same species as that of the donor of the serum protein, would be highly specific in the sense that it would be directed only to the particular determinant by which individuals of this species differ from each other. Such an antibody would not react with the serum of animals of a different species. The reactivity of antibody to MuB1 is, therefore, of considerable interest in that it does not conform to this general rule. This isologous antibody reacts not only with the serum of other rodents but also with the serum of many distantly related mammalian species.

The above exception to the general rule of narrow specificity, when the donor of the antigen is closely related to the donor of the antibody, constitutes important evidence that animals which do not possess the molecule, MuB1, completely lack all of its determinants.

(*c*) DIFFERENTIATION BETWEEN VARIOUS TYPES OF POLYMORPHISM

Thus there are several independent lines of evidence which lead us to the conclusion that some mice possess an antigen MuB1 and that other mice lack this antigen and any molecule structurally related to it.

In the foregoing, criteria have been developed which should be of general use in the identification of eniotypy. Wide cross-reactivity of antibodies, obtained when donors of antigen and antibody are of the same species, would be one of the most useful of these criteria. This approach might contribute to the analysis of many inborn metabolic errors, such as haemophilia, in which repeated transfusions have resulted in "resistance" to restoration of clotting ability by haemophilic globulins, or hypopituitary dwarfism, where antibody formation to human growth hormone occurs as a consequence of treatment with human growth hormone (52). In these situations, additional evidence distinguishing *eniotypy* from *allotypy* must be obtained; this can be furnished by quantitative studies with serum, raised in a species other than that of the donor of antigen (see (*b*), p. 207). If the activity of such an antiserum cannot be reduced, at least in part, by absorption with serum or tissue from an individual allegedly completely deficient in this factor, then it may be concluded that the deficiency is total. The sensitivity of this test can be increased by employing a concentrated fraction for the absorption. Such a preparation may be obtained by a method that is known to yield a concentrate of the factor, if applied to the serum of a normal animal.

The application of this second criterion is of decisive importance in the analysis of the polymorphism of molecules, such as hormones, which are normally present in extremely low concentrations. When this is the case, it must be envisaged that the immune apparatus *might* not have been appreciably affected by the molecules, so that the animal is neither immune nor tolerant to the autologous macromolecule. Any substantial fluctuation in the concentration of such a substance, whether through pathological processes or as a consequence of passive administration, may elicit antibody formation without hindrance by a tolerance barrier. The specificity of the resulting auto-antibody would have the same broad cross-reactivity as observed with eniotypic antibody. However, this would not be due to the absence of a molecule, but to its low level of concentration and consequent failure to induce tolerance. In these circumstances, discrimination between *eniotypy* and *allotypy* could not be achieved by the specificity of the isologous antibody and must thus depend on the second above-mentioned criterion, based on the absorption of heterologous antibody. These considerations are also relevant in considering the immune response in a situation where the same molecule is produced by all animals, but where individuals differ from one another in the synthesized *quantity* of the antigen (*plethotypy*). In some extreme cases of this type, the deficient animals may produce a quantity of antigen which is below the threshold that induces tolerance and thus may respond to passive administration of the antigen with production of an antibody of wide cross-reactivity. The test, based on absorption of heterologous serum with concentrates, might allow discrimination between variations of this type and *eniotypy*. It is clear, however, that, for extremely low production, the differentiation from *eniotypy* is impossible and the classification becomes meaningless.

It is clear, from the foregoing, that the two criteria, based on isologous and heterologous antibodies ((*a*) and (*b*), p. 207), make it possible to determine whether or not tolerance to an autologous macromolecule has been induced. In the absence of autologous tolerance, one might find broad reactivity of isologous antibody as well as removal of a fraction of heterologous antibody by absorption with the concentrated factor obtained from an animal allegedly deficient but, in fact, containing an allotypic antigen.

5. MuB1 AS A COMPONENT OF THE COMPLEMENT SYSTEM

Having established that MuB1 is an antigen, present in some mice, and that there is no detectable product of a gene allelic to MuB1 in other inbred strains of mice, we turned next to a search for the functions of this antigen. Our attention was directed to the relation between MuB1 and complement, since Rosenberg and Tachibana (53) and Herzenberg, Tachibana, Herzenberg, and Rosenberg (28) had demonstrated that some mice have an incomplete complement system, while others have a complete complement system.

We first surveyed the distribution of both MuB1 and the complete haemolytic complement system in some 24 inbred strains of mice and found that, wherever MuB1 could be detected in the serum of animals, a complete haemolytic complement system could be demonstrated. This indicated a link between MuB1 and the complement system. To test this further, we examined the offspring from back-crosses between MuB1-negative animals and hybrids resulting from matings between MuB1-negative and MuB1-positive mice. The animals so obtained were tested for the presence of MuB1 and of a competent haemolytic complement system. Fifty per cent of the offspring were MuB1 positive, and also contained a complete haemolytic complement system (Table III). It may be concluded from these observations that MuB1 is determined by a single gene and inherited in a dominant way; the same conclusion can be drawn from the distribution of haemolytic complement. Furthermore, it is evident from the experimental data that the genes controlling the synthesis of MuB1 and of complete haemolytic complement are closely linked. In fact, the evidence is compatible with the view that the synthesis of MuB1 and of a complement factor is controlled by the same gene.

TABLE III

CORRELATION BETWEEN THE PRESENCE OF MuB1 AND OF HAEMO-
LYTIC COMPLEMENT
(Tests were done on offspring from double backcrosses:
A/J × (C57L/J × A/J) and A/J × (C57BL/6J × A/J))

| | Haemolytic complement | | |
	Present	Absent	Total
MuB1 present	75 (38.7)	0 (36.3)	75
MuB1 absent	7 (43.3)	77 (40.7)	84
TOTAL	82	77	159

The figures in brackets give the expected numbers calculated on the assumption that there is no correlation between MuB1 and haemolytic complement. The probability for this assumption is $P < 0.005$ ($\chi^2 = 133.16$).

Yet another set of data supported the view that a connection existed between MuB1 and the complement system. If in any one strain the antigen concentration in MuB1-positive male and female individuals was followed as a function of age and sex, it was found that the antigen concentration increased with age and that it was always higher in the male than in the female (Fig. 3). Similarly, the number of haemolytic complement units in the serum of male and female individuals of the same strain was different and was always greater in the male than in the female. This observation was very suggestive, though not conclusive, since the ratio of antigen concentration in the serum of male and female mice of strain BALB/cJ was approximately 1.4, and that of the haemolytic units was close to 5.

We could examine some of the properties of MuB1 in terms of its reaction with antibody. Since the mouse antibody to this antigen reacted with a molecule analogous to MuB1 in a number of species other than the mouse, we could examine the properties of the antigen present in the serum of mammals other than the mouse, and in particular in the guinea pig and in man, about whose complement components much more is known than about those of the mouse. These tests showed that MuB1 and its other mammalian analogues were all insoluble in distilled water, that the antigen was fairly heat labile, that it was not destroyed by ammonia or hydrazine, that it had a molecular weight (as shown by gel filtration) similar to that of gamma globulin, and that its electrophoretic mobility was within the range of the slow alpha and fast beta globulins. On the basis of these properties it appeared to us that MuB1, if it was identical with a component of complement, was probably identical with one of the components that interacted subsequent to the reaction of the classical C'3 component. The work of Linscott and Nishioka (41) with partially

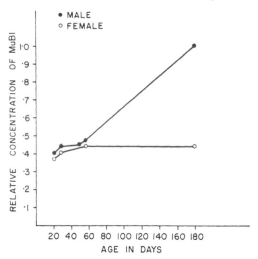

F<small>IG</small>. 3. Change in concentration of antigen MuB1 as a function of age. Mice of strain DBA/1J; concentration of MuB1 measured by single diffusion and expressed as a fraction of the concentration of MuB1 in the serum of 6-month-old male mice of strain DBA/1J.

purified components of the complement system of the guinea pig, suggested that MuB1 might be identical with C'3d (15).

The most convincing evidence of the identity of MuB1 with a constituent of the haemolytic complement system, and the identification of a complement component with MuB1, was due to Nilsson and Müller-Eberhard (46). While the work described in the preceding paragraphs was in progress, these workers identified a component in the human complement system which followed the action of a C'3 and which they designated as C'5 (Table IV). They succeeded in isolating this component from the serum of humans and raised a rabbit antibody to it. This antibody reacted with only one component in the purified preparation. When this antibody and the antibody to MuB1 were allowed to react with the human C'5 component, the two antibodies gave a reaction of partial identity, thus providing very good evidence that the human component, corresponding to MuB1, was the C'5 component of the haemolytic complement system (46).

The discovery of MuB1 and of its identity with the C'5 component of complement has opened the way for exploration of the role of complement *in vivo*.

6. THE COMPLEMENT-DEFICIENT MOUSE AS A RESEARCH TOOL

Some inbred mice possess all the constituents of the complex chain of interacting molecules which constitute the haemolytic complement system

TABLE IV

SEQUENCE AND MECHANISM OF IMMUNE HAEMOLYSIS

E = sheep erythrocyte   E* = injured erythrocyte

A = rabbit antibody directed against sheep erythrocyte

C'1, C'4, etc. designate serum proteins interacting in a sequence of reactions resulting in immune haemolysis. C'1a, C'2a, etc. refer to enzymatically active forms of the corresponding component, either known or postulated

C'1 = macromolecular complex, containing subunits designated C'1q (11S factor), C'1r, and C'1s (C'1 proesterase). The intact complex of all these molecules functions as C'1

Immuno-electrophoretic designation of some components of complement:

C'3 = β_{1C} globulin (converted in free solution to β_{1G} globulin under the influence of the C'4-2a complex)

C'4 = β_{1E} globulin

C'5 = β_{1F} globulin

Reaction	Biochemical event
$E + A \rightleftharpoons EA$ (Ca^{++})	
$EA + C'1 \longrightarrow EAC'1a$	Attachment of C'1 at a site on C'1q to a receptor on A; activation of a catalytic centre at a site on C'1s
$EAC'1a + C'4 \longrightarrow EAC'1a, 4$	Enzymatic attack of C'1a on C'4, creating a site on C'4 which attaches to a receptor on E
$EAC'1a, 4 + C'2 \xrightarrow{Mg^{++}} EAC'1a, 4, 2a$ ↑ ↑ Thermal decay	Attachment of C'2 to a receptor on C'4; enzymatic attack of C'1a on C'2, creating a catalytic centre on C'2; fulfilment of functions of C'1a
$EAC'1a, 4, 2a + C'3 \longrightarrow EAC'1a, 4, 2a, 3a$	Activation of C'3 and attachment to a receptor on E
$EAC'1a, 4, 2a, 3a + C'5 + C'6 + C'7 \longrightarrow EAC'1a, 4, 2a, 3a, 5, 6, 7a$	Formation of a stable intermediate no longer susceptible to thermal decay; activation of C'5-C'6-C'7
$EAC'1a, 4, 2a, 5, 6, 7a + C'8 + C'9 \longrightarrow E^*$	Unknown events leading to 80–100 Å holes in the erythrocyte membrane
$E^* \longrightarrow$ ghost + haemoglobin	Lysis of erythrocyte and release of haemoglobin

(Table IV). Other inbred mice lack one type of molecule, so that only the first four of the seven recognized reactions of the haemolytic complement system can occur. The relative reactivity of these two types of animals can be used to investigate the considerable range of complex *in vivo* reactions (i.e. tumour rejection, hypersensitivity, etc.) in which the complement system seems to be involved, in the hope of finding out whether the complete haemolytic complement system is involved.

It is quite possible that only the initial portion of the long chain of reactions resulting in immune haemolysis is of importance in some complement-mediated reactions. This may be the case in antibody-promoted phagocytosis. Support for this view emerges from the work of Stiffel *et al.* (63), who studied phagocytosis of bacteria and the opsonizing effect of antibody in different strains of mice. There were no differences between the phagocytic capacity of mice possessing the complete haemolytic complement system and that of complement-deficient animals. On the other hand, both types of mice showed a considerable reduction in the opsonizing effect of specific antibodies after experimental decomplementation *in vivo*. Furthermore, the rates of phagocytosis *in vivo* were similar in both groups of animals, before as well as after the experimental decomplementation. Thus, it seems that phagocytosis *in vivo* does not involve any of the circulating components of complement, whereas opsonization clearly does not involve the component missing from the sera of MuB1-negative mice.

As far as opsonization and phagocytosis are concerned, both MuB1-positive and MuB1-negative mice seem to have equal ability to resist bacterial invasion. It may, nevertheless, be expected that some differences between these two groups of animals, connected directly or indirectly with the haemolytic complement activity, will soon be encountered.

In at least one respect, a difference in reactivity of MuB1-positive and MuB1-negative animals has already been demonstrated. In a study of cutaneous response to antigen–antibody interaction, as judged by permeability increase, Ben-Efraim and Cinader (5) found that, with certain antisera, two phases of the cutaneous reaction were discernible in MuB1-positive animals and only one of these in MuB1-negative animals. It is quite clear that the reaction occurring in both MuB1-positive and MuB1-negative animals cannot involve the complete haemolytic complement system. The question arises whether this reaction involves the first stages of the chain of complement reactions which would proceed quite normally up to the point at which the deficient complement factor becomes involved, or whether a system completely independent of complement exists.

The problem of resistance to infection is even more complex than the cutaneous reaction. It involves many mechanisms, some of them complement-dependent, such as bacteriolysis, some not involving complement, such as neutralization of bacterial toxins, and others in which neither antibody nor complement takes part The analysis of this complex phenomenon may be aided by continued studies of the different reactivity of MuB1-positive and MuB1-negative animals in simplified systems concerned with each of these many processes.

ACKNOWLEDGMENTS

The authors are indebted to Dr. I. H. Lepow of Western Reserve University, Cleveland, Ohio, and to Dr. H. J. Müller-Eberhard of Scripps Clinic and Research Foundation, La Jolla, California, for valuable discussion. We are grateful to Dr. I. H. Lepow for summarizing the information in Table IV, to Dr. H. Parry of York University for suggesting the term "eniotypy," and to Dr. L. Woodbury of the University of Toronto for suggesting the term "plethotypy." We also wish to thank our colleagues who have generously provided inbred mice and sera of mammalian species, to whom we have acknowledged our indebtedness in detail elsewhere (15). Furthermore, we wish to thank Dr. I. Broder and Dr. L. Siminovitch for useful criticism of the manuscript.

The work was supported by grants from the Banting Research Foundation, the Canadian Arthritis and Rheumatism Society (Grant No. 7-7064), the Medical Research Council (Grants No. MT-835, MA-1580, ME-1543), the National Cancer Institute of Canada, and the (United States) National Institutes of Health (Grant No. 5T1 GM-506-03).

REFERENCES

1. AEBI, H., HEINIGER, J. P., BUTLER, R., and HÄSSIG, A. Two cases of acatalasia in Switzerland. Experientia, *17*: 466 (1961).
2. ALLEN, J. C., KUNKEL, H. G., and KABAT, E. A. Studies on human antibodies. II. Distribution of genetic factors. J. Exper. Med. *119*: 453 (1964).
3. BAUR, E. W. Catalase abnormality in a Caucasian family in the United States. Science, 140: 816 (1963).
4. BECKMAN, L. Associations between human serum alkaline phosphatases and blood groups. Acta genet. *14*: 286 (1964).
5. BEN-EFRAIM, S., and CINADER, B. The role of complement in the passive cutaneous reaction of mice. J. Exper. Med. *120*: 925 (1964).
6. BERG, K. A new serum type system in man—The Lp system. Acta path. et microbiol. scandinav. *59*: 369 (1963).
7. BERG, K., and EGEBERG, O. Individual antigenic differences of a human serum lipoprotein revealed by a "cold-precipitin" in the serum of a transfused patient. Nature, *206*: 312 (1965).
8. BIGGS, R., and MACFARLANE, R. G. Human Blood Coagulation and Its Disorders, 3rd ed. (Blackwell Scientific Publications, Oxford, 1962).
9. BLUMBERG, B. S., DRAY, S., and ROBINSON, J. C. Antigen polymorphism of a low density beta lipoprotein allotypy in human serum. Nature, *194*: 656 (1962).
10. CINADER, B. Dependence of antibody responses on structure and polymorphism of autologous macromolecules. Brit. M. Bull. *19*: 219 (1963).
11. ——— Specificity and inheritance of antibody response: A possible steering mechanism. Nature, *188*: 619 (1960).
12. CINADER, B., and DUBISKI, S. An alpha globulin allotype in the mouse. Nature, *200*: 781 (1963).
13. ——— Effect of autologous protein on the specificity of the antibody response: Mouse and rabbit antibody to MuB1. Nature, *202*: 102 (1964).
14. ——— The effect of immunogencity of acquired immunological tolerance. *In* Colloque sur la tolérance acquise et la tolérance naturelle a l'égard de substances antigéniques définies. Colloq. int. Cent. Nat. Rech. Sci. *116*: 225 (1963).
15. CINADER, B., DUBISKI, S., and WARDLAW, A. C. Distribution, inheritance, and properties of an antigen, MuB1, and its relation to hemolytic complement. J. Exper. Med. *120*: 897 (1964).
16. CLEVE, H., and BEARN, A. G. The group specific component of serum; genetic and chemical considerations. *In* Progress in Medical Genetics, *edited by* A. G. Steinberg and A. G. Bearn (Grune and Stratton, New York and London, 1962), vol. 2, p. 64.
17. COHEN, B. L., and SCHREFFLER, D. C. A revised nomenclature for the mouse transferrin locus. Genet. Res. *2*: 306 (1961).
18. DRAY, S., DUBISKI, S., KELUS, A., LENNOX, E. S., and OUDIN, J. A notation for allotypy. Nature, *195*: 785 (1962).

19. DUBISKI, S., and CINADER, B.   A new allotypic specificity in the mouse (MuA2). Nature, *197*: 705 (1962).
20. EARLE, P. D., HUTT, M. P., SCHMID, K., and GITLIN, D.   Observations on double albumin—A genetically transmitted serum protein anomaly. J. Clin. Invest. *38*: 1412 (1959).
21. FEINSTEIN, R. N., SEAHOLM, J. E., HOWARD, J. F., and RUSSEL, W. L.   Acatalasemic mice. Proc. Nat. Acad. Sci. U.S. *52*: 661 (1964).
22. GELL, P. G. H., and KELUS, A.   Deletions of allotypic gamma-globulins in antibodies. Nature, *195*: 44 (1962).
23. GIBLETT, E. R.   The plasma transferrins. *In* Progress in Medical Genetics, *edited by* A. G. Steinberg and A. G. Bearn (Grune and Stratton, New York and London, 1959), vol. 2, p. 34.
24. GOEDDE, H. W. and BAITSCH, H.   On nomenclature of pseudocholinesterase polymorphism. Acta genet. *14*: 366 (1964).
25. HARRIS, H.   Human Biochemical Genetics (Cambridge University Press, London, 1963).
26. HERZENBERG, L. A.   A chromosome region for gamma$_2$ and beta$_{2A}$ globulin H chains isoantigens in the mouse. Cold Spring Harbor Symp. Quant. Biol. *29*: 455 (1964).
27. ——— Personal communication (1965).
28. HERZENBERG, L. A., TACHIBANA, D. K., HERZENBERG, L. A., and ROSENBERG, L. T.   A gene locus concerned with hemolytic complement in Mus musculus. Genetics, *48*: 711 (1963).
29. HERZENBERG, L. A., WARNER, N. L., and HERZENBERG, L. A.   Immunoglobulin isoantigens (allotypes) in the mouse. I. Genetics and cross-reactions of the 7S γ_{2A}-isoantigens controlled by alleles at the Ig-1 locus. J. Exper. Med. *121*: 415 (1965).
30. HIRSCHFELD, J., and BLOMBÄCK, M.   A new anti-Ag serum (L.L.). Nature, *201*: 1337 (1964).
31. HOPKINSON, D. A., SPENCER, N., and HARRIS, H.   Red cell acid phosphatase variants: A new human polymorphism. Nature, *199*: 969 (1963).
32. HSIA, D. Y.   Inborn Errors of Metabolism (Year Book Publishers, Chicago, 1959).
33. KELUS, A. S., and GELL, P. G. H.   An allotypic determinant specific to rabbit macroglobulin. Nature, *206*: 313 (1965).
34. KELUS, A., and MOOR-JANKOWSKI, J. K.   An iso-antigen (γB^A) of mouse γ-globulin present in inbred strains. Nature, *188*: 673 (1960).
35. KIRKMAN, H. N., McCURDY, P. R., and NAIMAN, J. L.   Functionally abnormal glucose-6-phosphate dehydrogenase. Cold Spring Harbor Symp. Quant. Biol. *29*: 391 (1964).
36. KNEDEL, M.   Über eine neue vererbte Proteinanomalie. Clin. Chim. Acta, *3*: 72 (1958).
37. KUNKEL, H. G., MANNIK, M., and WILLIAMS, R. C.   Individual antigenic specificity of isolated antibodies. Science, *140*: 1218 (1964).
38. LANDSTEINER, K.   The Specificity of Immunological Reactions, rev. ed. (Dover Publ., New York, 1962).
39. LIEBERMAN, R., and DRAY, S.   Five allelic genes at the Asa locus which control γ-globulin allotypic specificities in mice. J. Immunol. *93*: 584 (1964).
40. LEHMANN, H., and LIDDELL, J.   Genetical variations of human serum pseudocholinesterase. *In* Progress in Medical Genetics, *edited by* A. G. Steinberg and A. G. Bearn (Grune and Stratton, New York and London, 1964), vol. 3, pp. 75–105.
41. LINSCOTT, W. D., and NISHIOKA, K.   Components of guinea pig complement. II. Separation of serum fractions essential for immune hemolysis. J. Exper. Med. *118*: 795 (1963).
42. MARTENSSON, L.   On the relationship between the gamma-globulin genes of the Gm system. J. Exper. Med. *120*: 1169 (1964).
43. MORTON, N. E.   Genetic studies of Northeastern Brazil. Cold Spring Harbor Symp. Quant. Biol. *29*: 69 (1964).
44. NANCE, W. E., and SMITHIES, O.   New haptoglobin alleles: A prediction confirmed. Nature, *198*: 869 (1963).
45. NEIDERS, M. E., ROWLEY, D. A., and FITCH, F. W.   The sustained suppression of hemolysin response in passively immunized rats. J. Immunol. *88*: 718 (1962).

46. NILSSON, V., and MÜLLER-EBERHARD, H. J. Immunologic reaction between human β 1F-globulin and mouse MuB1 (HC). Fed. Proc. *24*, pt. I: 620 (1965).
47. OUDIN, J. L' "allotypie" de certains antigènes protéidiques du sérum. Compt. rend. Acad. sci. *242*: 2606 (1956).
48. PAIGEN, K., and NOEL, W. K. Two linked genes showing a similar timing of expression in mice. Nature, *190*: 148 (1961).
49. PELZER, C. F. Erythrocytic esterase in Mus musculus. Mouse News Letter, *31*: 33 (1964).
50. PETRAS, M. Genetic control of a serum esterase component in Mus musculus. Proc. Nat. Acad. Sci. U.S. *50*: 112 (1963).
51. POPP, R. A. Inheritance of different serum esterase patterns among inbred strains of mice. Genetics, *46*: 89 (1961).
52. PRADER, A., SZÉKY, J., WAGNER, H., ILLIG, R., TOUBER, J. L., and MAINGAY, D. Acquired resistance to human growth hormone caused by specific antibodies. Lancet, *2*: 378 (1964).
53. ROSENBERG, L. T., and TACHIBANA, D. K. Activity of mouse complement, J. Immunol. *89*: 861 (1962).
54. ROWLEY, D. A., and FITCH, F. W. Homeostatis of antibody formation in the adult rat. J. Exper. Med. *120*: 987 (1964).
55. RUDDLE, F. H., and RODERICK, T. H. The genetic control of three kidney esterases in C57BL/6J and RF/J mice, Genetics, *51*: 445 (1965).
56. RUSSEL, R. L., and COLEMAN, D. L. Genetic control of hepatic δ-aminolevulinate dehydratase in mice. Genetics, *48*: 1033 (1963).
57. SHAW, C. R., SYNER, F. N., and TASHIAN, R. E. New genetically determined molecular form of erythrocyte esterase in man. Science, *138*: 31 (1962).
58. SMITHIES, O., CONNELL, G. E., and DIXON, G. H. Chromosomal rearrangement and the evolution of haptoglobin genes. Nature, *196*: 232 (1962).
59. SPENCER, N., HOPKINSON, D. A., and HARRIS, H. Phosphoglucomutase polymorphism in man. Nature, *204*: 742 (1964).
60. STEFANINI, M., and DAMESHEK, W. Hemorrhagic Disorders, 2nd ed. (Grune and Stratton, Inc., New York, 1962).
61. STEINBERG, A. G. Progress in the study of genetically determined human gamma globulin types (the Gm and InV groups). *In* Progress in Medical Genetics, *edited by* A. G. Steinberg and A. G. Bearn (Grune and Stratton, New York and London, 1962), vol. 2, p. 1.
62. STEINBERG, A. G. Personal communication (1965).
63. STIFFEL, C., BIOZZI, G., MOUTON, D., BOUTHILLIER, Y., and DECRESEFOND, C. Studies on phagocytosis of bacteria by the reticulo-endothelial system in a strain of mice lacking hemolytic complement. J. Immunol. *93*: 246 (1964).
64. TAKAHARA, S. Progressive oral gangrene probably due to lack of catalase in the blood (acatalasaemia), Lancet, *2*: 1101 (1952).
65. UHR, J. W., and BAUMAN, J. B. Antibody formation. I. The suppression of antibody formation by passively administered antibody. J. Exper. Med. *113*: 935 (1961).

PART VI

Connective Tissue Biochemistry

Chairman: Professor C. S. Hanes, Toronto

Brief Survey of the
Biochemistry of Connective Tissues*

CHARLES S. HANES

THE PURPOSE of this brief introduction is to provide some setting for the different communications which are to follow, and also to supplement them by referring to some outstanding biochemical features of one major constituent of connective tissues, namely collagen, which is the best characterized of all, but which has not found a place in the communications.

It is almost a truism to say that in the case of large organisms, both plant and animal, the gross features of the parts of the body and the physical properties of these (i.e. strength, texture, firmness, flexibility, etc.) depend not upon substances present inside the living cells, but upon anatomical structures laid down outside the protoplasts in characteristic fashion in the extra- or inter-cellular spaces. Thus the form and physical properties of a tree and its organs, as well as the internal demarcation of its specialized tissues, reflect the localized deposition of cell-wall material, composed largely of polysaccharides but with other encrusting and cementing materials of macromolecular nature. This is somewhat analogous to the dependence of the animal body for its physical properties and the mechanical support of its complicated and jointed structures upon the localized deposition by the mesenchymal cells of a remarkable range of macromolecular substances which occupy the intercellular spaces of the connective tissues of the animal body.

The past decade has seen considerable clarification of the chemical nature of these substances, which are synthesized within but secreted from the connective tissue cells into the intercellular spaces, thus forming the specialized realms or habitats which connective tissue cells create for themselves and in which they live and die. These peculiar systems comprising living cells plus non-living matrices have been selected presumably in the course of evolution for their suitability for the various supportive functions of the complex body; they present a great profusion of types ranging from limpid fluids to fibrous structures embedded in matrices which vary in consistency from soft gels to mineralized deposits of geological hardness. The intercellular spaces contain

*From the Department of Biochemistry, University of Toronto, Toronto.

an interesting range of macromolecules of which the chemical nature is becoming rapidly elucidated. Apart from the connective tissue cells (fibroblasts, macrophages, chondrocytes, fat cells, osteocytes, etc.), the major constituents of connective tissues present in the intercellular spaces are the fibrous structures and the ground substances.

THE FIBROUS STRUCTURES OF CONNECTIVE TISSUES

The fibrous structures are of great mechanical importance and chemical interest. They consist mainly of insoluble proteins but include also associated carbohydrates and lipids. The principal fibrous structures are: (1) collagenic fibres, (2) reticular fibres, (3) elastic fibres, and (4) other fibres recognized histologically or by electron microscope but of unknown chemical nature. Of these, collagen from collagenic fibres is the best characterized and, at the same time, the most prominent. It is the main protein of white connective tissue, comprising up to 90 per cent of the organic matter of tendon and bone, and a high percentage of the derma. (It is a striking fact that collagen comprises as much as one-third of the total body protein of the mammal.) I shall refer later to the macromolecular structure and properties of collagen, which mark it as a fascinating example of a structural protein. By comparison, little is known of the chemistry of the reticular fibres, which form a delicate network of fine fibres and which may be related to collagen. Elastic fibres, on the other hand, are prominent in yellow connective tissue and comprise varying proportions of the dry matter, e.g. about 80 per cent in ligamentum nuchae, 30 per cent in aorta, and 3–10 per cent in elastic cartilage.

It is appropriate to compare briefly the collagenic and elastic fibres, which, as you are aware, are readily distinguishable microscopically and also by their chemical properties. The collagen fibre is highly structured, showing a regular pattern of transverse bands which, in electron micrographs, are seen to recur at intervals of 640 Å along the fibre. The regularity of structure at the molecular level is demonstrated also in the X-ray diffraction pattern of collagen, which will be referred to below. In contrast, the elastic fibre shows no evidence of "crystallinity" in either the electron-micrograph or X-ray diffraction examination. Both proteins are insoluble under physiological conditions, but very different in that collagen can be disaggregated and dissolved in hot water (yielding gelatin) whilst elastin is extremely insoluble. In fact, elastin can be dissolved only by treatments that induce extensive chemical degradation.

The amino acid compositions of collagen and elastin are compared in Table I. They are both proteins of very unusual composition. The tabulation is made in such a way as to indicate peculiarities that are common to collagen and elastin and other features that distinguish them. The striking common features are that glycine makes up one-third and proline one-eighth of the total residues in each, and that cystine/cysteine and tryptophan are absent from both.

TABLE I

COMPARISON OF AMINO ACID COMPOSITIONS OF COLLAGEN AND ELASTIN

		Residues per 1000 residues		
		Collagen	Elastin	
	Alanine	99	234	Prominent in both
	Glycine	334	350	
	Proline	120	126	
	Leucine	39	60	
	Cystine/2	0	Trace	Absent or low in both
	Tryptophan	0	0	
	Tyrosine	6	5	
Basic	Methionine	5	0	
	Hydroxylysine	7	0	
	Histidine	5	0	
	Arginine	45	5	Very different in the two
	Lysine	29	2	
Acidic	Aspartic acid	43	6	
	Glutamic acid	71	17	
	Hydroxyproline	99	7	
	Serine	30	9	
	Threonine	21	9	
	Valine	27	130	
	Phenylalanine	14	30	

There are marked differences in the content of the two proteins in respect of the 12 other amino acids listed at the bottom of Table I. It must be borne in mind that the purity of insoluble proteins is difficult to establish, and this is especially true of elastin, as we shall see in a later paper. Despite this fact, however, the difference in the amino acid composition of the two seems to render quite untenable the view sometimes advanced that these two proteins may represent interconvertible forms of one protein. The exact structural relationship between them remains a most interesting chemical problem for the future. Comments on the chemical structure of collagen in relation to its macromolecular properties will be made below, and in one of the papers to follow a speculative model of elastin structure is to be presented.

MACROMOLECULAR CONSTITUENTS OF THE GROUND SUBSTANCES

Apart from the fibrous structures which, depending on their type, patterns of organization, and the presence or absence of mineralization, are the principal determinants of the strength and physical properties of connective tissues, the colloidal constituents of the ground substance are of great interest. Amongst these, as will be seen from Table II, polysaccharides are prominent, these being present in considerable variety and the types and distribution varying from one connective tissue to another. I should refer here to the

TABLE II
Constituents of the Ground Substance

I. Mucopolysaccharides (acidic heteropolysaccharides)
II. Mucopolysaccharide–protein complexes (dissociable)
III. Mucoproteins—chemically-linked complexes with 10–60 per cent carbohydrate
IV. Glycoproteins—chemically-linked complexes with 10-15 per cent carbohydrate
V. Free soluble proteins and other compounds diffusing between cells and plasma

Mucopolysaccharides and their Structure

	Abbrev. below	Repeating disaccharide unit
(a) Hyaluronic acid (D-glucuronic acid + N-acetyl-D-glucosamine)	H-A	[structure]
(b) Chondroitin-4-sulphate (A) (c) Chondroitin-6-sulphate (C) (d) Chondroitin (no sulphate) (D-glucuronic acid + N-acetyl-D-galactosamine + sulphate)	C-4-S C-6-S C	[structure]
(e) Dermatan sulphate (B) (L-iduronic acid + N-acetyl-D-galactosamine + sulphate)	D-S	[structure]
(f) Keratan sulphate (D-galactose + N-acetyl-D-galactosamine + sulphate)	K-S	[structure]

Occurrence of Mucopolysaccharides in Some Connective Tissues*

	H-A	C-4-S	C-6-S	C	D-S	K-S	Other
Skin	+	.	.	.	+	.	.
Embryo cartilage	.	+	+	+	.	.	.
Cartilage	.	+	+	.	.	+	.
Tendon	+	.	+	.	+	.	.
Vitreous and synovial fluid	+	.	.	.	.	.	.
Bone	.	+	.	.	.	.	.
Calf bone	.	+	+	.	.	+	+
Cornea	.	+	.	+	.	+	.
Aorta	+	+	.	.	+	.	+
Umbilical cord	+	.	.	.	+	.	.

*The dots indicate merely that the presence has not been reported.

dominance of polysaccharides in the intercellular deposits of plants as well as animals. In plants the fibrous structures are, of course, cellulosic in nature (cellulose being a homopolysaccharide of glucose) rather than protein but, as in animals, the encrusting or embedding medium contains usually a variety of heteropolysaccharides (the hemicelluloses, gums, etc.) which are in many ways analogous to the mucopolysaccharides of the ground substance of animal connective tissues. The acidic heteropolysaccharides as a group are outstanding in their hydrophilic and gel-forming capacity.

An attempt is made in Table II to give a glimpse of the present state of knowledge of these major constituents of the ground substance. Four categories of polysaccharide constituent are listed, differentiated on the basis of their relationship with protein moieties.

Many of the mucopolysaccharide molecules that have been isolated and characterized consist of chains of sugar residues joined together by saccharide linkages of different kinds but in which there is a repeating disaccharide unit. Examples of this basic structure of the mucopolysaccharides are given in the middle portion of Table II. It appears, however, that only in the case of vitreous and synovial fluids are there mucopolysaccharides not associated with proteins. It seems usual for the mucopolysaccharide to be linked with a protein moiety, but neither the proteins nor the mode of linkage are well characterized although this is a very active field of study. In the chondroitin-4-sulphate of cartilage, available evidence indicates that some 25–50 chains of the mucopolysaccharide of a mean molecular weight of about 40,000 are joined to a single protein core of about 170,000 M.W., the total aggregate having a molecular weight of about 2×10^6.

It will be noticed that the monosaccharides (or monosaccharide derivatives) which form the building units in these best-known examples include D-glucuronic acid, N-acetyl-D-glucosamine, N-acetyl-D-galactosamine, N-acetyl-D-galactosamine sulphated in either the 4 or 6 position, L-iduronic acid (a very unusual sugar), and D-galactose. There are many other mucopolysaccharides built on this general plan of repeating disaccharide units; it seems that more complex heteropolysaccharides such as the plant gums, which appear to contain four or five different kinds of monosaccharide units in a single macromolecule, may occur more rarely in animals. However, as we shall find in a communication to follow, the glycoprotein group of which the submaxillary gland glycoprotein is an example is built upon a quite different structural plan; in this particular example a large number of individual disaccharide moieties (made up of N-acetylneuraminic acid and N-acetyl-D-galactosamine residues) are attached to a single polypeptide chain.

The known occurrences of different mucopolysaccharides in a number of different tissues are indicated in the lower portion of Table II. While the absences of reported occurrences must be interpreted with caution, there seems little doubt that these constituents show specialized profiles of occurrence in the different tissues.

COLLAGEN, A FIBRE-FORMING MACROMOLECULE

The papers comprising this session deal mainly with elastin and mucoproteins and little, if at all, with collagen, which is not only the best characterized of all connective tissue constituents but also a most dramatic macromolecule in its inherent fibre-forming propensity. I shall refer here briefly to only two of the special features of the collagen molecule, namely, its very special three-dimensional structure, which reflects its peculiar amino acid composition, and the fact that collagen fibres can be dispersed into subunits which retain the capacity to re-form the native structure under appropriate conditions.

It was noted above in reference to Table I that collagen has a very unusual amino acid composition. Even though the full sequence of amino acids in collagen has not been established, knowledge of the chemical structure and organization of the constituent polypeptide chains is well advanced as a result mainly of studies by X-ray diffraction and the electron microscope supplemented by physicochemical studies. Pioneering X-ray studies beginning 25 years ago pointed to a high degree of crystallinity in collagen fibres, i.e. the presence of many accurately repeating spacings. Within recent years the triple-stranded spiral model of the collagen molecule, proposed and elaborated by Ramachandran in Madras and by Crick and Rich, has gained wide acceptance. Each strand of the triple helix consists of a single polypeptide chain itself coiled in a tight helix with about three amino acid residues per turn (the pitch being about 8.6 Å) and about 3000 Å in length. The triple helix consists of three of these minor helices coiled together with a pitch of 86 Å, these being bonded together by hydrogen bonding and apparently in mature tissues by ester-linkages involving aspartic and glutamic acid side-chains.

The triple helix consists of an end-to-end assembly of segments 2800 Å long and about 14 Å in diameter; these constitute tropocollagen molecules, which have a molecular weight of about 350,000 and are the most asymmetric molecules observed in nature. When collagen is "dissolved" in hot water it is broken down further than the trimeric tropocollagen stage, the soluble products consistsing of monomers and dimers of the individual polypeptide chains. But if the skins of very young animals are extracted with cold water or salt solution a clear solution of tropocollagen in the form of the individual trimeric helix is obtained. (A somewhat similar preparation can be obtained from insoluble adult collagen by prolonged extractions with dilute acid.)

Tropocollagen molecules, the rigid rod-like individual segments of the triple helix, readily undergo aggregation under a variety of conditions. On simple warming of the solution (in dilute salt) to 40° C. collagen fibres that appear to be identical to natural fibres are formed. In addition to the native type of fibrous aggregate showing the typical 640 Å recurrent pattern in the electron micrograph, a number of other types of aggregate can be induced to form under other conditions. It is now clear from many studies that the tropocollagen molecules are able to aggregate by end-to-end splicing of the triple helices as well as by lateral bonding. Much work designed to elucidate the exact bonds involved is proceeding, since this provides a most interesting example of morphogenesis at the molecular level.

We are accustomed to the remarkable specificity of complexing sites on protein molecules in connection with enzyme catalysis. The complex between enzyme and substrate results in a labilization of particular bonds in the substrate and the result is catalytic action. We see in the case of collagen how the existence of specific and complementary complexing sites on the two ends of the rod-like tropocollagen molecule leads to the formation of a stable complex which is the basis of the native fibre of collagen.

The collagen story presents many additional facets of great biological interest, which are described in review articles to which references will be appended below.

IMPLICATIONS

I have reviewed briefly these non-living chemical substances present in the intercellular spaces of connective tissues, and in conclusion I should now like to turn more directly to the main point of our conference. So far as rheumatoid diseases are concerned, I have confined my remarks merely to a sketchy description of the inanimate setting of the crime, a general glimpse of the chemical neighbourhood in which it takes place.

In the past two days we have had stimulating reviews of the behaviour of the living inhabitants of connective tissue and emphasis on the probable part played by the immune mechanisms in rheumatic disease. The growing conviction of the immunological basis of rheumatoid arthritis and the involvement of auto-immune reactions, which has been emphasized by various speakers, throws emphasis upon the importance of the fullest possible knowledge of the chemistry and biology of the substances peculiar to the tissues of the joints. These must be regarded as potential sources of auto-antigens special to joints.

I would point out that we have been considering, amongst connective tissue constituents, some of the least-soluble constituents of the body with which living cells come into contact and I would suggest that some group or component present in one of the insoluble macromolecular structures in (say) synovial cartilage should be regarded as a potential source of the mysterious auto-antigen. It may not be unreasonable to suggest that the very mode of origin of the insoluble fibrous structures, whereby they appear to be secreted in the form of precursor molecules which then aggregate outside the cells into the larger complexes, could be a factor in preventing the acquirement of immune tolerance to such components; this might be all the more likely if, as is suggested in the case of collagen, new cross-linkages are formed after deposition in insoluble form. If indeed the fibrous structures of connective tissues contain antigenic configurations which have been shielded from reaction with the immune system either because of the rapid removal of potential antigen by deposition in an insoluble form or because of the formation of new antigenic sites after extracellular deposition, then indeed such structures might be expected to constitute a potential source of auto-antigens if subsequently such insoluble structures are brought into solution, as a result for example of enzymic degradation accompanying some microbiological infection.

This may be far-fetched but I have been encouraged to mention the concept by the trend of thinking at this conference. For some time we have planned the testing of the auto-antigenicity of elastin breakdown products on these grounds, and the preparation of rabbit ear elastin to be described later by Dr. Anwar was made with this object in view.*

ACKNOWLEDGMENTS

I wish to thank various colleagues, especially Drs. R. K. Murray, R. A. Anwar, and R. G. Donovan, who have given valuable advice in the formulation of this little review, but who are free from responsibility for errors of fact or judgment which remain.

Our work on this subject in the Department of Biochemistry, University of Toronto, has received generous financial support from the National Research Council of Canada and the Medical Research Council of Canada.

REFERENCES

General Biochemical Background

WHITE, A., HANDLER, P., and SMITH, E. L. Principles of Biochemistry, 3rd ed. (McGraw-Hill, New York, 1964).

Fibrous Proteins

AYER, J. P. Elatsic tissue. Internat. Rev. Conn. Tissue Res. 2: 33 (1964).

GALLOP, P. M. Structural features of the collagen molecule. Connective Tissue: Intercellular Macromolecules (Little, Brown & Co., Boston, 1964), p. 79.

GROSS, J. Organization and disorganization of collagen. *Ibid.*, p. 63.

RAMACHANDRAN, G. N. Molecular structure of collagen. Internat. Rev. Conn. Tissue Res. 1: 127 (1963).

VERZAR, F. Aging of the collagen fibre. Internat. Rev. Conn. Tissue Res. 2: 243 (1964).

WOOD, G. C. The precipitation of collagen fibres from solution. Internat. Rev. Conn. Tissue Res. 2: 1 (1964).

Mucopolysaccharides

MUIR, H. Chemistry and metabolism of connective tissue. Connective Tissue: Intercellular Macromolecules (Little, Brown & Co., Boston, 1964), p. 101.

Note added in proof. Subsequent to the presentation of this paper, Stein, Pezess, Robert, and Poullain (Nature, 207: 312 [1965]) demonstrated antigenicity of soluble peptides from bovine aortic elastin.

A Picture of the
Breakdown of Elastin
under the Action of Elastase[*]

R. G. DONOVAN,[†]
R. A. ANWAR, and C. S. HANES

ELASTIN is a protein with an unusual complement of amino acids, and with unusual physical and chemical properties. From its amino acid composition (cf. p. 225) it is clear that the elastin macromolecule possesses few charged groups and many neutral groups; it is a very insoluble protein, and a high degree of intra- and inter-molecular hydrophobic bonding may be inferred.

The present paper deals with observations on the process of enzymic degradation of elastin, and with a hypothetical structure for elastin which is in accord with these observations and with many of its physical and chemical properties.

The degradation of elastin has been followed most commonly by the measurement of its dissolution. It is possible, however, to have extensive degradation with little dissolution. Thus, the intact fibre of elastin is insoluble in water even at 100° C. but after restricted attack by elastase, much of the insoluble residue becomes soluble in boiling water; furthermore, the portion not dissolved by this treatment is much more readily attacked by elastase than is the original fibre.

Two methods of following the dissolution of elastin were employed extensively in the present study. The first, with Congo-red-dyed elastin (2) as substrate, involved measuring the appearance of dye in the solution. The second, with undyed elastin, involved following by the biuret method the amount of protein solubilized.

With either dyed elastin or undyed elastin as substrate, the progress of dissolution is sigmoidal with time, but the shape of the sigmoid differs in the two cases. The shape also differs with different preparations of enzyme or with different amounts of the same enzyme. A single number is obviously inadequate to describe the enzymic activity in such a complex system. Accordingly an

[*]From the Department of Biochemistry, University of Toronto, Toronto.
[†]Present address: Research Laboratories, Canada Packers Ltd., Toronto, Ontario.

R. G. DONOVAN, R. A. ANWAR, C. S. HANES

empirical system of evaluation of activity was evolved in which a figure for the "average" rate (r) in a particular assay is supplemented by two additional figures indicating the initial rate (i) and the maximum rate (m) relative to the "average" rate. Thus, the activity of the enzyme used in a particular assay would be described by the figures $r(i, m)$, where r = the reciprocal of the time taken for 50 per cent dissolution,

$$i = (\text{initial rate})/r,$$

and

$$m = (\text{maximum rate})/r.$$

On the basis of the results indicated below, as well as much information about elastin described in the literature (1), a hypothetical picture of the structure of this protein has been constructed. This picture, shown in Fig. 1, provides a reasonable basis for explaining the salient physical and chemical characteristics of elastin, and its behaviour as a substrate for elastases.

The fibre of elastin is conceived as a bundle of fibrils held together perhaps through hydrophobic forces. Each fibril is conceived as an assembly of four filaments as illustrated in Fig. 1. The upper part of the figure depicts a single fibril in the stretched or extended state; this is shown in both side and end views. Only three of the four longitudinal filaments are visible in the side view because filament IV is envisaged as lying directly behind filament II. Each filament will be seen to consist of a longitudinal series of the poly-functional cross-linking bodies joined together by two peptide chains. In

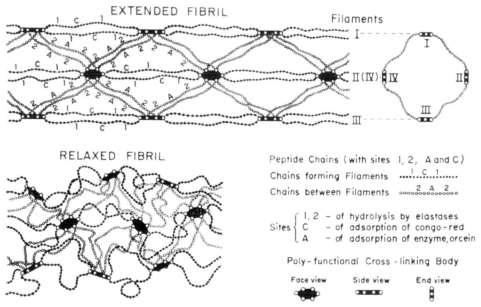

FIG. 1. Hypothetical model of elastin.

addition, the cross-linking bodies of each filament are connected to those of the adjacent filaments by additional pairs of peptide chains to form a quasi-tubular structure. In the lower part of Fig. 1 the same length of fibril is shown in the relaxed state; this indicates much folding and coiling of polypeptide chains and much interaction between individual chains.

The "cross-linking body" is shown as containing six sites at which C-termini and N-termini of peptide chains can be attached. These six sites are pictured as being six out of the eight amino-acyl groups of desmosine and isodesmosine. Thus our tentative suggestion is that the cross-linking body contains one residue of desmosine, one residue of isodesmosine, and possibly some chromogenic and/or fluorescent structure.*

It has been concluded that elastin contains *at least* two categories of sites on the polypeptide chains which are attacked by elastase. Two such categories (labelled 1 and 2 in the illustration) are adequate to explain the observed phenomena but there may be additional categories of hydrolysable sites. Sites of category 1, located on the longitudinal chains forming the filaments, bind enzyme strongly, but are cleaved slowly, while sites of category 2, on the chains between filaments, adsorb enzyme weakly but are cleaved rapidly. Congo red molecules (which are adsorbed at sites C) seem to interfere with the access of the enzyme to category 1 sites in the intact fibre of elastin, and cleavage of these sites appears to be necessary for solubilization of the dye. In addition to sites of cleavage, elastin may adsorb elastase at sites A which are not hydrolysable by the enzyme, and which may not involve the active centre of the enzyme; the same or other sites on the interfilament chains are responsible for the adsorption of the dye orcein. The evidence that will be adduced in support of this model is summarized under seven headings as follows:

1. *Influence of enzyme concentration on rates of dissolution.* Initial rates of dissolution of elastin are not proportional to the amount of enzyme in the system. Dyed elastin and undyed elastin show opposite departures from linearity, indicating a selective effect of Congo red on one category of sites of enzymic action.

2. *Influence of enzyme concentration on rates of liberation of amino groups.* The initial rate of release of free amino groups from undyed elastin increases with increasing amount of enzyme in a more-than-proportional manner. Thus as sites of category 1 become saturated, more enzyme will be available for action at sites of category 2, resulting in a more-than-proportional rise in the initial rate of release of amino groups even though the rate of solubilization of protein proved to be less-than-proportional to the amount of enzyme.

3. *Effects of dyeing elastin with Congo red.* Congo red causes an apparent

Note added in proof. In a recent paper, Partridge (Fed. Proc. 25: 1023 [1966]) has proposed a generally similar structure for elastin. This differs primarily in suggesting that the units of the network are deformable corpuscular polypeptide structures joined by cross-linkages involving the desmosines.

decrease in initial rates of dissolution, whereas it increases the "average" and maximum rates of dissolution. Obstruction of sites of category 1 by the Congo red results in more action at sites of category 2 (for a given amount of enzyme). This results in *greater* solubilization of protein, but *less* solubilization of dye, initially. Later in the degradation, with many of the sites of category 2 already cleaved, relatively more enzyme is available for cleavage of the rate-limiting sites of category 1. At the same time these sites may become more accessible through the opening up of the three-dimensional structure, and their cleavage may be more effective in releasing soluble fragments.

4. *Relation of rate of dissolution to concentration of elastin.* For a given amount of enzyme the relationships of the rates of dissolution to the concentrations of elastin differ for dyed and undyed elastin. With dyed elastin, maximum values of the initial rates occur at moderate concentrations of elastin; lower initial rates occur as the concentration of elastin is increased or decreased from this "optimum" level. With undyed elastin, however, the relationship is simpler; the initial rate increases to an asymptotic maximum as the concentration of elastin is increased. These observed effects are not surprising inasmuch as an insoluble substrate such as elastin may have only a small proportion of its reactive groups exposed, all of which may be saturated at low ratios of enzyme to substrate. Consider the initial rates in a series of digests under these conditions. At low concentrations of either substrate, all the available sites of categories 1 and 2 will be saturated, and the initial rate of dissolution will increase with increasing concentration of substrate. At very high levels of substrate, all of the available enzyme will be bound; with dyed elastin it will act primarily at sites of category 2, while with the undyed elastin it will act primarily at sites of category 1. Since the site of action on undyed elastin is also the site of the rate-limiting cleavage, decreasing the concentration of substrate will cause a drop in initial rates when the enzyme is no longer saturated. With dyed elastin, however, as the concentration of substrate is decreased, more enzyme will become available for action at the sites of the rate-limiting cleavages (i.e. sites of category 1). This will produce an increase in initial rates at intermediate concentrations of dyed elastin, as observed.

5. *Carboxyl and amino-terminal groups liberated.* Soluble products from the enzymic degradation of elastin contained a variety of C-terminal and N-terminal amino acids, corroborating the conclusion that more than one category of site of cleavage exists in elastin.

6. *Synergistic action of separated elastase components.* Chromatography of crude elastase on carboxymethylcellulose resulted in the separation of five fractions showing some activity on elastin. Of these, two gave low initial rates when acting separately on dyed elastin. When combined, however, a four-fold increase in initial rate was observed. This synergesis can be explained only on the basis of the attack of two different sites for which the two elastase peaks show some degree of selectivity.

7. *Effects of soluble products of elastin.* Low levels of soluble products of elastin caused activation of elastase, while high levels caused inhibition. These effects were observed at all stages of the degradation of the substrate. They can be explained on the basis of the non-hydrolysable sites (A), assumed to exist on elastin, which bind some of the enzyme in non-effective complexes. Direct evidence was obtained that soluble products of elastin possess sites at which elastase can be adsorbed. Thus soluble products were able to elute appreciable quantities of elastase from adsorption on fibrous elastin. Soluble products, therefore, may adsorb enzyme in competition with the insoluble fibre. Such enzyme would be more effective, because of its mobility, than that found on the fibre. In the presence of large amounts of soluble products, however, the efficiency of the enzyme might be decreased by virtue of the large number of non-hydrolysable sites of binding.

CONCLUSION

The proposed model of elastin is highly speculative but it provides explanations of the various phenomena observed during the present study, and of pertinent observations contained in the literature. It may not be unique, however, in these properties.

ACKNOWLEDGMENTS

Our work on this subject in the Department of Biochemistry, University of Toronto, has received generous financial support from the National Research Council of Canada and the Medical Research Council of Canada. One of us (R.G.D.) wishes to acknowledge support by Canada Packers Ltd. and the Collis Leather Co. Ltd. We thank Mrs. C. Grauer for her careful technical assistance.

REFERENCES

1. PARTRIDGE, S. M.   Advances Protein Chem. *17*: 227 (1962).
2. NAUGHTON, M. A. and SANGER, F.   Biochem. J. *78*: 156 (1961).

Separation of the
Fluorescent Components of Elastin *

DONALD P. THORNHILL, PH.D.,† and
FRANK S. LaBELLA, PH.D.‡

ELASTIN, as the name implies, is the protein responsible for the elastic properties of certain connective tissues. There is some resemblance between the
molecular structure of elastin and that of rubber-like polymers. About 80 per
cent of the amino acids constituting the peptide chain are non-polar. The
chains are considered to be randomly coiled with sufficient cross-links to make
the protein elastic.

Some pathological changes in connective tissue, such as arteriosclerosis, are
associated with loss of elasticity. It has been suggested that loss of elasticity is
due to a progressive cross-linking of the peptide chains, analogous to excessive
vulcanization of rubber which results in brittleness. No doubt the mineral
deposition in the arterial wall, usually associated with arteriosclerosis, might
also be expected to contribute to a decrease in elasticity.

The cross-links in elastin are considered to be strong covalent linkages in
view of the fact that elastin is soluble only in reagents that break peptide
bonds. Elastin is one of the most insoluble proteins known and is not attacked
by most proteolytic enzymes. It is solubilized by the pancreatic enzyme
elastase, but is only slightly degraded to dialysable fragments. Complete hydrolysis has been reported after a minimum of 72 hours of treatment with $6N$
hydrochloric acid at $100°$ (1).

Partridge and co-workers (2) have isolated an isomeric pair of hitherto
undescribed amino acids, desmosine and isodesmosine. The schematic structure of these is shown in Fig. 1. These appear to fulfil the requirements of a
cross-linking species in elastin on account of their polyfunctional nature. It is
not clear, however, to what extent these components contribute to the yellow

*From the Department of Pharmacology and Therapeutics, University of Manitoba
Faculty of Medicine, Winnipeg, Manitoba.
Supported by grants from the Canadian Arthritis and Rheumatism Society and the
American Heart Association.
†Canadian Arthritis and Rheumatism Society Medical Research Fellow.
‡Established Investigator of the American Heart Association.

colour and fluorescence of elastin. The peptide fragment containing these residues is yellow and fluorescent (3), but the isolated desmosines are virtually colourless and only weakly fluorescent. It has been postulated that these structures are formed by the condensation of four lysine residues, possibly involving an oxidative deamination (4). This poses an intriguing problem as elastin contains only two or three per cent of lysine, and it is difficult to envisage how four lysine residues could have sufficient proximity to combine in this way. Nevertheless, very recent work by Piez and co-workers (1) has convincingly demonstrated that lysine is a precursor of these cross-links.

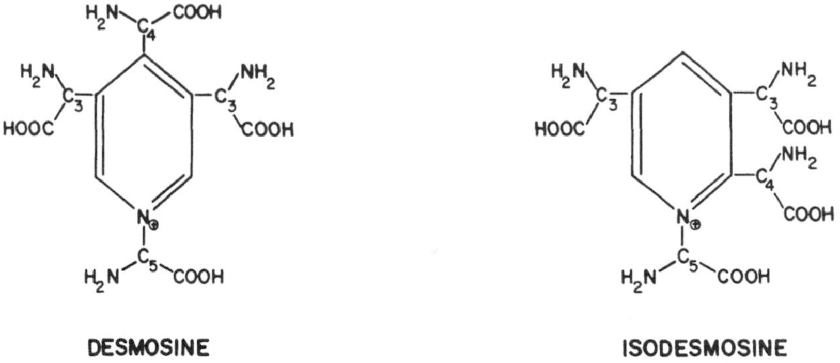

DESMOSINE

ISODESMOSINE

Fig. 1. Schematic structure of desmosine and isodesmosine.

The study of connective tissue is important from the viewpoint of biological aging. Deterioration of bodily function and eventual death have been accepted as inevitable until relatively recently. However, with the advent of modern medicine the chances of mortality due to old age, in contrast to disease, have increased, and greater emphasis is being focused on gerontology. One theory of the aging process states that connective tissue becomes progressively more cross-linked with age. There is considerable evidence indicating an increase in cross-linking of collagen and elastin with age. In this laboratory LaBella has shown, for example, that human Achilles tendon collagen and human aortic elastin become more resistant to solubilization with age (5). It was also shown that there is a concomitant increase in fluorescence of these proteins with age suggesting that cross-linking and fluorescence are associated.

There appears to be a direct converse of the aging process in the disease osteolathyrism, a condition characterized by a decrease in the tensile strength of connective tissue and resulting from a defect in protein cross-linking. For example, dissecting aortic aneurysm has been achieved in a matter of days by feeding lathyrogens to young turkeys (6). The agents causing this condition include compounds that can combine with aldehydes (7), and there has been some speculation that cross-linking may in some manner be associated with functional aldehyde groups in the peptide chains. While it is generally agreed that aldehydic residues may be present in collagen and elastin, no definite species have yet been identified (8, 9).

Paper or thin layer chromatography on silica gel, of acid hydrolysates of elastin, indicates that at least two fluorescent species are present, and previous work by LaBella (10) and Loomeijer (11) have shown the existence of a yellow pigment in elastin. The present work was carried out in an attempt to determine the relationship, if any, between the yellow constituents, pigment, and fluorescent components.

EXPERIMENTAL

PURIFICATION AND HYDROLYSIS OF ELASTIN

Bovine ligamentum nuchae was purified as described previously (12).

Total hydrolysis was carried out by refluxing for 72 hours in 6N HCl under a nitrogen atmosphere. The acid had previously been deoxygenated by bubbling nitrogen through it for 30 minutes. The ratio of protein to liquor was 10 gm. to 600 ml. The product was taken to dryness on a rotary evaporator after several additions of water.

CHROMATOGRAPHY ON ALUMINA

A portion of the hydrolysate equivalent to 1 gm. elastin in 5 ml. water was then chromatographed through a 3 cm. by 50 cm. alumina column. The alumina had been washed extensively with water, 1N HCl, and again with water. Elution was carried out with water, 0.005M NH$_4$OH, 0.5M NH$_4$OH, and NaOH in that order. The fraction volume collected was 15 ml.

FLUORESCENCE AND ABSORPTION SPECTRA MEASUREMENTS

Fluorescence activation and emission data were determined on an Aminco Bowman spectrophotofluorometer using a 0.5 cm. cuvette.

Ultraviolet absorption was determined on a Beckman DK2 recording spectrophotometer using a 1 cm. cell.

The infrared absorption spectrum of the aldehyde was obtained with a Perkin-Elmer double-beam instrument, using carbon tetrachloride as solvent in an NaCl cell.

Paper chromatography was carried out on Whatman No. 1 paper. Development was carried out using the upper layer of a butanol/acetic acid/water mixture (4:1:5). After drying, the developed chromatograms were examined in a dark room using a mercury vapour lamp fitted with a Wood's filter. The papers were sprayed with polychromatic ninhydrin (13) to locate amino acids.

RESULTS AND DISCUSSION

The separation illustrated in Fig. 2 indicates that four fluorescent fractions were resolved by this method. Three of these fractions were associated with

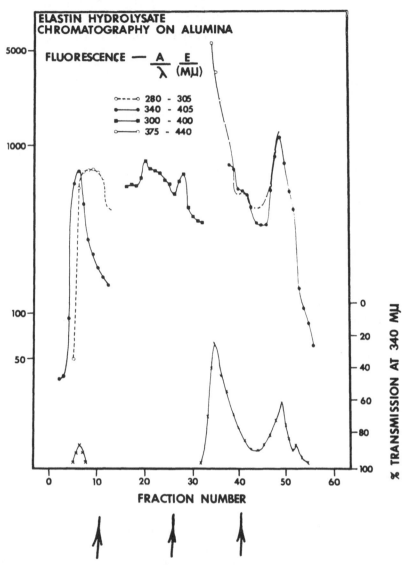

FIG. 2. Appearance of fluorescent and coloured fractions after chromatography on alumina. Arrows indicate change of influent.

yellow colour. Fluorescence in proteins is generally associated only with tryptophan, tyrosine, and phenylalanine, the relevant data being shown in Table I (14). Phenylalanine is only feebly fluorescent anyd tryptophan is not present in elastin. The excitation (280 mμ) and emission (305 mμ) maxima of the first fluorescent fraction corresponded to tyrosine. Paper chromatography showed that all the major neutral amino acids and tyrosine were eluted in this

TABLE I

FLUORESCENCE CHARACTERISTICS OF AMINO ACIDS

Amino acid	Excitation max. (mμ)	Emission max. (mμ)
Tyrosine	275	303
Phenylalanine	260	282
Tryptophan	287	348

region. The three subsequent fractions showed fluorescence at a longer wavelength, which corresponded to that of the native protein. The first of these was associated with a small amount of yellow colour and may represent a neutral degradation product, because browning becomes visibly more pronounced during acid hydrolysis. The second fluorescent fraction was colourless and, after chromatography on paper, gave a faint ninhydrin reaction at the origin. The ultraviolet absorption spectra of the fractions separated on alumina are illustrated in Fig. 3. It is seen that a chromophore absorbing strongly at a wavelength less than 220 mμ was present in all fractions. The third fluorescent fraction shows a well-defined peak at 275 mμ. Although absorbing maximally at the same wavelength as desmosine, this fraction was brilliantly fluorescent and also coloured. The effect of sodium borohydride on the ultraviolet absorption is illustrated in Fig. 4. It is difficult to interpret the change in the spectrum but it may represent the presence of two species in equilibrium to form an isosbestic point. Although not evident from Fig. 2, the fraction with the maximum optical density and that with the maximum fluorescence intensity did not quite coincide, the former following the latter by one tube, under the conditions of the experiment. This difference could be explained either by assuming that a deeper-coloured solution tended to quench the fluorescence, or that two species were eluted simultaneously. The latter explanation would be in accordance with the observed effect of borohydride.

It is of interest to compare the separation on alumina with the appearance of a one-dimensional paper chromatogram of an acid hydrolysate of elastin. After development on paper there were two regions of visible fluorescence, one at the origin due to desmosine plus isodesmosine, which gave a greyish brown colour with polychromatic ninhydrin, and another situated near proline.

This work has demonstrated that there is more than one fluorescent species present in elastin. Chromatography on alumina was examined because ion exchange resins tend, to a very minor extent, to contribute fluorescent impurities to the eluate. Unfortunately, separation on alumina did not appear suitable for preparative scale work. If the main yellow fraction was rechromatographed, the recovery was unsatisfactory and, subsequently, a brown material could be eluted with NaOH. This indicated that a component in the fraction was labile and the nature of the adsorbent was such that oxidation may have taken place.

The brown material could not be eluted from Dowex 50 with HCl. This

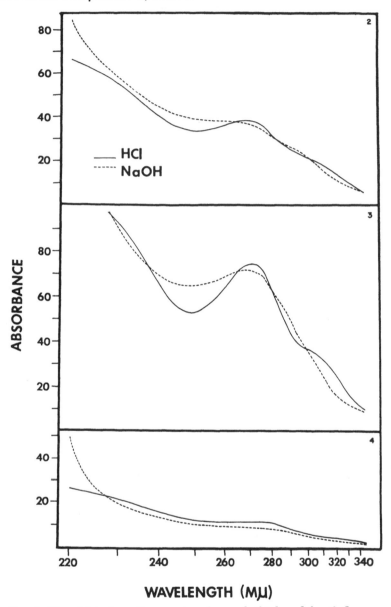

FIG. 3. Ultraviolet absorption spectra of second, third, and fourth fluorescent fractions eluted from alumina. ——— HCl, — — — NaOH.

fraction could, however, be isolated by means of an aliphatic carboxylic acid resin, Bio Rex 70. The resin was titrated and a pK value of 5.4 was indicated. When an elastin hydrolysate buffered at pH 5.4 was placed on this resin, the amino acids and the main yellow fraction were not retained. Subsequent

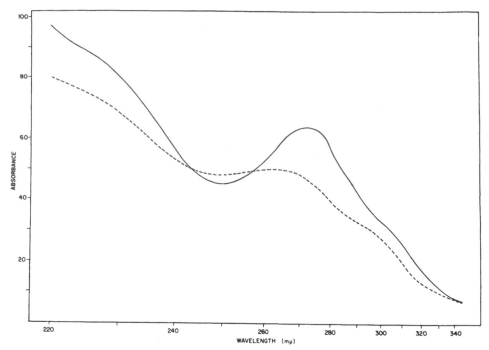

FIG. 4. Effect of borohydride on ultraviolet spectrum of third fluorescent fraction.
—— NaOH, – – – NaOH + NaBH$_4$.

elution using 2N acetic acid followed by 2N formic acid gave rise to two
fluorescent fractions. The fluorescence spectra of these fractions and a comparison with desmosine are illustrated in Fig. 5. The acetic acid eluate appeared
to be similar to desmosine, but the formic acid eluate shows an emission
maximum at a longer wavelength.

An additional fluorescent material has been isolated that appeared to be an
aldehydic or ketonic compound probably related to a plasmalogen. Elastic
fibres are characteristically Schiff positive, and there is evidence that a plasma-
logen-like substance is present. For instance, it has been shown that Schiff
staining is enhanced by prior treatment with mercuric chloride and blocked
by prior treatment with iodine (15). Elastin powder was stirred overnight at
room temperature with 1 per cent mercuric chloride and the product extracted
with ether. An ether-soluble material was obtained which migrated as a
discrete fluorescent spot when examined by thin layer chromatography on
silica gel. The spot stained yellow with 2,4-dinitrophenylhydrazine. The infrared absorption spectrum of this material is shown in Fig. 6. The compound was
saturated, exhibited a relatively intense CH$_2$ band indicating a long aliphatic
chain, and possessed either an aldehydic or ketonic carbonyl group. There is
relatively weak absorption at 7.3 microns (1380 cm.$^{-1}$), which may be due to

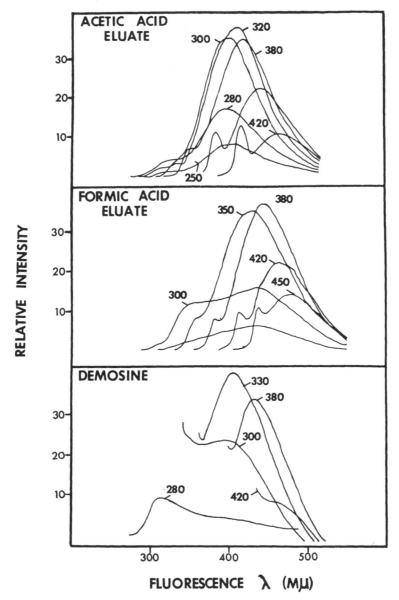

Fig. 5. Fluorescence spectra of fractions eluted from Bio Rex 70 and of desmosine.

two equivalent methyl groups, indicating a branched structure, but absorption in this region is by no means diagnostic.

The properties of the lipid-like substance were very similar to those of the fluorescent polar organic acid isolated by Loomeijer (16), which was reported

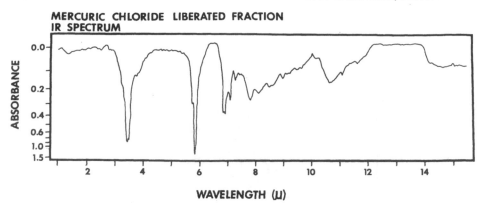

FIG. 6. Infrared absorption spectrum of lipid-like material isolated after mercuric chloride treatment.

to have a chain length of 12 carbon atoms and was considered to be derived from a lipopeptide. It is likely that this aldehyde or ketone, isolated under the conditions employed by Loomeijer, i.e. by refluxing in hot acid, would be partly oxidized to a carboxylic acid. Depending on the extent of oxidation, our results would be compatible with those of the latter author noting infrared absorption corresponding to a carboxyl function, which was absent from our spectrum, and also an inconclusive reaction with 2,4-dinitrophenylhydrazine. The fact that our material was saturated is of considerable interest in view of the fact that plasmalogens of the vinyl ether type give rise to an unsaturated aldehyde on hydrolysis. The action of mercuric chloride has been reported to be specific in cleaving an unsaturated ether (17) but the compound obtained by us was definitely saturated, as evidenced by its infrared spectrum. The possibility is being investigated that the compound may have contained mercury, analogous to the β chloromercuriacetaldehyde obtained by Norton (17) from the action of mercuric chloride on butyl vinyl ether.

It is possible that prolonged digestion of elastin in hot, strong acid would result in polymerization or modification of the fatty aldehyde, giving rise to fluorescent artifacts. Before attempting to characterize the unknown fluorescent species demonstrated by the separation on alumina, alternative methods of hydrolysis have to be investigated to establish their actual existence in elastin.

SUMMARY

Chromatography of acid hydrolysates of elastin using an acid-washed alumina column resolved four fluorescent fractions. The fluorescence of one of these fractions was due to tyrosine and that of another appeared to be due to the desmosines. The remaining two fractions appeared to be due to hitherto uncharacterized constituents. Two of these fractions were associated with yellow colour. A lipid-soluble compound was isolated from mercuric-chloride-treated elastin and its infrared absorption spectrum indicated that it was a long-chain saturated aldehyde or ketone which may have had a branched structure.

REFERENCES

1. Piez, K. A., *et al.* Biochem. Biophys. Res. Comm. *17*: 248 (1964).
2. Partridge, S. M., *et al.* Nature, *200*: 651 (1963).
3. ——— Nature, *197*: 1297 (1963).
4. ——— Biochem. J. *93*: 30c (1964).
5. LaBella, F. S., and Paul, G. J. Gerontol. *20*: 54 (1965).
6. Waibel, P. E., *et al.* Metabolism, *13*: 473 (1964).
7. Levene, C. I. J. Exper. Med. *116*: 119 (1962).
8. Landucci, J. M., *et al. In* Recent Advances in Gelatine and Glue Research (Pergamon Press, London, 1957).
9. Gallop, P. M., *et al.* Biochem. Biophys. Res. Comm. *17*: 320 (1964).
10. LaBella, F. S. J. Gerontol. *17*: 8 (1962).
11. Loomeijer, F. J. Nature, *182*: 182 (1958).
12. LaBella, F. S. Arch. Biochem. *93*: 72 (1961).
13. Moffat, E. D., and Lytle, R. I. Anal. Chem. *31*: 927 (1959).
14. Teale, F. W. J., and Weber, G. Biochem. J. *65*: 476 (1956).
15. LaBella, F. S. J. Histochem. *6*: 260 (1958).
16. Loomeijer, F. J. J. Atheroscler. Res. *1*: 62 (1961).
17. Norton, W. T. Nature, *184*: 1144 (1959).

Effects of Ultraviolet
Irradiation on Human and Bovine
Collagen and Elastin:
Relationship of Tyrosine to
Native Fluorescence*

FRANK S. LaBELLA, PH.D.,† and
DONALD P. THORNHILL, PH.D.‡

CROSS-LINKING of peptide chains appears to be fundamental in the maturation, aging, and degeneration of the fibrous connective tissue proteins. There appear to be several different types of cross-links involving covalent bonding between two or more reactive sites within chains and on adjacent peptide chains comprising the proteins. The nature of only a few of the apparent cross-links has been indicated. Gallop and his group (1) have provided convincing evidence that γ-glutamyl groups in collagen form intrachain ester bonds with as yet unknown groups. Partridge (2) has isolated two polyamino, polycarboxylic compounds from elastin which appear to represent sites of multiple cross-links among several peptide chains.

We have recently determined in human collagen a decrease in tyrosine content with age and a concomitant increase in a fluorescent compound, the nature of which is not yet definitely established (3). Previous work from our laboratory has provided evidence suggesting that the fluorescence is associated with cross-linking in elastin (4). The increase in fluorescence of human collagen and elastin with age parallels the increasing resistance of these proteins to solubilization or hydrolysis (3, 5), an observation compatible with the cross-linking hypothesis.

A role for tyrosine has been proposed in the "tanning" of the developing cuticle of certain insects (6). Tyrosine and other phenols are believed to become

*From the Department of Pharmacology and Therapeutics, Faculty of Medicine, University of Manitoba, Winnipeg, Manitoba.

Supported by grants from the Canadian Arthritis and Rheumatism Society and the American Heart Association.

†Established Investigator of the American Heart Association.

‡Canadian Arthritis and Rheumatism Society Medical Research Fellow.

oxidized to chemically reactive quinone or quinone-like structures, which can subsequently serve as cross-linking species between protein chains in the cuticle. The cross-linking process renders the protein–chitin complex hard, insoluble, and inert. Andersen (7) has provided evidence that dityrosine is a cross-linking agent in resilin, an elastin-like protein from insect ligaments. The present report describes studies designed to determine whether tyrosine derivatives can serve as cross-links in mammalian collagen and elastin.

METHODS

Elastin and collagen were prepared as described previously (3–5). Human aortic elastin was treated with 90 per cent formic acid at 40° C. for 16 hours in order to remove inorganic material. Bovine ligamentum elastin, unlike old human elastin, leaves no residue after dissolution by elastase. One gram of elastin powder was iodinated by suspending it in a solution consisting of 50 ml. of $0.2M$ Tris buffer pH 8.2, 1 ml. of $0.1N$ I_2 in 5 per cent KI, and 1 ml. of NaI^{131} (200 μc./ml.). The mixture was shaken at 4° C. for 30 minutes, washed thoroughly with boiling water, $0.01N$ NaOH, boiling water, acetone, and dried at 100°. Ultraviolet irradiation was carried out on suspensions of purified collagen and elastin powders in $0.05M$ phosphate buffer pH 7.4 at 37° with a Sylvania germicidal lamp consisting of two 15-watt bulbs, placed 15 cm. above the suspension. After irradiation the powder was washed extensively with water, then acetone, and dried at 100°. Control preparations were incubated under identical conditions except for being shielded from the ultraviolet irradiation. Hydrolysis of elastin was carried out with $6N$ HCl in sealed vials for 48 hours in an autoclave at 120° C. HCl was then removed *in vacuo* and the residue taken up in water. I^{131} was measured in test tubes in a scintillation well-counter containing a NaI crystal. For enzyme hydrolysis studies, 1 ml. of aqueous suspension containing 10 mg. of elastin powder was mixed with 3 ml. borate buffer pH 8.9, and 200 μg elastase (Sigma) was added. The rate of hydrolysis was determined by measuring the decrease in turbidity of elastin preparations which were suspended with a tissue homogenizer to the same initial turbidity. Optically clear solutions resulted eventually for all preparations. For absorption and fluorescence measurements the powders were dissolved in hot $6N$ HCl, neutralized, and made up to volume with appropriate buffers. Absorption measurements were carried out with a Beckman DK2 spectrophotometer and fluorescence with an Aminco-Bowman spectrophotofluorometer.

RESULTS

Irradiation of collagen and elastin resulted in a progressive visible yellowing of the powders with time. Absorption in the ultraviolet (ca. 275 mμ) also increased with time of irradiation, as did fluorescence (405 mμ) and Schiff positivity (studied on elastin only). Tyrosine content, as measured by fluorescence at 305 mμ, diminished with duration of irradiation (Table I). Fluorescence, which increased upon exposure to ultraviolet light, exhibited a spectrum

TABLE I

EFFECTS OF ULTRAVIOLET IRRADIATION ON ELASTIN*

| | Days of u.v. | | | |
	0	1	2	3
Rel. fluor. (305 mμ)	44	37	31	27
Rel. fluor. (405 mμ)	57	69	88	94
Yellowing	+1	+2	+3	+4
Schiff reaction†	+1	+2	+3	+4
Rel. absorbance (275 mμ)	0.76	0.83	0.86	0.88

*Similar results were obtained with collagen except that Schiff positivity was not determined.

†Solubilization of elastin with acid or with elastase causes disappearance of the colour and prevents quantitation.

identical with that present in the non-irradiated proteins (Figs. 1 and 2). To determine whether tyrosine was a precursor of the substance fluorescing at 405 mμ, iodination of tyrosine residues in elastin with I^{131} was carried out on irradiated and non-irradiated samples which were subsequently hydrolysed and fractionated on alumina (Fig. 3). I^{131} was recovered both in the water and NH_3 eluates, peak radioactivity being obtained one fraction earlier than tyrosine, and one fraction earlier than the substance fluorescing at 405 mμ. Ultraviolet treatment of the I^{131}-labelled protein resulted in a marked decrease in the amount of tyrosine, a marked increase in the amount of material fluorescing at 405 mμ, and a greater proportion of I^{131} associated with the NH_3 eluate. The susceptibility of elastin to elastase was found to be directly proportional to the duration of exposure to ultraviolet irradiation, as determined by the rate of solubilization, although the degree of elastin degradation to dialysable fragments during the brief exposure to elastase was similar for all preparations (Fig. 4). All elastin preparations were eventually dissolved completely.

DISCUSSION

That tyrosine may be implicated in cross-linking of collagen is suggested by the work of Schmitt (8), who found that the removal of tyrosine-rich peptides at the ends of collagen chains prevents end-to-end aggregation, and, more directly, by Bensusan (9) who reported increased aggregation of procollagen by prior iodination of the protein.

The present findings tend to support the hypothesis that a fluorescent component, common to collagen and elastin, is derived from the oxidation of tyrosine. Iodination of proteins under the conditions described is generally

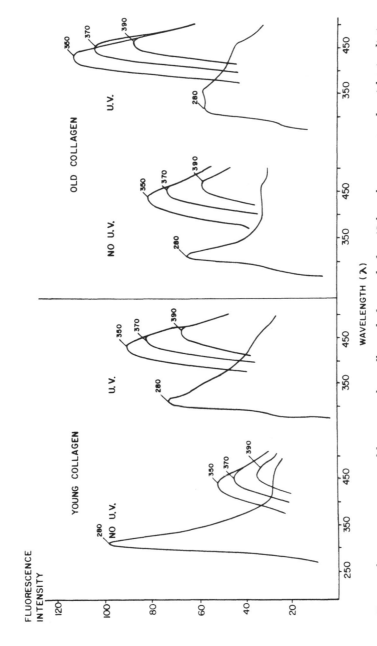

Fɪɢ. 1. Fluorescence spectra of human tendon collagen before and after 48 hours' exposure to ultraviolet irradiation. Young: Pooled specimens from males aged 11–20 years. Old: Pooled specimens from males aged 81–90 years.

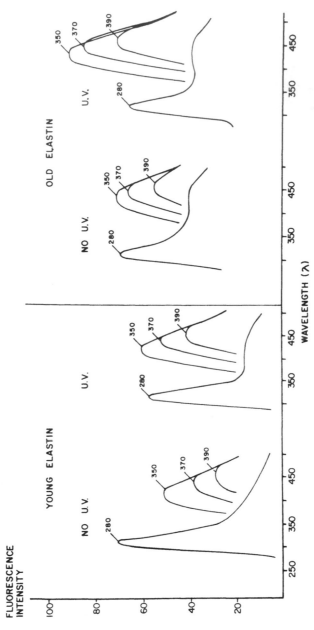

FIG. 2. Fluorescence spectra of human aortic elastin before and after 48 hours' exposure to ultraviolet irradiation. Young: Pooled specimens from males aged 11–20 years. Old: Pooled specimens from males aged 81–90 years.

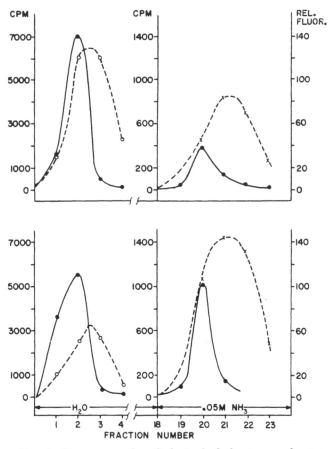

Fig. 3. Chromatography of elastin hydrolysates on alumina. An acid hydrolysate equivalent to 100 mg. of bovine ligamentum elastin was placed on an alumina column and eluted with water followed by 0.05M NH$_4$OH. Seventeen millilitre fractions were collected. Upper curves: I^{131}-elastin. Lower curves: Elastin treated with ultraviolet light for 48 hours and then iodinated with I^{131}; c.p.m.; o, fluorescence at 305 mμ; x, fluorescence at 405 mμ.

believed to occur at tyrosine (phenolic) residues with high specificity (9). Therefore, I^{131} associated with the fluorescent fractions eluted from alumina with ammonia would be expected to be substituted on a molecule related to tyrosine. The iodinated tyrosine and presumed iodinated tyrosine derivative appear to be eluted slightly earlier than the non-iodinated compounds. Ultraviolet treatment of the iodinated protein causes a shift of I^{131} from iodinated tyrosine in the water eluate to the presumed derivative in the NH$_3$ eluate, observations again consistent with the stated hypothesis of tyrosine transformation.

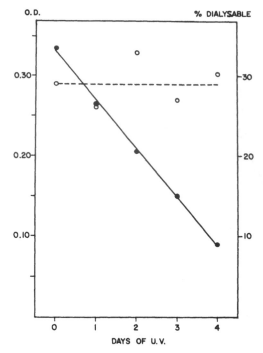

Fig. 4. Effect of 15-minute incubation with elastin on the solubilization (O.D.) and degradation (dialysable nitrogen) of elastin treated with ultraviolet light for varying periods. ●, O.D.; o, % nitrogen dialysable.

There are several fluorescent substances in elastin (10, 11), but at least one of these is also present in collagen, i.e., the presumed tyrosine derivative. In human collagen, the fluorescent component increases with age, whereas the tyrosine content diminishes, suggesting a relationship between the two (3). In human elastin, however, although this same fluorescence accumulates with age (5), tyrosine content is unaltered or even elevated in older preparations. One might speculate that the particular fluorescent substance in collagen is derived exclusively from tyrosine residues protruding from the protein molecule, whereas deposition of circulating tyrosine on elastin and its subsequent oxidation could account for the apparent lack of relationship between tyrosine content and fluorescence.

Quinones are known to be extremely reactive and to combine, for example, with NH_2 and SH groups (12). Benzoquinone-2-acetic acid, a metabolite of tyrosine, has been reported to add amino acids and amines at 1,4 positions *in vitro* (13). Tyrosine residues in peptides could presumably cross-link adjacent peptide chains as shown schematically in Fig. 5. A similar reaction might take place through incorporation of circulating phenols into collagen and elastin.

Accelerated cross-linking by ultraviolet irradiation might be expected to produce a protein substrate more resistant to enzyme attack. Ultraviolet-treated elastin, however, was more readily solubilized; increased susceptibility to proteolysis has been reported for other proteins, presumably due to rupture of some peptide bonds and unfolding of the peptide chains (14). Any possible increased cross-linking through tyrosine oxidation could be masked by the other actions of ultraviolet irradiation on powdered elastin.

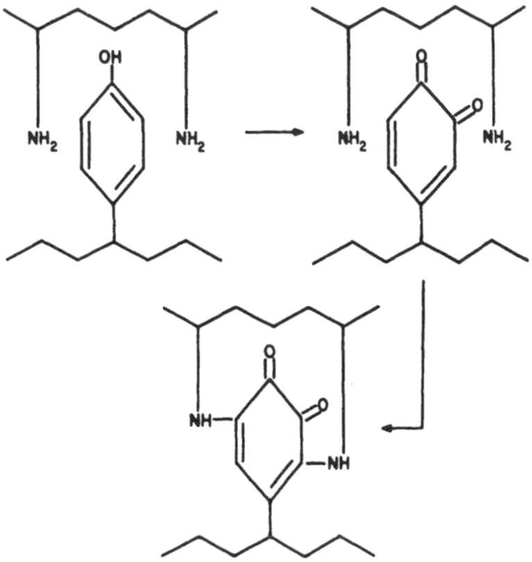

FIG. 5. Hypothetical reaction between derivative of a tyrosine residue of one peptide chain and functional groups on adjacent chains.

Collagen and elastin appear to be two distinct proteins as exemplified by their general amino acid compositions and their physical-chemical properties. However, there has long been the underlying suspicion that some relationship exists, more specifically that collagen may be a precursor for elastin synthesis. In any event, one definite similarity is found in the presence of a particular fluorescent compound referred to in this report. Although certain cross-linking mechanisms may be specific for one or the other protein, tyrosine oxidation to a reactive derivative may be common to both.

Mature collagen and elastin, once laid down, are essentially inert and may serve as a framework for the deposition of reactive, circulating metabolites such as quinones, phenols, aldehydes, unsaturated lipids, lipid peroxides, and others. All of these substances have been shown effectively to cross-link fibrous proteins *in vitro*, and support is accumulating for corresponding processes *in vivo*. Degenerative changes in the fibrous connective tissue proteins are prominent in many disease processes affecting animals and man. It seems likely that if, indeed, multiple chemical substances are concerned with cross-linking of collagen and elastin, then a number of metabolic defects could result in a premature or disorganized elaboration of the fibrous proteins. The processes responsible for the development as well as the degeneration of collagen and elastin may in fact be continuous processes. Certain pieces of evidence suggest this. The elucidation of the mechanism or mechanisms concerned with chemical modification of collagen and elastin *in vivo* seems to be essential for understanding diseases of connective tissue in general.

REFERENCES

1. GALLOP, P.   New York Heart Assoc. Symp. on Connective Tissue: Intercellular Macromolecules (Little, Brown & Co., Boston, 1964), p. 79.
2. THOMAS, J., ELSDEN, D. F., and PARTRIDGE, S. M.   Nature, *200*: 651 (1963).
3. LABELLA, F. S., and PAUL, G.   J. Gerontol. *20*: 54 (1965).
4. LABELLA, F. S.   Arch. Biochem. *93*: 72 (1961).
5. LABELLA, F. S., and LINDSAY, W. G.   J. Gerontol. *18*: 111 (1963).
6. PRYOR, M. G. M.   Proc. Roy. Soc. (London), Ser. B, *128*: 393 (1940).
7. ANDERSEN, S. O.   Biochem. et biophys. acta, *93*: 213 (1964).
8. SCHMITT, F. O.   Fed. Proc. *23*: 618 (1964).
9. BENSUSAN, H. B., and SCANU, A.   J. Am. Chem. Soc. *82*: 4990 (1960).
10. LABELLA, F. S.   J. Gerontol. *17*: 8 (1962).
11. THORNHILL, D. P., and LABELLA, F. S.   This Conference, preceding article.
12. GUSTAVSON, K. H.   The Chemistry of Tanning Processes (Academic Press, New York, 1956).
13. STONES, R., and BLIVASS, B. B.   Fed. Proc. *24*: 656 (1965).
14. GIESE, A. C.   Physiol. Rev. *30*: 431 (1950).

Comparison of Elastins from Various Sources[*]

R. A. ANWAR,
R. G. DONOVAN, and C. S. HANES

THERE ARE mainly two types of load-bearing protein fibres in animal connective tissue. One is collagenous in type and the other elastic. The amount and proportion of these two types of fibres vary from tissue to tissue. Further, these fibres are embedded in an amorphous ground substance which varies in composition from tissue to tissue.

The protein comprising the elastic fibre is called elastin. It is a very inert protein and is not known to go into solution in any solvent unless degraded. Because of its insolubility, the procedure for its isolation from any tissue is to remove everything possible by dissolution in different solvents and under various treatments; the material that remains insoluble after all these treatments is taken as elastin.

The proteins thus isolated from different tissues show differences in amino acid composition. For example, the protein isolated from bovine ligamentum nuchae is very low in acidic and basic amino acids, whereas the protein isolated from bovine aorta is higher in acidic and basic amino acids, while the amount of these amino acids is even higher in a protein isolated from bovine external ear (1, 2). These differences in amino acid composition and other minor differences have led to the suggestion that the structure of elastin from different tissues may be different.

But it can be argued that these differences may be due to incomplete removal of non-elastin components. For this purpose an analogy can be drawn between cellulose and elastin. Cellulose, as you are aware, is an important component of plants. Its structure and composition are well established. Isolation of cellulose is similar to that of elastin in the sense that non-cellulosic material is removed by dissolution under various treatments and the material left undissolved in cellulose. The degree of purity of the cellulose varies with the source and method of isolation. It is now a well-established fact that the differences between different cellulose preparations are due to incomplete removal of non-cellulosic components.

The same could be true in the case of elastin. The probability of this being

[*]From the Department of Biochemistry, University of Toronto, Toronto.

the case increases if important structural similarities can be shown to exist among the elastins isolated from different sources. The results of experiments carried out in our laboratory show that structural similarities among the proteins isolated from different sources do exist.

Experiments were carried out on elastins fom bovine ligamentum nuchae, human aorta, and rabbit ear. The amino acid composition of the three preparations is shown in the accompanying table (Table I). In all three specimens the most prominent amino acids in order of abundance were glycine, alanine, valine, proline, leucine (phenylalanine, isoleucine). It will be seen that the ligamentum nuchae elastin showed very low amounts of histidine, lysine, hydroxyproline, arginine, aspartic acid, threonine, and serine and no cystine or methionine. In contrast the human aorta and rabbit ear elastin showed considerably higher amounts of these amino acids. Incidentally the composition of the rabbit ear elastin in Table I is very similar to that reported for bovine ear elastin by Gotte *et al.* (2).

Recently, Partridge *et al.* (3, 4) have reported the isolation from bovine ligamentum nuchae elastin of two polyfunctional amino acids, namely desmosine and isodesmosine. These two amino acids are not known to be present in other proteins and they probably serve as cross-linking bodies in elastin. These amino acids can cross-link four polypeptide chains.

In the present work a method for the isolation of desmosine and isodesmosine has been developed. The application of this method to human aorta and rabbit ear elastin yielded in both cases desmosine and isodesmosine identical with those obtained from bovine ligamentum nuchae elastin. The desmosine obtained from these three different sources showed a characteristic ultraviolet absorption spectrum with maxima at 269 and 235 mμ and an inflexion at 275 mμ. Similarly, the ultraviolet absorption spectra of isodesmosine obtained from these three different sources were identical with a maximum at 280 mμ and an inflexion at 285μ in each case.

It is clear, therefore, that the elastin obtained from three different species and three different tissues contains both the desmosines, which are thought to be the cross-linking bodies.

Gotte *et al.* (2), using bovine ligamentum, bovine aorta, and bovine ear cartilage elastins, observed that after 72 hours' treatment with 0.5N NaOH at 25° C. the whole of the ear cartilage elastin had gone into solution, but during this period only 60 per cent of the aorta and 30 per cent of the ligamentum nuchae elastin had dissolved. These differences in the rates of hydrolysis were taken to suggest differences in the degree of cross-linking of the protein concerned. They felt that to release soluble peptide, more peptide bonds would have to be hydrolysed in a highly cross-linked protein than in one less highly cross-linked. If this explanation is correct, it should be valid also for the action of elastase on these different elastins. On the basis of this argument the pattern of dissolution of elastins from different sources with dilute alkali and with the enzyme elastase should be similar.

TABLE I

THE AMINO ACID COMPOSITION OF ELASTIN (RESIDUES/1000 RESIDUES)

Amino acid	Bovine ligamentum		Human aorta		Rabbit ear	
	Autoclaved	Solubilized with elastase	Autoclaved	Solubilized with elastase	Autoclaved	Solubilized with elastase
Glycine	332	356	301	304	284	277
Alanine	237	232	247	245	170	198
Valine	153	146	135	132	99	102
Proline	96	90	86	86	83	75
Leucine	63	61	63	64	76	76
Isoleucine	28	26	32	30	29	29
Phenylalanine	30	29	22	24	29	28
Glutamic acid	16	18	29	28	55	52
Aspartic acid	8	9	13	13	33	38
Serine	9	8	11	10	24	24
Threonine	9	9	19	16	24	25
Tyrosine	2	7	10	24	34	31
Arginine	7	5	13	12	24	18
Lysine	4	4	8	8	20	19
Histidine	1	Trace	4	1	8	6
Methionine	—	—	2	2	7	2
Cystine	—	—	—	—	—	—
Hydroxyproline	4	—	6	—	6	—

Investigations carried out with our three preparations of elastin (i.e. bovine ligamentum nuchae, human aorta, and rabbit ear) showed that the rates of dissolution in dilute alkali were similar to those observed by Gotte *et al.* The rate was highest with rabbit ear elastin, followed by human aorta elastin. Elastin from bovine ligamentum, which was solubilized most slowly in dilute alkali, however, was the only one of the three which was completely solubilized by elastase. A portion of the protein from human aorta elastin could not be solubilized and the amount left undissolved after the action of elastase was greatest from rabbit ear elastin. These observations suggest that the observed differences are probably not due to a different degree of cross-linking, but may reflect the presence of non-elastin component or components, which can be easily solubilized by dilute alkali and some of which cannot be acted upon by elastase.

When the values of desmosine and isodesmosine obtained from human aorta and rabbit ear elastin are corrected for components which may well be mere contaminants, they approach those obtained from bovine ligamentum nuchae elastin (i.e. desmosine 1.9 moles/1000 residues and isodesmosine 1.6 moles/1000 residues).

The peptides obtained after the action of elastase on three preparations of elastins were subjected to high-voltage electrophoresis on Whatman No. 3 paper, pH 3.5. On electrophoresis, each sample separated into the same number of bands.

It is not intended to suggest that the elastins from these three sources were identical. Some differences in different species can be expected and indeed peptide maps, obtained by electrophoresis in one direction and chromatography in the other, show minor differences among the three preparations. Although the peptide maps are not identical, yet they show many common major features.

In conclusion, all the above observations taken together suggest that elastins from three different organs and from three different species have chemical structures which are probably similar but not identical. It will be interesting to determine whether elastins prepared from different organs of the same species are identical.

ACKNOWLEDGMENTS

Our work on this subject in the Department of Biochemistry, University of Toronto, has received generous financial support from the National Research Council of Canada and the Medical Research Council of Canada.

REFERENCES

1. PARTRIDGE, S. M.   Advances Protein Chem. *17*: 227 (1962).
2. GOTTE, L., STERN, P., ELSDEN, M., and PARTRIDGE, S. M.   Biochem. J. *87*: 344 (1963).
3. PARTRIDGE, S. M., ELSDEN, D. F., and THOMAS, J.   Nature, *197*: 1297 (1963).
4. THOMAS, J., ELSDEN, D. F., and PARTRIDGE, S. M.   Nature, *200*: 651 (1963).

The Biosynthesis of Bovine
Submaxillary Mucin*

G. ROSS LAWFORD, B.A., and
HARRY SCHACHTER, B.A., M.D., PH.D.

THERE EXIST in animal tissues a great variety of hexosamine-containing macromolecules or mucosubstances (see Table I), composed of a polysaccharide moiety linked in various ways to a polypeptide backbone (1). The acidic mucopolysaccharides consist of polymers of hexuronic acid and N-acetylhexosamine linked to polypeptide by weak ionic forces or by labile covalent bonds; a recent report (2) has provided good evidence for an alkali-labile O-serine glycosidic linkage between chondroitin sulphate and polypeptide. In glycoproteins the carbohydrate moiety does not contain hexuronic acid or sulphate esters and can vary considerably in composition from one glycoprotein to another. The carbohydrate of glycoproteins is firmly linked to the protein backbone by covalent bonds; several glycoproteins have now been shown to contain an alkali-stable amide link between the beta-carboxyl group of asparagine and the first carbon of N-acetylglucosamine (1, 3–7).

TABLE I

MUCOSUBSTANCES DERIVED FROM ANIMAL TISSUES

1. Connective tissue acid mucopolysaccharides:
   Hyaluronic acid, chondroitin sulphates, heparin, keratosulphate

2. Glycoproteins:
   (a) Plasma glycoproteins:
       Orosomucoid, fetuin, haptoglobin, ceruloplasmin, 7S and 19S gamma globulins, transferrin, prothrombin, fibrinogen, etc.
   (b) Glycoprotein hormones:
       Interstitial-cell-stimulating hormone, follicle-stimulating hormone, the gonadotrophins, thyroid-stimulating hormone, thyroglobulin
   (c) Egg white glycoproteins:
       Ovalbumin, ovomucoid

3. Epithelially derived mucins:
   Mucins can be isolated from the mucous secretions of the salivary glands, tracheobronchial glands, gastro-intestinal mucous glands, and genito-urinary mucous glands

4. Blood group substances:
   Occur in red blood cells, ovarian cysts, meconium, etc.

*From the Department of Biochemistry, University of Toronto, Toronto.

The third group of mucosubstances listed in Table I is the mucins, a group of glycoproteins which usually contain more carbohydrate than the plasma glycoproteins and are usually highly viscous. The salivary mucins have been studied in several laboratories (8–10), and it appears that the predominant carbohydrate-protein link in the bovine and ovine submaxillary mucins is an alkali-labile glycosidic bond between hexosamine and the hydroxyl groups of serine and threonine; such a bond has also been reported for chrondroitin sulphate (2).

Figure 1 summarizes the present state of knowledge on the biosynthesis of mucosubstances (11, 12). It has been shown that the acidic mucopoly-saccharides are polydisperse molecules (13) which are synthesized from nucleotide sugar precursors by a non-template mechanism under the catalytic influence of various polymerase enzymes (11, 14, 15). Proteins, on the other hand, are synthesized on polyribosomes with messenger-RNA serving as a template (16). Little is known about the biosynthesis of glycoproteins although several laboratories have reported on the incorporation of label into glyco-

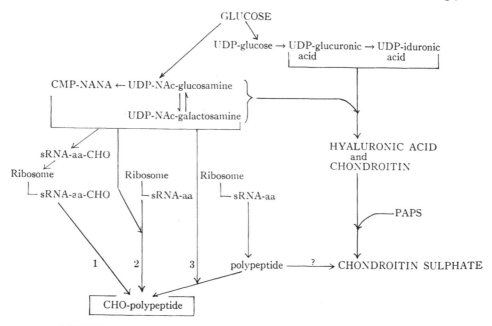

MUCINS & GLYCOPROTEINS

Fig. 1. A simplified scheme of the biosynthesis of mucosubstances (see references 1 and 12 for a more complete outline). The nucleotide sugars (of which only a few are shown in the figure) are probably the precursors of the polysaccharide moieties of glycoproteins. Three routes of attachment of carbohydrate to protein are possible: (1) pre-ribosomal, (2) ribosomal, (3) post-ribosomal (see text). Abbreviations: UDP = uridine diphosphate, PAPS = phosphoadenosinephosphosulphate, CMP = cytidine monophosphate, NANA = N-acetylneuraminic acid, N-Ac = N-acetyl, sRNA = soluble RNA, aa = amino acid, CHO = carbohydrate.

proteins by liver (1, 17–21) and by tumour cells (22, 23). We have studied the biosynthesis of a typical mucin, bovine submaxillary mucin (BSM), by gland slices (24) in an attempt to determine the subcellular sites of biosynthesis. Figure 1 indicates the three general routes by which polysaccharide (or, for that matter, any prosthetic group) can be attached to protein. First, carbohydrate may be attached to amino acid *before* the amino acid arrives at the polyribosome to be incorporated into protein (pre-ribosomal attachment). Second, carbohydrate may be attached to amino acid while the amino acid is being incorporated into protein on the polyribosome (ribosomal attachment). Third, carbohydrate may be attached to amino acid *after* the completed protein has left the polyribosome (post-ribosomal attachment). We have attempted to determine which of these three routes is followed in the biosynthesis of BSM, a well-characterized mucin (8, 25). Slices of submaxillary gland (500 mg. wet weight) were incubated for varying periods of time at 37° C. in 2.0 ml. of Krebs medium III (pH 7.4) containing 0.25 mM complete amino acid mixture and either ^{14}C-threonine or ^{14}C-glucosamine. The incubation was stopped by washing the slices with ice-cold 0.9 per cent saline solution, the slices were homogenized in a buffered 0.25M sucrose medium with an all-glass Duall tissue grinder, and the incorporation of label into various subcellular fractions was determined.

Figure 2 shows the incorporation of ^{14}C-threonine into BSM prepared by the Cetavlon (cetyl trimethylammonium bromide) method of Tsuiki *et al.* (25) at various times after the addition of tracer. Slice homogenates were also subjected to differential centrifugation (900g for 10 minutes, 16,000g for 15 minutes, and 105,000g for 60 minutes). The soluble supernatant was treated with trichloroacetic acid (TCA) at a final concentration of 6 per cent and a protein pellet obtained. This TCA-insoluble pellet and the three pellets obtained by differential centrifugation were washed with 12 per cent TCA followed by a chloroform–methanol–ether wash to remove lipid. The washed pellets were dissolved in 1N NaOH and aliquots were counted with a Packard TRI-CARB liquid scintillation counter. Figure 2 shows the total counts incorporated into these various fractions by 500-mg. slices. It is seen that BSM synthesis represents about a third of the total soluble protein synthesis. The incorporation is time-dependent and is still linear 60 minutes after addition of tracer. The intracellular concentration of TCA-soluble ^{14}C-threonine levels off within 10 minutes, indicating that diffusion of tracer into the cell occurs rapidly and is not limiting incorporation into protein. Tissue homogenates do not incorporate ^{14}C-threonine into protein under the conditions of these experiments.

Figure 2 shows that the 900g pellet is the only pellet showing significant incorporation of tracer into protein. The 900g pellet contains 85 per cent of the cell's particulate ribonucleic acid (RNA), and electron microscopy of this pellet revealed the presence of large amounts of rough endoplasmic reticulum

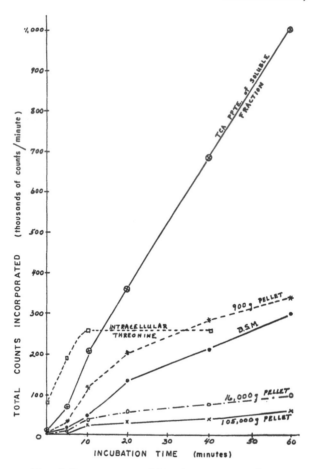

FIG. 2. Incorporation of ^{14}C-threonine into the protein
of various submaxillary gland fractions prepared as
described in the text.

(we are indebted to Drs. P. D. Sadowski and J. W. Steiner of the Pathology
Department, University of Toronto, for the electron micrographs). We concluded that the rough endoplasmic reticulum of bovine submaxillary gland is
tightly bound to the nuclei and sediments with the nuclei in the 900g pellet.
On treatment of the 900g pellet with sodium deoxycholate (DOC), it is
possible to isolate the subcellular fractions indicated in Fig. 3. Soluble BSM
(fraction C) and total soluble protein (fraction P) were prepared as described
above except that a mixture of TCA and phosphotungstic acid (PTA) was
used for all precipitations and acid washings instead of TCA alone. The DOC-
treated pellet was fractionated into a ribosomal fraction R, a "debris" fraction
D, and a DOC-soluble fraction S. Fraction S represents membrane-bound

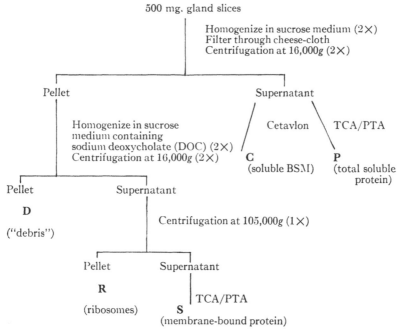

FIG. 3. Fractionation of bovine submaxillary gland slices into subcellular components.

material solubilized by the action of DOC on the membrane. Fractions P, D, R, and S were washed with TCA/PTA and with chloroform–methanol–ether. The resulting protein pellets and fraction C were counted and analysed for protein (26) in the case of ^{14}C-threonine incorporation and for hexosamine (27) in the case of ^{14}C-glucosamine incorporation; the specific activities of these fractions were calculated from the data. Table II shows that fraction R contains 41 per cent of the cell's particulate RNA. The ratio of optical densities at 260 and 280 mμ for fraction R was found to be between 1.7 and 1.8. Electron microscopy (by Drs. Sadowski and Steiner) indicated that fraction R contained mainly ribosomes 160 Å in diameter.

Figure 4 shows the results of ^{14}C-threonine incorporation into the protein of these fractions. Fractions R and S are rapidly labelled, indicating the presence of protein pools undergoing rapid turnover. Some recent unpublished experiments have indicated that protein is synthesized on the ribosomal fraction R, is subsequently transferred to the membrane fraction S, and from there enters the soluble protein pool. This sequence of events is analogous to the biosynthetic pathway of the secretory proteins of the exocrine pancreas (28).

Figure 5 shows that ^{14}C-glucosamine is incorporated at identical rates into both R and S, suggesting that both ribosomal and post-ribosomal attachment

TABLE II

CHEMICAL COMPOSITION OF SUBCELLULAR FRACTIONS OF BOVINE SUBMAXILLARY GLAND

Subcellular fraction	% particulate DNA	% particulate RNA	mg. protein (Prot.) in 500-mg. slices	mg. hexosamine (HA) in 500-mg. slices	HA/Prot.
105,000g pellet	8	12	—	—	—
16,000g pellet	92	88	6.9	0.29	—
D	55	34	4.1	0.06	0.016
S	27	13	1.7	0.19	0.11
R	10	41	1.1	0.04	0.037
C	—	—	2.5	0.95	0.38
P	—	—	10.8	0.86	0.080

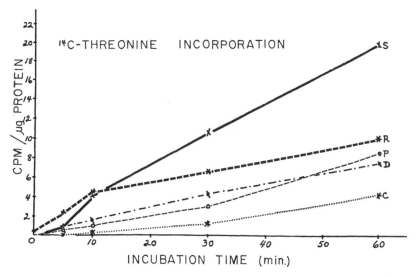

Fig. 4. Incorporation of ^{14}C-threonine into the protein of various submaxillary gland fractions prepared as described in the text. Radioactivity is expressed as counts per minute in the protein pellet per microgram of protein.

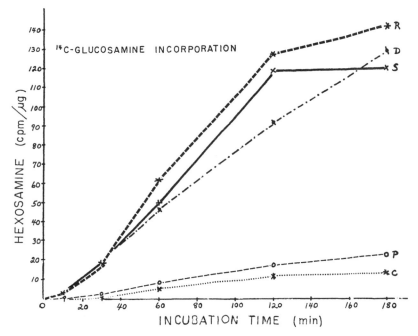

Fig. 5. Incorporation of ^{14}C-glucosamine into the protein of various submaxillary gland fractions prepared as described in the text. Radioactivity is expressed as counts per minute in protein-bound hexosamine per microgram of hexosamine.

of carbohydrate to protein may be occurring. This conclusion will remain tentative until the purity of the ribosomal fraction can be established.

Table III indicates that puromycin (29) inhibits both ^{14}C-threonine and ^{14}C-glucosamine incorporation into the protein of all fractions. This finding is compatible with all three routes of carbohydrate attachment to protein. However, Table III does suggest that the above incorporation studies represent *de novo* synthesis rather than an exchange phenomenon.

TABLE III

PER CENT INHIBITION OF INCORPORATION BY PUROMYCIN

Subcellular fraction	% inhibition of ^{14}C-glucosamine incorporation			% inhibition of ^{14}C-threonine incorporation		
C	73	81	94	76		90
P	62	61	84	68		78
R	56	56	93			
S	52	42	95	73†		99†
D	54	40	86			
Puromycin concentration* (μg./ml.)	25	25	50	25		100

*Puromycin was added 15 minutes prior to the addition of tracer.
†These figures were obtained with a fraction containing a mixture of R, S, and D.

In conclusion, we have described a system capable of synthesizing BSM, and our preliminary data indicate that protein is synthesized on ribosomes and then transferred to some sort of membrane before entering the soluble protein pool. Glucosamine is apparently incorporated both at the ribosomal and post-ribosomal stages of protein biosynthesis. We hope that elucidation of the pathways involved in the biosynthesis of glycoproteins may be of great importance to the understanding of connective tissue diseases.

REFERENCES

1. SPIRO, R. G.   New England J. Med. 269: 566, 616 (1963).
2. ANDERSON, B., HOFFMAN, P., and MEYER, K.   J. Biol. Chem. 240: 156 (1965); Biochim. et biophys. acta, 74: 309 (1963).
3. FLETCHER, A. P., MARKS, G. S., MARSHALL, R. D., and NEUBERGER, A.   Biochem. J. 87: 265 (1963).
4. MARKS, G. S., MARSHALL, R. D., and NEUBERGER, A.   Biochem. J. 87: 274 (1963); MARSHALL, R. D., and NEUBERGER, A., Biochemistry, 3: 1596 (1964).
5. YAMASHINA, I., and MAKINO, M.   J. Biochem. (Tokyo), 51: 359 (1962).
6. BOURRILON, R., GOT, R., and MEYER, D.   Biochim. et biophys. acta, 74: 255 (1963); 83: 178 (1964).
7. ROTHFUS, J. A., and SMITH, E. L.   J. Biol. Chem. 238: 1402 (1963).
8. HASHIMOTO, Y., and PIGMAN, W.   Ann. New York Acad. Sci. 93: 541 (1962); TANAKA, K., BERTOLINI, M., and PIGMAN, W.   Biochem. Biophys. Res. Comm. 16: 404 (1964); TANAKA, K., and PIGMAN, W.   J. Biol. Chem. 240: PC 1487 (1965).

9. BHAVANANDAN, V. P., BUDDECKE, E., CARUBELLI, R., and GOTTSCHALK, A.   Biochem. Biophys. Res. Comm. *16*: 353 (1964).
10. HARBON, S., HERMAN, G., ROSSIGNOL, B., JOLLÉS, P., and CLAUSER, H.   Biochem. Biophys. Res. Comm. *17*: 57 (1964).
11. DORFMAN, A.   Fed. Proc. *21*: 1070 (1962).
12. ROSEMAN, S.   Fed. Proc. *21*: 1075 (1962).
13. TANFORD, C., MARLER, E., JURY, E., and DAVIDSON, E. A.   J. Biol. Chem. *239*: 4034 (1964).
14. SILBERT, J. E.   J. Biol. Chem. *239*: 1310 (1964).
15. PERLMAN, R. L., TELSER, A., and DORFMAN, A.   J. Biol. Chem. *239*: 3623 (1964).
16. WATSON, J. D.   Bull. Soc. chim. biol. *46*: 1399 (1964).
17. SPIRO, R. G.   J. Biol. Chem. *234*; 742 (1959).
18. SARCIONE, E. J.   Biochemistry, *1*: 1132 (1962); J. Biol. Chem. *239*: 1686 (1964); SARCIONE, E. J., BOHNE, M., and LEAHY, M.   Biochemistry, *3*: 1973 (1964).
19. RICHMOND, J. E.   Biochemistry, *2*: 676 (1963).
20. SHETLAR, M. R., CAPPS, J. C., and HERN, D. L.   Biochim. et biophys. acta, *83*: 93 (1964).
21. ROBINSON, G. B., MOLNAR, J., and WINZLER, R. J.   J. Biol. Chem. *239*: 1134 (1964); MOLNAR, J., ROBINSON, G. B., and WINZLER, R. J.   J. Biol. Chem. *239*: 3157 (1964).
22. COOK, G. M. W., LAICO, M. T., and EYLAR, E. H.   Fed. Proc. *24*: 230 (1965).
23. SU-CHEN LI, YU-TEH LI, GEK-LIEN OEI, and SHETLAR, M. R.   Fed. Proc. *24*: 231 (1965).
24. LAWFORD, R., and SCHACHTER, H.   Fed. Proc. *24*: 231 (1965).
25. TSUIKI, S., HASHIMOTO, Y., and PIGMAN, W.   J. Biol. Chem. *236*: 2172 (1961).
26. LOWRY, O. H., ROSEBROUGH, N. J., FARR, A. L., and RANDALL, R. J.   J. Biol. Chem. *193*: 265 (1951).
27. BOAS, N. F.   J. Biol. Chem. *204*: 533 (1953).
28. CARO, L. G., and PALADE, G. E.   J. Cell Biol. *20*: 473 (1964).
29. NATHANS, D.   Fed. Proc. *23*: 984 (1964).

Effect of Inhibitors of
Protein Synthesis on the Plasma
Seromucoid and
Haptoglobin Levels of
Rats during Inflammation*

M. MAUNG, D. G. BAKER, and R. K. MURRAY

WINZLER (1) has defined the seromucoid fraction of plasma as that fraction not precipitable by 0.6M perchloric acid, but precipitable by 5 per cent phosphotungstic acid. This fraction contains a complex mixture of glycoproteins, and its clinical importance has recently been reviewed by Keyser (2). In his review, Keyser points out that elevations of this fraction have been reported in patients with cancer, rheumatoid arthritis, rheumatic fever, pulmonary tuberculosis, pneumonia, acute infections, trauma and myocardial infarction. Greenspan (3), in an earlier review, suggested that the concentration of seromucoid is dependent on the one hand on tissue responses such as inflammation, degeneration, or trauma, which raise the seromucoid concentration, and on the other on hepatic or endocrine hypofunction, which is associated with low concentrations. Of relevance to the present conference is the fact that in both rheumatoid arthritis and rheumatic fever a fairly characteristic elevation of this fraction is found, and Shetlar and Payne (4) have shown that this elevation may parallel the activity of rheumatoid arthritis. For this reason, measurement of the seromucoid fraction has been advocated by some clinicians as a test for following the activity of various rheumatic conditions.

Our laboratory has been interested for some time in the metabolism of this fraction in experimental animals. Neuhaus and Liu (5) have demonstrated that the seromucoid fraction of rat plasma contains six or seven glycoproteins, including haptoglobin. It has been our belief that further advances in understanding the mechanism and significance of the seromucoid changes during various disease processes will come largely from studies, both metabolic and structural, on the individual components of the fraction. Some years ago we

*From the Department of Biochemistry, University of Toronto, and Brookhaven National Laboratory, Long Island, New York.

showed that the subcutaneous injection of turpentine into rabbits produced a marked rise of plasma haptoglobin and also of total protein-bound carbohydrate (6). We have analysed purified rabbit haptoglobin and found it to be a typical plasma glycoprotein, containing 22 per cent carbohydrate, comprising galactose, mannose, glucosamine, and N-acetylneuraminic acid (7). Recent studies in our laboratory indicate that when rabbit haptoglobin is split into its constituent polypeptide chains by reduction of disulphide bonds in 8*M* urea, mercaptoethanol, and iodoacetamide (the method used by Smithies *et al.* (8) to separate the constituent chains of human haptoglobin) almost all of the carbohydrate is located in the larger of the two polypeptide chains (β chain). When the β chain is treated with pronase, a proteolytic enzyme of broad specificity, glycopeptides of relatively low molecular weight can be obtained by subjecting the incubation mixture to gel filtration. We hope to be able to determine the nature of the linkage of the carbohydrate to peptide in these fragments.

The problem we have attempted to answer in the present work is whether the increases of the total seromucoid fraction and of haptoglobin during experimental inflammation are due to *de novo* synthesis of these plasma glycoproteins or are due to release of them from damaged tissue. Work by Neuhaus (9), in which he studied amino acid incorporation into the seromucoid fraction *in vivo* suggested the former explanation. Our approach to this problem has been to study the effect of various inhibitors of protein synthesis on the response of the seromucoid fraction and of haptoglobin to experimental inflammation. The three agents selected for use were actinomycin D, ethionine, and puromycin. Actinomycin D is believed to inhibit protein synthesis by binding to DNA and thus interfering with DNA-directed messenger RNA formation (10). It may thus be used to evaluate the half-life of messenger RNA species for specific proteins and enzymes (11). Ethionine depletes the cellular level of ATP and thus inhibits protein synthesis by interfering with amino acid activation and messenger RNA formation (12). Puromycin has been shown to interfere with protein synthesis at the stage of involvement of soluble RNA (13).

The procedure for the experiments in which the effect of the three inhibitors of protein synthesis on the seromucoid response to subcutaneous injection of turpentine was studied is shown in Table I. The procedure for the similar experiments in which only the haptoglobin response was studied is given in Table II.

The dosages of the three agents used to inhibit protein synthesis were based on those used by Weber and Singhal (15).

The results we have obtained from the experiments on the effect of administration of actinomycin D, ethionine, or puromycin on the seromucoid response to experimental inflammation are shown in Table III. The normal level of the seromucoid fraction in rats was found to be 12.2 ± 2.4 mg. %

TABLE I

PROCEDURE OF EXPERIMENTS IN WHICH THE EFFECT OF INHIBITORS OF PROTEIN SYNTHESIS
ON THE SEROMUCOID RESPONSE TO INFLAMMATION WAS STUDIED

1. 200–220 gm. male Wistar rats used

2. All animals starved for 24 hours prior to the experiment

3. (a) Control rats injected with 0.5 ml. of turpentine subcutaneously
   (b) Test rats injected with 0.5 ml. of turpentine subcutaneously plus one of:
   1. Actinomycin D
   2. Ethionine
   3. Puromycin

4. All rats starved for a further 24 hours and then exsanguinated

5. Seromucoid fractions prepared and measured by the method of Winzler (1) and expressed as mg. % of hexose

TABLE II

PROCEDURE OF EXPERIMENTS IN WHICH THE EFFECT OF INHIBITORS OF PROTEIN SYNTHESIS
ON THE HAPTOGLOBIN RESPONSE TO INFLAMMATION WAS STUDIED

1. 80–100 gm. male Wistar rats used

2. All animals starved for 24 hours prior to the experiment

3. 0.5 ml. of blood taken by intracardiac puncture from all rats for initial plasma haptoglobin level

4. (a) Control rats injected with 0.2 ml. of turpentine subcutaneously
   (b) Test rats injected with 0.2 ml. of turpentine subcutaneously plus one of:
   1. Actinomycin D
   2. Ethionine
   3. Puromycin

5. All rats starved for another 24 hours and then exsanguinated

6. Haptoglobin levels determined on the final plasma sample

7. Haptoglobin levels determined by the method of Owen *et al.* (14) utilizing the peroxidatic activity of haemoglobin–haptoglobin complexes

TABLE III

EFFECT OF INHIBITORS OF PROTEIN SYNTHESIS ON THE SEROMUCOID
RESPONSE TO EXPERIMENTAL INFLAMMATION

	No. of rats	Mean seromucoid level*	P value
Normal	8	12.2±2.4	<0.001
Turpentine	7	38.1±6.1	
Turpentine + actinomycin D	19	27.5±7.5	≃0.001
Turpentine	11	36.3±3.2	
Turpentine + ethionine	7	9.9±2.9	<0.001
Turpentine	8	36.4±4.7	
Turpentine + puromycin	9	18.0±3.3	<0.001
Turpentine	22	34.3±5.3	

*The seromucoid level is expressed as mg. % hexose.

hexose. At 24 hours after the subcutaneous injection of turpentine the level had risen to 38.1 ± 6.1 mg. %. The corresponding values after administration of turpentine plus actinomycin D, ethionine, and puromycin were 27.5 ± 7.5, 9.9 ± 2.9, and 18.0 ± 3.3 mg. % respectively. Thus all three inhibitors inhibited the seromucoid response significantly.

In Table IV are shown the results from the experiments in which the effect of the three inhibitors on the haptoglobin response to turpentine injection was studied. The normal haptoglobin level was found to be approximately 60 mg. of haemoglobin-binding capacity %. At 24 hours after turpentine injection the plasma haptoglobin level had increased by approximately 75 mg. %. All three inhibitors completely suppressed this increase, puromycin actually producing a marked drop below the initial level.

TABLE IV

EFFECT OF INHIBITORS OF PROTEIN SYNTHESIS ON THE HAPTOGLOBIN (HP) RESPONSE TO EXPERIMENTAL INFLAMMATION

	No. of rats	Initial Hp*	24 hr. Hp	Δ 24 hr.
Turpentine	8	46.8±10.5	128.6±9.3	+81.8
Turpentine + actinomycin D	8	51.3±11.1	47.4±7.7	− 3.9
Turpentine	6	75.2±8.4	142.4±8.4	+67.2
Turpentine + ethionine	8	70.0±5.4	53.0±6.0	−17.0
Turpentine	6	64.0±6.0	140.0±8.5	+76.0
Turpentine + puromycin	7	81.0±12.8	38.0±7.9	−43.0

*Hp level expressed in mg. of haemoglobin-binding capacity %.
†Δ (24 hr.) = mean increase of Hp level after 24 hours.

These results demonstrate that whereas ethionine completely suppressed the seromucoid response to experimental inflammation, puromycin partially suppressed it and actinomycin D only affected it to a minor extent. The fact that ethionine could achieve such a complete inhibition suggests that the response was in fact due to increased protein synthesis rather than release from damaged tissue. This interpretation is supported by results from preliminary experiments in which the seromucoid response to injection of turpentine and ethionine was compared to the response to injection of turpentine alone. No significant difference in final seromucoid levels was found in these two groups of animals, indicating that the suppression of the seromucoid response by ethionine is not due solely to inhibition of the basal rate of synthesis of this fraction. This type of experiment is being extended to include the other two inhibitors and also the comparable effect on the haptoglobin response. The lesser inhibitions of the seromucoid response produced by the other two agents may reflect the fact that the doses of these agents were not sufficient to inhibit protein synthesis completely. Higher doses than that used in this group of experiments were found to result in a very high mortality. On the other hand, the only partial inhibition produced by actinomycin D may also be due to the possibility that the template stabilities of the messenger RNA species for most of the seromucoid fraction proteins are relatively stable (11).

All three inhibitors completely blocked the haptoglobin response, puromycin being the most effective. The dosage of actinomycin D and puromycin used in these experiments was slightly higher than that used in the corresponding studies on the seromucoid response, as it was found that the 80–100-gm. rats used for the haptoglobin studies could tolerate somewhat higher doses of these agents than could the 200-gm. rats used for the seromucoid studies. This fact may account for their greater efficacy in blocking the haptoglobin response.

We interpret the above results in the light of the following experimental findings by other workers. First, work by Neuhaus and Liu (6) indicates that the synthesis of the seromucoid fraction and of haptoglobin occurs primarily in the liver. Secondly, Neuhaus (9) has shown, by analysis of the specific activity of the plasma seromucoid fraction following injection of glycine-C^{14} into normal and injured rats, that the increase of this fraction in injured rats is probably due to increased synthesis in the liver. Thirdly, Zeldis et al. (16) have demonstrated that liver cell fractions from turpentine-treated rats show increased amino acid incorporation into protein in comparison with normal cell fractions in an in vitro system. Taken in conjunction with our present experiments in which the increase of both the seromucoid fraction and of haptoglobin was suppressed by inhibitors of protein synthesis, it would appear that during experimental inflammation the synthesis of glycoproteins in the liver is specifically stimulated.

What is the nature of this stimulus to glycoprotein synthesis? In their studies, Zeldis et al. (16) found that prednisone, a synthetic adrenal steroid, reproduced some of the features of stimulation of amino acid incorporation produced by turpentine injection. However, Krauss (17) has shown that the plasma level of haptoglobin of adrenalectomized rats increases after turpentine injection so that factors other than solely increased adrenocortical activity must be involved in the stimulation of haptoglobin production. Very recently, Sarcione et al. (18) have obtained evidence for the presence in acute phase plasma of a factor that markedly stimulates incorporation of radioactive amino acids and sugars into the seromucoid fraction by the isolated perfused rat liver. Characterization of the nature and source of this material, tentatively called seromucoprotein, will be an important contribution to the understanding of the mechanism of increase of the seromucoid fraction in clinical and experimental inflammatory conditions.

This work was supported by the Medical Research Council of Canada and at BNL by the U.S. Atomic Energy Commission.

REFERENCES

1. WINZLER, R. Methods of Biochemical Analysis, vol. 2 (Interscience Publications, New York, 1955), p. 279.
2. KEYSER, J. W. Postgrad. Med. J. *40*: 184 (1964).
3. GREENSPAN, E. M. Advances Int. Med. 7: 101 (1955).
4. SHETLAR, M. R., and PAYNE, R. W. J. Lab. Clin. Med. *51*: 588 (1958).
5. NEUHAUS, O. W., and LIU, A. Y. Proc. Soc. Biol. & Exper. Med. *117*: 244 (1964).
6. MURRAY, R. K., and CONNELL, G. E. Nature, *186*: 86 (1960).
7. MAUNG, M., BAKER, D. G., and MURRAY, R. K. Proc. Can. Fed. Biol. Sci. 7 (No. 39): 18 (1964).
8. SMITHIES, O., CONNELL, G. E., and DIXON, G. H. Am. J. Human Genet. *14*: 14 (1962).
9. NEUHAUS, O. W. Fed. Proc. 22: 238 (1963).
10. GOLDBERG, I. H., and REICH, E. Fed. Proc. 23: 958 (1964).
11. PITOT, H. C. Perspectives Biol. & Med. *8*: 50 (1964).
12. FARBER, E., SHULL, K. H., VILLA-TREVINO, S., LOMBARDI, B., and THOMAS, M. Nature, *203*: 34 (1964).
13. NATHANS, D. Fed. Proc. 23: 984 (1964).
14. OWEN, J. A., BETTER, F. C., and HOBAN, J. J. Clin. Path. *13*: 163 (1960).
15. WEBER, G., and SINGHAL, R. Metabolism, *13*: 8 (1964).
16. ZELDIS, L. J., SMITH, G. S., MOYER, D. L., and MADDEN, S. C. Am. J. Path. *44*: 29a (1964).
17. KRAUSS, S. Proc. Soc. Biol. & Exper. Med. *112*: 552 (1962).
18. SARCIONE, E. J., BOHNE, M., and KRAUSS, S. Fed. Proc. 24: 230 (1965).

PART VII

Clinical Studies and Methods of Therapy
Chairman: Dr. J. A. Blais, Montreal

Involvement of the Pulmonary
Parenchyma in Rheumatoid Arthritis[*]

S. KIM, A. U. SARGENT, R. E. DONEVAN,
M. BOISVERT, M. NEWHOUSE, and L. JOHNSON

NUMEROUS CASE REPORTS and autopsy studies documenting the involvement of the pulmonary parenchyma by the rheumatoid process have been published (1–5). Despite these studies, the lung manifestations of rheumatoid arthritis remain one of the most controversial of the constitutional manifestations associated with this disease. While there have been several reports of pulmonary function in rheumatoid patients selected on the basis of X-ray involvement (3, 4), to our knowledge there exists no report on the status of the pulmonary function of a general population of patients with rheumatoid disease selected irrespective of lung involvement. We have, therefore, studied 43 such patients, whose rheumatoid arthritis fulfilled the criteria established by the American Arthritis Association, from the outpatient clinic of the Royal Victoria Hospital. This group contained 15 men and 28 women ranging in age from 17 to 69 years, 81 per cent of whom had received steroid therapy during the course of their illness.

A chest X-ray was obtained on each patient, and the sera of each subject was examined for rheumatoid factor. Cellulose acetate electrophoresis was performed on sera obtained from 33 of the 43 patients. The following function studies were performed: forced expiration volume (referred to as $F.E.V._{0.75} \times 40$), maximal mid-expiratory flow rate (M.M.F.R.), and diffusing capacity (DCO) at rest. If the patient was capable of exercise on a bicycle ergometer, a diffusing capacity on exercise was also obtained.

Rheumatoid factor could be demonstrated in the sera of 40 of the 43 patients. Pulmonary fibrosis was diagnosed by chest X-ray in 5 of the 43 patients, 2 women and 3 men. In each instance the signs and symptoms referable to this condition preceded those of rheumatoid arthritis by at least one year. Positive L.E. cell tests could never be demonstrated with sera obtained from any one of the five patients. This incidence of fibrosis is higher than that reported by

[*]From the Division of Rheumatology, the Joint Cardiorespiratory Unit, and the Division of Immunochemistry, McGill University Clinic, Royal Victoria Hospital, Montreal.

other workers (4–7). It is possible that, as our hospital is recognized as a chest centre, our patient population may be biased in this regard.

A total of four patients (3 men and 1 woman) showed a resting diffusing capacity reduced by four units or more. The female was known to have bronchiectasis, while the X-rays of the three males showed pulmonary fibrosis. Two of these men also exhibited a reduced diffusing capacity on exercise; the other was not capable of exercise. In the 27 other patients in whom an exercise DCO could be performed, no such reduction could be detected. With the exception of those rheumatoid patients in whom the changes were radiologically demonstrable, the diffusing capacity did not reveal evidence of diffuse lung involvement.

The predominant abnormality in pulmonary function was a significant reduction in one or both measures of ventilatory function. Twenty-five per cent of our patients showed a significant reduction in M.M.F.R. and $F.E.V._{-0.75}$ $\times$ 40, thus suggesting the presence of obstructive lung disease. This was particularly striking among the women, in whom 32 per cent showed such reduction. A preliminary survey of the smoking habits of the patients revealed that, at least in women, our findings are unlikely to be due to smoking alone. No correlation existed between the duration of the disease and the degree of reduction of $F.E.V._{-0.75} \times 40$.

It is significant that Aronoff *et al.* (5), in a study of case histories, chest X-rays, and autopsy material derived from rheumatoid patients and carefully matched with non-rheumatoid controls, showed a greater incidence of lung disease (bronchitis, bronchiectasis, emphysema) in rheumatoid patients than in the control population. It should be noted that these disease states may be associated with abnormalities of ventilatory function similar to those we have reported.

While it is true that a clinic population may not be representative of rheumatoids in general, it is interesting that, employing two entirely different experimental approaches in two widely separated areas of the world, an increased incidence of obstructive lung disease in subjects with rheumatoid arthritis has been suggested.

REFERENCES

1. RUBIN, E. H.   Am. J. Med. *19*: 569 (1955).
2. NEWCOMER, A. D., MILLER, R. D., HEPPER, N. G., and CARTER, E. T.   Dis. Chest, *46*: 562 (1964).
3. CUDKOWICZ, L., MADOFF, I. M., and ABELMANN, W. H.   Brit. J. Dis. Chest, 55: 1 (1961).
4. PATTERSON, W. T., HORVILLE, W., and PIERCE, J.   Ann. Int. Med. *62*: 685 (1965).
5. ARONOFF, A., BYWATERS, E. G. L., and FEARNLEY, G. R.   Brit. M. J. *1*: 228 (1955).
6. TALBOTT, J. A., and CALKINS, E.   J.A.M.A. *189*: 911 (1964).
7. BRANNAN, H. M., GOOD, C. A., DIVERTIE, M. B., and BAGGENSTOSS, A. H.   J.A.M.A. *189*: 138 (1964).

DISCUSSION

Dr. Hart: Mr. Chairman, at the Sunnybrook Hospital we have been very much interested for the past one and a half years in the incidence of pulmonary fibrosis in rheumatoid arthritis, and we have studied two groups: one group of patients with rheumatoid arthritis and radiological evidence of pulmonary fibrosis, and for comparison a control group of rheumatoid arthritics who matched these patients in every respect, except that they had no pulmonary fibrosis. In many aspects I think that our studies agree with what Dr. Sargent has shown in his patients.

There were 20 patients in each group and there was a highly significant difference between the mean of their diffusions of carbon monoxide. The radiological picture is, we think, characteristic, although not pathognomonic, since it is known that there are certain conditions that can give rise to this sort of picture. In the absence of other provable disease, one must attribute it to the rheumatoid disease. This is a picture of a diffuse net-like fibrosis that usually starts in the lower lung fields in the lateral aspect of the lungs, and then seems to work its way medially.

The objections raised against the idea that pulmonary fibrosis is a part of the rheumatoid disease process seem to have been valid up to now, because there is still no good study of the prevalence in a large group of rheumatoid arthritics. We found that about 10 per cent of our selected patients with rheumatoid arthritis have pulmonary fibrosis.

Rheumatoid Pleural and Pulmonary Disease

C. A. GORDON, C. P. HANDFORTH, and
J. F. L. WOODBURY

SINCE 1947 it has been appreciated that pleural effusions and parenchymal pulmonary lesions of a rheumatoid nature occur in patients suffering from rheumatoid arthritis. The purpose of this presentation is to describe the types of pleural pulmonary disease encountered in 14 patients studied by us. We were surprised to recognize rheumatoid pneumoconiosis in over 1 per cent of the patients examined because of claims of industrial pulmonary disease.

RADIOLOGICAL FINDINGS

On radiological examination three main patterns of disease are recognized. First, when pleuritis is accompanied by effusion, this may be evident in the chest X-ray. Secondly, the radiograph may show what appears to be diffuse interstitial pulmonary fibrosis, and this may, or may not, be accompanied by small nodular shadows up to 4 mm. in diameter. This appearance is non-specific, and its identification with the rheumatoid disease process can only be confirmed by microscopic examination of the tissue. Examples of cavitary disease in these patients could lead to a suspicion of pulmonary tuberculosis based on an erroneous interpretation of the radiological finding. Thirdly, there may be evidence of the large nodules described by Caplan (1) in association with pneumoconiosis.

PATHOLOGICAL FINDINGS

A pathological study of patients exhibiting pleuritis may demonstrate nodules located on visceral pleura and in the subjacent lung, with histological features similar to those of rheumatoid nodules occurring in subcutaneous tissues.

In cases showing evidence of parenchymatous pulmonary change, diffuse interstitial fibrosis of the lung may be present, and biopsy or autopsy may also demonstrate granulomatous lesions in the lung, identical in appearance with rheumatoid nodules. This microscopic appearance is not sufficiently specific to warrant a diagnosis of rheumatoid disease, although it strongly suggests it. Other forms of granulomatous inflammation, particularly the so-called collagen diseases and pulmonary tuberculosis, can produce similar appearances and must be excluded by culture for *Mycobacterium tuberculosis* and consideration of the over-all clinical picture.

CASE PRESENTATIONS

Two patients had *pleural effusions without radiological evidence of associated lung disease*. One had bilateral pleural effusion necessitating the repeated removal of very large quantities of pleural fluid. Tests of the pleura fluid were negative for *M. tuberculosis*, punch biopsy of the pleura revealed non-specific inflammatory cells, and histological and cultural examination of the tissue failed to reveal evidence of tuberculosis or malignancy.

Pleural effusion without radiological evidence of pulmonary parenchymal disease occurred in a second patient. It was suspected that he was suffering from the arteritis of rheumatoid disease. Tart cells but no true L.E. cells were demonstrated.

APPARENT FIBROSIS WITH OR WITHOUT NODULATION

Figure 1 shows diffuse nodulation in the lungs of a patient whose pulmonary disease was present for several years before his subcutaneous nodules (proven by biopsy) and his peripheral joint arthritis made their appearance. This man has been followed up; his arthritis has improved during gold salt therapy, and the X-ray picture has shown improvement. His vital capacity and the mechanics of his breathing have also improved, but his slight alveolocapillary diffusion defect persists unaltered.

In one other patient suffering from diffuse nodular lung disease, evidence of improvement has been demonstrated in the chest X-rays coinciding with lessening of the activity of peripheral joint arthritis during gold salt therapy.

PNEUMOCONIOSIS

Pneumoconiosis is apparently modified by the presence of rheumatoid disease. Some of the patients develop multiple well-defined round radio-opacities measuring from ½ to 5 cm. in diameter throughout both lung fields. This X-ray finding was first identified with rheumatoid disease by Caplan in 1953 (1). These opacities are often quite apparent, while in the background the evidence of pneumoconiosis may be slight or absent. The opacities tend to increase in size and number, fresh crops appearing very quickly at intervals of

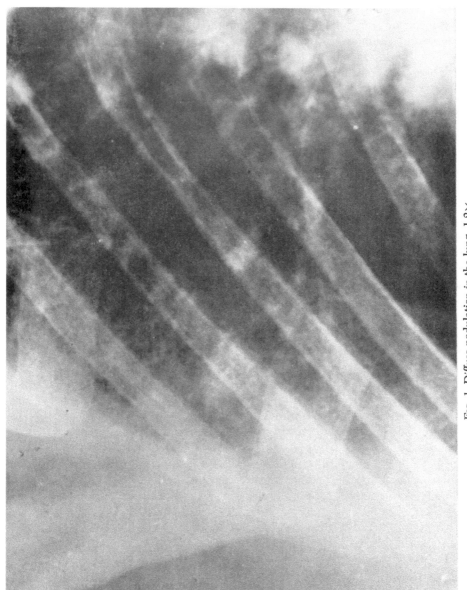

Fig. 1. Diffuse nodulation in the lung. 1.2×.

a few months. It is not uncommon for the lesions to cavitate, sometimes disappearing completely in the process. Calcification of lesions may occur, and if the cases are followed it is discovered that massive fibrosis develops.

A Cape Breton coal-miner had a long history of exposure to silica-rock dust. His chest X-ray when first observed by us showed large nodular opacities as well as the diffuse small nodules seen in silicosis. X-rays of his wrists showed extreme erosions of the bones. He had axillary and epitrochlear lymphadenopathy. Biopsy of the lymph nodes revealed only non-specific fibrosis. The sheep-cell agglutination test for rheumatoid arthritis was positive. The patient was hospitalized for rest, physiotherapy, and treatment with chloroquine and salicylates. Although great improvement in general health and in his joint inflammations ensued, the pulmonary findings did not change. Prednisone was given in a dose of 60 mg. per day, in an effort to determine whether the size of the radio-opacities could be decreased, but the pulmonary lesions appeared not to change. A chest X-ray taken four years after he came under our observation (Fig. 2) shows progression to the late stage of Caplan's syndrome with diffuse fibrosis, large nodules, and cavitation in the left upper lobe. Two years later the patient died of respiratory failure. A most assiduous search for morphological and cultural evidence of tuberculosis yielded entirely negative results.

NON-PULMONARY ASPECTS

Every one of our 14 patients was a white male, and, with one exception, the age of onset was over 40 years (Table I). The exception was the patient with arteritis, pleural effusion, tart cells, and no evidence of parenchymatous lung disease.

TABLE I

NUMBER OF PATIENTS WITH RHEUMATOID PULMONARY DISEASE (OUT OF A TOTAL OF 14) WITH INFLAMED PERIPHERAL JOINTS, POSITIVITY OF LATEX PARTICLE AND SENSITIZED SHEEP-CELL AGGLUTINATION TESTS, AND SUBCUTANEOUS RHEUMATOID NODULES

	Present	Absent
Inflamed peripheral joints	14	0
Age at onset over 40	13	1
Positive latex agglutination test	9	0
Positive sheep-cell agglutination test	9	1
Subcutaneous rheumatoid nodules	8	3

Some of the early cases were studied primarily from the pulmonary standpoint. Agglutination tests were not being done when some first came under observation; however, in all patients in whom the tests were carried out, an agglutination test was positive. All had involvement of the peripheral joints, and in eight cases the cervical spine was also affected. None had Marie

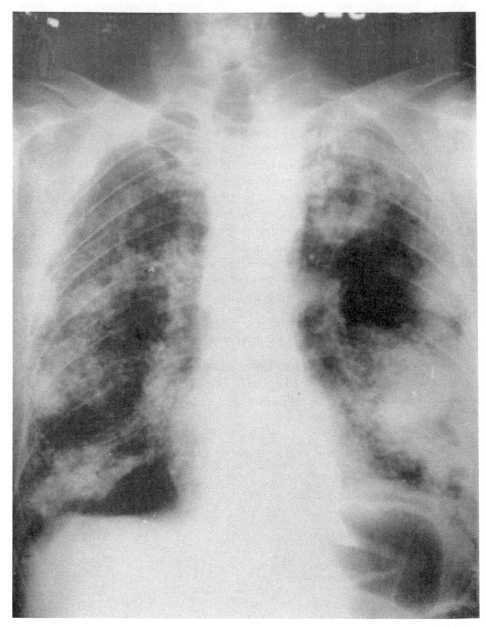

FIG. 2. Caplan's syndrome (late stage), showing diffuse fibrosis, large nodules, and cavitation in the left upper lobe.

Strumpell spondylitis, none showed true L.E. cells, and all had an elevated erythrocyte sedimentation rate.

PULMONARY FUNCTION STUDIES

These studies showed a reduction in vital capacity and in the mechanics of breathing with some diffusion defect. (The presence of alveolocapillary block is demonstrated by the employment of the steady-state carbon monoxide method of Krogh in a modified form.)

SUMMARY

1. Rheumatoid pulmonary disease is likely to occur in males with positive agglutination tests for rheumatoid disease and arthritis of the peripheral joints. Pleural effusions or parenchymatous lung lesions of several types occur and appear to be an integral part of the rheumatoid disease process. The pleuropulmonary respiratory manifestation may even be the presenting feature.

2. Diffuse interstitial pulmonary fibrosis is non-specific, and when encountered in arthritic patients its rheumatoid identity can only be confirmed by examination of the tissue under a microscope. The presence of cavitation and/or calcification is compatible with rheumatoid pulmonary disease.

3. There may be clinical and radiological improvement in the lungs of patients with non-pneumoniotic rheumatoid lung disease. In these instances pulmonary-function studies may show improvement in the lung volumes and mechanics of breathing, but the diffusion defect persists.

4. In workers exposed to various industrial dusts, pneumoconiosis appears to be altered by the presence of rheumatoid disease. Rheumatoid pneumoconiosis is progressive and will lead to respiratory failure and death.

REFERENCE

1. CAPLAN, A.   Certain unusual radiological appearances in the chest of coal-miners suffering from rheumatoid arthritis. Thorax, 8: 29 (1953).

Studies on the Anti-Inflammatory
Activity of
Alkoxyglycerols in Rats*

R. G. BURFORD† and C. W. GOWDEY

IN 1922 Japanese investigators (1) found three distinct compounds of the alkoxyglycerol configuration in the unsaponifiable fraction of certain fish-liver oils (notably the shark). They named these compounds batyl, selachyl, and chimyl alcohol.

Figure 1 shows the molecular structure of these oil-soluble alkoxyglycerols; it is apparent that each of these three compounds is made up of one molecule of glycerol and one of several long-chain fatty alcohols attached by a strong ether–oxygen link. Batyl alcohol contains a fully saturated C_{18} side chain and chimyl alcohol has a saturated C_{16} side chain, whereas the C_{18} side chain of

CHIMYL ALCOHOL (3-(hexadecyloxy)-1,2-propanediol)

$CH_2OCH_2(CH_2)_{14}CH_3$
|
$CHOH$
|
CH_2OH

BATYL ALCOHOL (3-(octadecyloxy)-1,2-propanediol)

$CH_2OCH_2(CH_2)_{16}CH_3$
|
$CHOH$
|
CH_2OH

SELACHYL ALCOHOL ("cis" 3-(9-(octadecenyloxy)-1,2-propanediol)

$CH_2OCH_2(CH_2)_7CH{=}CH(CH_2)_7CH_3$
|
$CHOH$
|
CH_2OH

FIG. 1. The molecular structure of alkoxyglycerols.

*From the Department of Pharmacology, University of Western Ontario, London, Ontario Supported by a grant-in-aid from the Medical Research Council of Canada.
†Present address: Bio-Research Laboratories, Pointe Claire, Quebec.

selachyl alcohol contains one double bond which makes this compound a liquid at room temperature.

Most of the work done so far on these compounds has been concerned with their chemistry and detection. Although the alkoxyglycerols were found first in the liver oils of Elasmobranch fishes, they have subsequently been found in the body-cavity fat of the rat, the egg yolks of the domestic hen, the yellow bone marrow of cattle, and the spleen of pigs, in erythrocytes and arteriosclerotic arteries of man and in human meconium, but not in human liver. It appears that these substances are found only in tissues of mesenchymal origin.

The detection of batyl and selachyl alcohol in the reticulo-endothelial system has led to a search for the possible role that these compounds might play in radiation-induced leucopenia and in leukaemia and inflammation. It is the possible anti-inflammatory action of these substances that we have investigated.

METHODS

There are many techniques for assessing anti-inflammatory activity, and all of them are plagued with inherent difficulties of interpretation. However, one of the most widely used methods is that of the rat granuloma pouch, first described by Selye (2) and later modified by Robert and Nezamis (3). To date we have carried out most of our anti-inflammatory studies using this technique with male rats of the Sprague–Dawley strain; food and water were provided ad libitum throughout the study. A pouch is made by injecting 30 ml. of air subcutaneously into the back of an anaesthetized rat so that the skin is lifted away from the muscle mass. As an irritant to the muscle layer 0.5 ml. of a 1 per cent solution of croton oil dissolved in cottonseed oil is injected into the pouch. The pouch, of course, provides a reasonably constant cavity size and facilitates spreading of the irritant. Forty-eight hours later the pouch is deflated and three days after that, the animals are sacrificed and the volume of fluid exudate in the cavity is carefully measured. Drugs to be tested were usually administered by gavage once a day for four days commencing within one hour of the pouch formation. Their anti-inflammatory activity was measured by the degree of suppression of the exudate compared with that in the control animals. The alkoxyglycerols were usually dissolved in olive or cottonseed oil and the control rats received similar amounts of these oil vehicles. However, for comparison with hydrocortisone acetate suspensions, saline controls were also used. For comparison of the alkoxyglycerols with other agents such as acetylsalicylic acid, phenylbutazone, etc., suspensions were made in Tween 80 and water and compared with the vehicle itself. Since preliminary experiments showed no detectable anti-inflammatory activity with any of the vehicles (olive oil or cottonseed, saline or Tween 80 in water), these various controls are not shown in the figures.

RESULTS

Figure 2 summarizes the results of treatment with batyl and selachyl alcohol using old, heavy rats. For comparison, hydrocortisone-treated animals are also shown. It can be seen immediately that all dosage levels tested of the three compounds were significantly anti-inflammatory when compared with controls, but there seemed to be no simple relation between the dose and the degree of effect. Furthermore, it is evident that at a dose of 0.7 mg./kg./day, both batyl and selachyl alcohol are as potent as hydrocortisone.

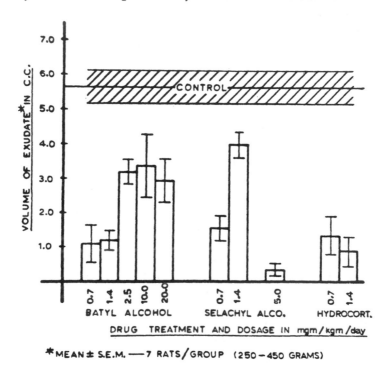

*MEAN ± S.E.M. ——7 RATS/GROUP (250-450 GRAMS)

FIG. 2. The effect of treatment on the seven-day granuloma pouch.

Figure 3 summarizes the effect of treatment on the four-day granuloma pouch and compares this effect in both young and old animals. In the young rats shown on the left, only selachyl alcohol was significantly anti-inflammatory at all dose levels. Because of the large standard errors, it is apparent that at low doses in young rats there is no significant difference, mg. for mg., in the anti-inflammatory activity of selachyl alcohol and hydrocortisone, but at the higher dose levels hydrocortisone does appear more effective.

In old rats depicted on the right-hand side, it is plain that all doses of all three compounds showed significant anti-inflammatory activity and all were

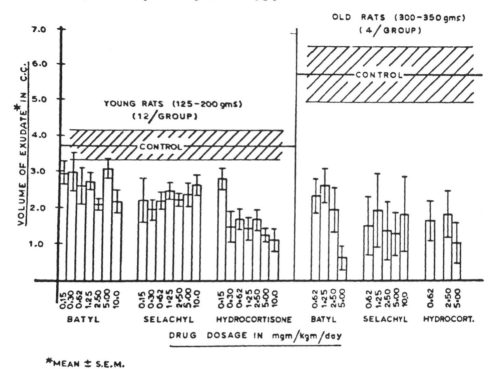

FIG. 3. The effect of treatment on the four-day granuloma pouch.

about equally potent. It is interesting to note that in the older animals selachyl alcohol is just as potent as hydrocortisone at any dose level.

If we now compare the response of the older animals to that of the younger animals, it is apparent that the exudate volume of the older controls is significantly larger than that of the younger animals. It is also apparent that most of the dose levels allowed about the same volume of exudate to be formed in both young and old animals. However, if we calculate the *per cent inhibition* of the inflammatory response, for 2.5 mg./kg./day of selachyl alcohol for example, we obtain a 39 per cent inhibition in young rats compared with a 76 per cent inhibition in the older animals. This, of course, is due to a seemingly greater inflammatory response of the older animals to the same dose of irritant. It may be seen that alkoxyglycerols, hydrocortisone, and phenylbutazone, as we shall see, do not completely suppress the inflammatory reaction, but that their relative degree of effectiveness is somehow related to the subject's own ability to counteract the inflammatory stimulus and, further, that this ability could be modified by an age factor.

Figure 4 shows the effects of salicylate alone and in combination with selachyl alcohol on the four-day granuloma pouch. In this experiment the

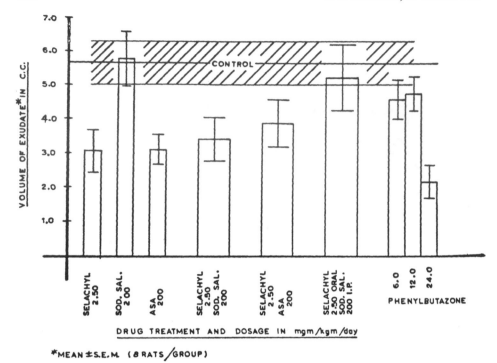

FIG. 4. The effect of various treatments on the four-day granuloma pouch.

treatment vehicle was Tween 80 and the rats weighed between 250 and 350 gm. Salicylate was administered in two different forms, as sodium salicylate and as acetylsalicylic acid, but in each case the dose administered was calculated in terms of salicylate. The dose chosen was 200 mg./kg./day salicylate. Also, all drug treatment, with the exception of phenylbutazone, was administered orally in divided doses, three times per day; the figures on the graph show the total dosage per day. Phenylbutazone was administered only once a day.

It is apparent from this chart that selachyl alcohol and acetylsalicylic acid alone significantly suppressed the induced inflammation, whereas sodium salicylate had no obvious effect. On the other hand, when selachyl alcohol and acetylsalicylic acid were combined and administered together orally, the effect was no greater, and was possibly even less than with either substance alone. The combination of selachyl alcohol and sodium salicylate, when administered together orally, also showed a significant anti-inflammatory effect, but it was not different from that of selachyl alcohol alone. For some unknown reason, when the selachyl alcohol was given orally and the sodium salicylate by intraperitoneal injection, the anti-inflammatory effect shown originally by oral administration of this combination disappeared.

The right-hand side of the figure shows the effect of phenylbutazone. Only the highest tested dose of this compound showed a significant effect, and by comparing this effect with that of selachyl alcohol on the extreme left-hand side, it can be seen that there is no real difference. Thus selachyl alcohol in this experiment was almost 10 times as effective, mg. for mg., as phenylbutazone on the granuloma-pouch inflammation.

Another test for anti-inflammatory activity described by Winter in 1962 (4) involves the production of local oedema by another irritant, carrageenan. In this test, 0.05 ml. of a 1 per cent solution of carrageenan (a mucopolysaccharide derived from Irish sea moss) is injected into the plantar tissue of the hind paw of the rat. The volume of the foot is measured immediately after injection of the phlogistic agent and again three hours later when maximum oedema has occurred. Drugs to be tested for their anti-inflammatory activity are usually administered orally one hour prior to injection of the carrageenan and the degree of inhibition of the oedematous response is a measure of the anti-inflammatory activity.

A number of experiments were carried out using various anti-inflammatory drugs at different dosages and given at various times in relation to the carrageenan injection. Since both oil- and water-soluble drugs were to be tested, the vehicle chosen was Tween 80 in water. In none of these experiments did either selachyl or batyl alcohol show significant anti-inflammatory activity, but hydrocortisone acetate suspensions in saline were effective. However, in

TABLE I

THE EFFECT OF TREATMENT ON THE RAT FOOT CARRAGEENAN INFLAMMATION
(Weight range: 175–225 gm.)

Pre-oral treatment 1 hour prior to carrageenan	Number of animals	Change in foot size at 3 hours (ml.), Mean ± S.E.M.	P value	Mean per cent inhibition
Controls, olive oil, 1 ml.	14	0.85±0.06	—	—
Batyl alcohol, 10 mg./kg.	15	0.85±0.19	—	—
Batyl alcohol, 20 mg./kg.	14	0.71±0.05	<0.05	16
Hydrocortisone acetate, 10 mg./kg.	15	0.68±0.06	<0.001	20

one experiment, shown in Table I, batyl alcohol was dissolved in olive oil and compared with olive oil controls and hydrocortisone acetate suspensions. It is evident from the results shown in this table that both the higher dose of batyl alcohol and the hydrocortisone were effective in reducing the inflammatory response. The per cent inhibition of the oedema by batyl alcohol was somewhat lower than that for the hydrocortisone, even though the dose of batyl alcohol was twice that of hydrocortisone. Further work using this test is planned.

SUMMARY

It is clear from our results that both batyl and selachyl alcohol have significant anti-inflammatory activity in the experimental rat granuloma pouch. Indeed selachyl alcohol is approximately as potent as hydrocortisone. From these results it appears that a clinical trial is warranted, but the prediction of efficacy in human subjects cannot be made with certainty from the results of experiments in animals. Experience in the past has shown that the granuloma-pouch assay, although it responds well to corticosteroids, is rather insensitive to non-steroids. Large doses of the latter are needed and the dose-response curves are rather flat.

No ideal reliable screening method yet exists. Most methods involve oedema of the rat paw induced by a host of irritants varying from formalin, egg powder, and foreign proteins to dextran, kaolin, and carrageenan. But, as Rosenkilde (5) says, many compounds with activities that are not anti-inflammatory are known to reduce the swelling and in some instances the method may fail to indicate anti-inflammatory activity. The fact is that in the laboratory anti-inflammatory drugs are elusive agents because so far we are unaware of any structural characteristics to which their activity can be attributed. Moreover, it hardly needs emphasizing that we lack precise knowledge of inflammation. Rosenkilde puts it this way: "in screening for anti-inflammatory activity we try to detect, without a clue to its identity, a compound that will suppress in a specific (and as yet wholly obscure) manner, signs of an acute or subacute inflammatory reaction artificially induced in laboratory animals. Thereby we demonstrate an action of questionable therapeutic usefulness but potentially valuable because of its empiric relationship to hitherto unexplained beneficial effects in patients suffering from chronic diseases with connective tissue manifestations of unknown etiology" (5, p. 492).

REFERENCES

1. Tsujimoto, M., and Toyama, Y.   Chem. Umschau, 29: 27–29, 43–45 (1922).
2. Selye, H.   J.A.M.A. 152: 1207, 1212 (1953).
3. Robert, A., and Nezamis, J. F.   Acta endocrinol. 25: 105–12 (1957).
4. Winter, C. A., Risley, E. A., and Nuss, G. W.   Proc. Soc. Exper. Biol. & Med. 111: 544–97 (1962).
5. Rosenkilde, H.   Animal techniques for evaluating anti-inflammatory drugs. In Animal and Clinical Pharmacologic Techniques in Drug Evaluation, edited by J. H. Nodine and P. E. Siegler (Year Book Medical Publishers, Chicago, 1964).

The Effect of
Chelation Therapy on
Rheumatoid Arthritis*

LYLA LEIPZIG, M.D.,† D. S. McCANN, PH.D.,
R. E. MOSHER, PH.D.,‡ and A. J. BOYLE, M.D., PH.D.

THE GROUPING TOGETHER of certain syndromes under the general heading of collagen diseases (or more recently connective tissue diseases) is about 20 years old (1). The common denominator associated with these maladies is fibrinoid changes of extracellular connective tissue, often accompanied or followed by calcification. Aside from the local changes in connective tissue, several of this group, such as rheumatoid arthritis and systemic lupus erthematosus, tend to show characteristic serum factors. These have not only been exploited rather successfully for diagnostic purposes, but have lent considerable support to the hypothesis that the diseases result from autosensitization.

Whether the aetiology of rheumatoid arthritis is due to an antigen producing a rheumatoid factor and whether this antigen is endogenous or exogenous remains the object of much research. It is our feeling that such an antigen may be the result of ground-substance abnormality which mechanically inhibits cellular metabolism which in turn gives rise to chronic cellular debris foreign to the normal protein of the organism. The suggestion is that rheumatoid arthritis is fundamentally a metabolic disturbance of connective tissue.

A successful permanent "cure" has not yet been found for rheumatoid arthritis. We would, nevertheless, like to add to the existing concepts some challenging observations that have been made through the use of a chelating compound, ethylenediaminetetracetic acid (EDTA).

Our laboratory interest in EDTA extends over a number of years. Very early in our experience with this compound it was recognized that it passes through the animal body virtually unchanged. Given orally it does not pass into the blood stream but remains in the faeces; given intravenously it remains in the extracellular fluid and is rapidly excreted in the urine. Sufficient experimentation with the compound suggested the sodium salt as a potential

*From the Department of Chemistry, Wayne State University, Detroit, Michigan.
†Public Health Service research fellow.
‡Providence Hospital, Detroit, Michigan.

parathyroid-stimulating agent since it binds or chelates calcium ion. The ion so bound becomes physiologically inactive and is subsequently excreted as the calcium EDTA. Theoretically, sodium EDTA introduced parenterally often enough and in sufficient quantities could have a stimulating influence on the parathyroid glands, which respond to lowered serum calcium ion.

Recent literature on parathyroid activity suggests that parathormone de-polymerizes mucopolysaccharides and that the influence of this hormone may be general over ground substance present in the animal organism and not specialized with respect to bone (2–8). The story of blood citrate levels and parathyroid activity is a relatively new one and it seems to be well founded. Phosphate exchange between cells and extracellular fluid encouraged by para-thormone may be indicative of some relation between the synthesis and degradation of connective tissue substance. Of particular interest to us has been the experimental observation that glucocorticoids depress blood citrate and calcium levels in animals otherwise stimulated by parathormone (9). The cystic bone disease of the hyperparathyroid patient and the gross tissue calcifi-cation of the hypoparathyroid subject represent the extremes of parathyroid influence on connective tissue. The level of optimum parathyroid activity appears to be worth investigating. As in all borderline abnormalities, shades of difference are difficult to detect. This remains for the development of more delicate tests and techniques. It seemed to us that in the instance of rheuma-toid arthritis one might obtain some clue as to whether the connective tissue involved would be benefited by parathyroid stimulation. It is well known that the pregnant patient suffering from rheumatoid arthritis may experience a remission of symptoms. This phenomenon was credited to the elaboration of placental corticoids. Relatively recently it has been demonstrated that the presence of transcortin in the blood of the pregnant female binds glucocorti-coids effectively, so that the functional availability of this substance approxi-mates that present in the non-pregnant subject. On the other hand, it has generally been overlooked that by about the third month of gestation when remission becomes apparent, the parathyroid glands have become hyper-trophied—probably a manifestation of foetal calcium demands (10–14). Often the remission continues for long periods after childbirth. Parenthetically, one is tempted to ask whether this remission is extended if the child is breast fed— a physiologic function requiring three times the amount of calcium demanded during a similar period of gestation. Assuming that sodium EDTA would, indeed, stimulate parathyroid activity, it was decided to try this compound in rheumatoid arthritis. First, a search for tissue changes in the experimental animal on long-term EDTA administration was undertaken.

The sodium salt of EDTA at body pH is an extremely irritating substance when given subcutaneously, but at this pH it is readily tolerated intravenously. In animals the intravenous route is not practical over long periods of time. The irritating influence of sodium EDTA given subcutaneously was thought to be due to the chelation of magnesium extracted from cells in which it is abundant. By administering the magnesium salt of EDTA adjusted to body pH with sodium hydroxide, the irritation on subcutaneous administration was obviated. Later this preparation proved of value in the treatment of juvenile arthritis in which one is faced with the problem of finding adequate veins for daily injections.

Some of the more gross changes in tissue which can be brought about with sodium or magnesium EDTA were found in rabbits with induced atherosclerosis. In the aorta of such animals the long-term administration of magnesium EDTA brings about a decrease in calcium, copper, phospholipids, and cholesterol (15). These are favourable changes which tend to make the artery normal in appearance and chemical composition.

Work in our own as well as some other laboratories suggests that the acid mucopolysaccharide (AMPS) metabolism of the atherosclerotic aorta is disturbed (16). Although hyaluronic acid remains unaffected, chondroitin sulphate content in early atherosclerosis is very much increased above normal. MgEDTA administration to atherosclerotic animals corrects this situation. Aside from the increase in chondroitin sulphate, changes were observed in the neutral sugar-containing polysaccharides of the aorta whose level was found to decrease in atherosclerosis and reverted back to normal after EDTA treatment. Although this fraction was not identified definitively, it undoubtedly included keratosulphate and perhaps some glycogen. In half-life studies of the sulphated mucopolysaccharides it was demonstrated that, at least in the serum, EDTA caused a reversion towards normal values of the very much accelerated sulphate turnover found in atherosclerosis as compared with control animals.

We attribute these findings to a physiologic stimulation of the parathyroid glands brought about by the EDTA chelation of extracellular calcium ion. As the administration of calcium EDTA elicits none of the responses listed above, we do not feel that trace metal chelation is responsible for them. All trace metals chelated by EDTA at body pH are bound more tightly than calcium, so it would matter little whether the sodium, magnesium, or calcium salt of EDTA was given if chelation of trace metals effected these changes. It should be emphasized that what appears to be of importance is the immediate, although temporary, lowering of extracellular ionic calcium and not the overall calcium balance.

The schedule of EDTA administration has been summarized in Table I. It is important to start the intravenous administration with a needle and syringe because neutral sodium EDTA is extremely painful when extravasation into the tissue occurs. Necrosis does not result and there is no residuum, but the immediate pain, which lasts for an hour or so, is extremely uncomfortable. The use of pyridoxine for supportive therapy is based on work which suggested that rheumatoid arthritis patients suffer from a functional pyridoxine

TABLE 1

TREATMENT SCHEDULE

1. Dosage: NaEDTA or MgEDTA 50 mg./kg. body weight in 250–500 ml. 5 per cent dextrose (The dosage is critical; lower levels are generally ineffective, and doses above 60 mg./kg. not recommended. This dosage is based on the EDTA portion of the molecule only.)

2. Route of administration: I.V., started with a syringe

3. Time per infusion: 60 ± 10 minutes

4. Treatment schedule: 3 to 4 courses each consisting of 1 infusion per day, 5 days per week for 2 weeks; one week off

5. Supportive therapy: Vitamin B_6, potassium chloride 10 grains/day

6. Laboratory control: Urinalysis, routine blood examination

deficiency which occasionally becomes apparent with EDTA treatment (17, 18). If the patient is on aspirin for the control of pain, we do not insist that this medication be discontinued immediately but only as the diminution of pain permits. This is a factor used in the evaluation of the patient's progress. Long-term EDTA administration results in an increased urinary excretion of potassium; hence the oral administration of this ion is encouraged either by prescribing potassium chloride during periods of EDTA administration or by encouraging the patient to drink orange juice.

The magnesium salt of EDTA may be prepared by the addition of magnesium sulphate (6 meq. Mg/gm. sodium EDTA) to the I.V. bottle containing 500 c.c. of 5 per cent glucose and sodium EDTA. This renders the infusion much less irritating if extravasation into tissue should occur and obviates a drawing sensation along the venous route of the drug of which some patients complain. However, it is not our usual practice to prepare the EDTA in this manner.

When dealing with very small children neutral magnesium EDTA may be given subcutaneously. This route is practicable only for dosages not exceeding 1 gm. Such small doses may be diluted with 35 c.c. water to which 2 c.c. of 2 per cent nesacaine has been added. Administration is made by the slow drip method directly into the lateral aspect of the thigh.

Because experience in the treatment of rheumatoid arthritis patients with EDTA is still very limited, it is difficult to make definitive decisions as to which patients will respond. Certain observations have been made which assist one to predict the therapeutic effectiveness of EDTA.

It appears that early as well as late cases of rheumatoid arthritis respond favourably to chelation therapy, although existing deformities will not be corrected.

Patients on corticoids do not respond to chelation treatment. This may be due to the abnormally long half-life of mucopolysaccharides under the influence of such hormones. In these cases we have had success by administer-

TABLE II

SUMMARY OF PRELIMINARY PATIENT TRIAL

Patient sex–age	First seen	Years of R.A. before EDTA	Initial courses of EDTA	Subsequent courses	EDTA salt used	Extent of involvement	Comment
S.B., M, 41	1956	2	5	0	Na	Bedridden	Followed for 3 years after EDTA. Remained symptom free
D.M., F, 31	1958	0	3	14	Na	Extensive during most exacerbations	No apparent joint damage by 1965
D.K., M, 9	1959	0.5	3	1	Na	Bedridden. On steroids when first seen (Cushing's synd.)	R.A. still arrested, 1965
K.V., F, 4.5	1961	2.5	3		Mg S.C.	Acutely ill, bedridden.	As of 1965, unlimited ambulation. Attending public school
	1962			1	Mg S.C.	Extensive involvement.	
	1963			1	Mg I.V.	Had never walked properly	
M.M., F, 42	1960/61	8	4		Na	Extensive involvement.	Off steroids by second 40 I.V.'s, 1965, continued remission
	1962			4		Bedridden. Steroids.	
	1963			2		Cushing's synd.	
S.S., F, 8	1962	3	4	2	Mg S.C.	All joints. Severest involvement, hips. By 1963 complete destruction of left hip joint (Cushing's Synd.)	At this time unable to get totally off steroids. G.H.
	1963			5	Mg I.V.		Off steroids
	1964			1	Mg I.V.		As of 1965, remission of fall of 1963 maintained. Limited ambulation but no pain

ing ACTH while tapering off the oral medication until the patient elaborates sufficient hormone on his own. EDTA infusions are then begun and the ACTH is withdrawn gradually over a two-week period. Cessation of ACTH is manifested by joint stiffness but usually little or no pain. The EDTA therapy is continued as described in Table I. Juvenile rheumatoids follow the same pattern as adults. In one case we were able to give human growth hormone* in conjunction with EDTA. This hormone is known to influence the metabolism of sulphated mucopolysaccharides (19). It was hoped that the EDTA and growth hormone might have a beneficial synergistic effect, since synergism has been described between parathormone and growth hormone (20). The child in question was short as a result of two years of corticoid treatment—a situation that was corrected by the growth hormone. It is difficult to assess what other benefits might be attributed to growth hormone in this instance. If exacerbations occur some time after the initial series of treatments, response to one or two courses of EDTA is usually rapid.

To date some dozen patients suffering from rheumatoid arthritis have been treated with EDTA. The case histories of the original six have been summarized in Table II. None of these patients is on any medication at this time. Encouraged by these results, a more systematic approach including Lansbury indices and range of motion studies by a physical therapist was

TABLE III
Summary of Current Patients

Patient, sex, age*	Years of diagnosed R.A. before EDTA	Courses of EDTA		EDTA salt used	Lansbury Index		
		Initial	Subs.		Time (months)	Articular	Systemic
J.N., M, 46	10	2.5	–	Na	0	103	92
					2	74	33
N.L., F, 15	2	3	–	Na	0	153	75
					2	86	67
G.B., F, 50	7	3	1	Mg	0	30	38
					3	31	4
					6	30	28
M.M., F, 18	1	3	1	Mg	0	126	70†
					3	67	52
H.D., F, 56	2	4	–	Mg	0	100	113
					3	77	89
M.K., F, 51	7	4		Mg	0	159	101
					3‡	58	81
			1		6	77	97

*Age corresponds to 0 times, i.e. when patient was first seen in our clinic and shortly before EDTA therapy was started.
†The patient received five courses of EDTA at approximately two-thirds of the recommended dosage before we saw her, with little apparent benefit.
‡Flared shortly thereafter; responded well to subsequent course.

*Obtained through the generosity of Dr. A. E. Wilhelmi, Emory University, and the Endrocrinology Study Section of the National Institutes of Health.

started last year. The information obtained from this group so far is contained in Table III.

CONCLUSION

While the laboratory research to elucidate the mechanism of EDTA action on metabolism is far from complete, and the clinical trials to date have been limited, we cannot help but feel that this compound is a promising agent in the armamentarium of drugs used to treat rheumatoid arthritis.

ACKNOWLEDGMENTS

This investigation was supported in part by (1) a Public Health Service fellowship No. 5F2 AM-19,928 from the National Institutes of Arthritis and Metabolic Diseases, (2) Public Health Service Research Grant No. HE-04543, and (3) Scientific Advisory Council to the Licensed Beverage Industries, Inc. grant on "Connective Tissue in Liver Cirrhosis."

REFERENCES

1. KLEMPERER, P., POLLACK, A. D., and BAEHR, G. J.A.M.A. *119*: 331 (1942).
2. NEUMAN, W. F., and NEUMAN, M. W. Am. J. Med. *22*: 123 (1957).
3. ––– The Chemical Dynamics of Bone Mineral (University of Chicago Press, Chicago, 1958).
4. SHETLAR, M. R., BRADFORD, R. H., JOEL, W., and HOWARD, R. P. *In* The Parathyroids, *edited by* R. O. Greep and R. V. Talmage (Charles Thomas, Springfield, Ill., 1961).
5. GAILLARD, P. J. Acta physiol et pharmacol. neerl. *8*: 287 (1959).
6. ––– Koninkl. Med. Aka. Wetensch. Proc. C, *63*: 26 (1963).
7. KROON, D. B. Acta. anat. *21*: (1) (1954).
8. –––Acta morphol. Neerl. *2*: 38 (1958).
9. WILLIAMS, R. H. Textbook of Endocrinology, 3rd ed. (W. B. Saunders Co., Philadelphia, 1962), p. 792.
10. GREEP, R. O. Physiology and Chemistry of Parathyroid Hormone (Academic Press, Inc., New York, 1948), vol. 1, chap. 7.
11. BODANSKY, M. Am. J. Clin. Path. *9*: 36 (1939).
12. BODANSKY, M., and DUFF, V. B. J.A.M.A. *112*: 223 (1939).
13. OPPER, L., and THALE, T. Am. J. Physiol. *139*: 406 (1943).
14. SINCLAIR, J. G. Anat. Rev. *80*: 479 (1941).
15. KOEN, A., McCANN, D. S., and BOYLE, A. J. J. Chron. Dis. *16*: 329 (1963).
16. LACSON, T., McCANN, D. S., and BOYLE, A. J. J. Atherosclerotic Res. *6*: 277 (1966).
17. FLINN, J. H., PRICE, J. M., YESS, N., and BROWN, R. R. Arth. & Rheum. 7: 201 (1964).
18. McKUSICK, A. B., SHERWIN, R. W., JONES, L. B., and HSU, J. M. Arth. & Rheum. 7: 636 (1964).
19. SCHILLER, S. J. Chron. Dis. *16*: 291 (1963).
20. FRASER, R., and HARRISON, M. Ciba Foundation Colloquia on Endocrinology, vol. 13 (Little Brown and Co., Boston, 1959), p. 135.

Alteration of Some Laboratory Tests in Patients Receiving Norethynodrel (Enovid) for the Treatment of Rheumatoid Arthritis *

ROGER DEMERS, M.D., F.R.C.P.(C),†
J. A. BLAIS, M.D.,‡ and H. PRETTY, M.D.§

NORETHYNODREL, commonly known as Enovid, is a synthetic progestogen free from anabolic, androgenic, or cortisone-like effect (1). It has a slight oestrogenic effect, which is about 5 to 7 per cent that of oestrone. The drug is known to produce a state of pseudo-pregnancy when administered continuously at a dosage of about 30 mg. a day.

The favourable influence of pregnancy on rheumatoid arthritis suggested to one of us (J. A. B.) the possibility of remission of the disease resulting from pseudo-pregnancy induced by norethynodrel. In an attempt to establish the value of this hypothesis, a clinical study was carried out on 44 female patients receiving norethynodrel, 30 mg. a day, for periods ranging from 7 to 24 months. Eleven patients were omitted from the clinical study for different reasons.

Since the primary aim of this paper is to report on some laboratory tests made before and during norethynodrel administration, the results of the clinical response will be very briefly summarized.

The predominant clinical response in the late stages seems to be the suspension of any further deterioration. At the less advanced stages, an objective and subjective improvement is noted. In the less severe forms, there is, to all

*From the Department of Medicine, Section of Rheumatology, Hotel Dieu Hospital, Montreal. This investigation was supported by G. D. Searle and Co. and by the Canadian Arthritis and Rheumatism Society.

†Section of Rheumatology; Assistant Professor of Medicine at the University of Montreal.

‡Previously Chief of the Section of Rheumatology; now Medical Director of the Canadian Arthritis and Rheumatism Society (Quebec Division).

§Resident in Medicine.

outward appearances at least, a remission of the disease. The numerous relapses occurring after discontinuation of the drug show that norethynodrel does not cure rheumatoid arthritis. Nevertheless, satisfactory results seem to be obtained in about 60 per cent of cases.

LABORATORY TESTS

Latex fixation. Latex fixation was determined in 35 patients. The results do not show any direct correlation between latex fixation and clinical improvement.

Erythrocyte sedimentation rate. Sufficient data are available, for comparison, from 23 patients. In short, norethynodrel does not seem to have a significant effect on the E.S.R., as it remained accelerated in more than half of the improved patients. The rate is physiologically accelerated during pregnancy and possibly during pseudo-pregnancy.

Haemoglobin value. Haemoglobin concentration was determined periodically in 37 of the patients. On the whole the haemoglobin concentration increased by 1 or 2 gm. in 13 of the 14 patients considered anaemic. In the others the haemoglobin concentration remained unchanged or improved further. Several weeks after the medication was stopped, the haemoglobin showed a tendency to revert to pre-treatment levels. Since during treatment the majority of the patients noted an increase in their appetite, it would appear that the improvement in the haemoglobin concentration may quite possibly be due to better nutrition.

Liver function test. Liver function tests were made on 36 of the 44 patients included in this study, both before and during therapy, except in nine for whom there was no pre-treatment control. These tests show: B.S.P. retention exceeding 12 per cent in 15 (41%) of the patients; an increase in SGO and SGP transaminases in 12 (33%) of the patients (it was less than 300 units in 12 but exceeded 300 units in one only); a rise in total bilirubin above 1.5 mg. % in 6 (16%); an increase in alkaline phosphatase of more than 12.4 but less than 15 Bodansky units in 5 (13.8%). Five liver biopsies by needle puncture showed no significant damage of the hepatic parenchyma except in one case in which mild chronic portal hepatitis was reported. Jaundice developed in three patients, which disappeared after discontinuation of the drug. Liver function tests returned to normal within four weeks in all cases.

COMMENTS ON LIVER FUNCTION TESTS

Norethynodrel is commonly used at 30 mg. a day for the treatment of endometriosis, and it is surprising that the current literature should carry no mention of changes in the liver function tests associated with this drug. Garcia and Pincus (2) claimed that no liver dysfunctions were noted during their long-term experience with norethynodrel, but they do not report any specific series or any function tests being made. Goldzieher (3) reported a non-significant rise in B.S.P. retention in his series but made no mention of any other test. If these statements are well founded, it can be presumed that in rheumatoid arthritis, which is a systemic disease associated with aberration in protein electrophoresis, norethynodrel should more readily cause changes in liver function test than in endometriosis, in which the general condition is intact.

TABLE I

ALTERATION OF ONE OR MORE LIVER FUNCTION TESTS IN 17 OUT OF 36 PATIENTS RECEIVING NORETHYNODREL FOR RHEUMATOID ARTHRITIS

Tests	No. of patients abnormal	Range of change during treatment	% of patients with abnormal tests
B.S.P. retention, 7%, 1 hr.	15	10–42%	41
Transaminases SGO, 5–40 units SGP, 5–35 units	12	62–710 50–420	33
Bilirubin Total: 1.2 mg. % Direct: 0.02–0.18	6	1.5 to 6.4 1.1 to 1.63	16
Alkaline phosphatase, 2.2 to 8.5 Bodansky units	5	12.4 to 14.4	13.8
Liver biopsy	5	4 cases; no lesion seen 1 case; slight chronic portal hepatitis	
Icterus	3		8.3

Moreover, hepatic impairment in rheumatoid arthritis has never been satisfactorily elucidated (4–7). Nevertheless, changes in liver function test following the administration of norethynodrel should not appear as an unexpected phenomena when considering the structural relationship of this compound with some 19-nor-17-alkylated anabolic agents, which according to the literature can modify liver function tests and in some cases can induce jaundice (8–13). While norethynodrel is not an anabolic agent, it is like most of the latter substances a 19-nor steroid except that there is an ethinyl group on carbon 17.

Discussion of the mechanism of the action of this compound on the liver falls outside the scope of the present study. However, hepatic dysfunction caused by norethynodrel corresponds to the same type of liver dysfunction and jaundice produced by the 17-alkylated anabolic steroids as reported by Zimmerman (14): "The dysfunction is of the canalicular type characterized biochemically by normal flocculation test, an alkaline phosphatase level of less than 15-Bodansky units, and transaminases not exceeding 300 units. Histologically, the liver parenchyma and portal spaces are normal. Jaundice is cholestatic, the prognosis is good and there are no sequelae." These statements are in full accordance with our clinical observations and laboratory data.

In view of the fact that infectious hepatitis usually results in remission of rheumatoid arthritis, the question has been raised whether patients with an abnormal liver function test might not show a better clinical improvement than those with normal tests. Yet, a comparative study of the results does not warrant the conclusion that either group, as a whole, showed greater improvement. The most that can be said is that the group with abnormal tests had a more severe type of arthritis.

From this study, it appears that norethynodrel administered at 30 mg. a day can affect liver function tests. In most cases, the changes are minimal and the tests tend to reach a plateau or return to normal even when administration of the drug is continued. All the tests return to normal after the medication is stopped. Liver impairment with norethynodrel does not differ from the canalicular type of liver dysfunction seen with some of the 17-alkylated anabolic agents.

PLASMA AND URINARY LEVELS OF 17-HYDROXYCORTICOSTEROIDS

Figure 1 shows the plasma and urinary levels of 17-hydroxycorticosteroids in three patients with rheumatoid arthritis aged respectively 23, 33, and 72 years and one patient with endometriosis as control, aged 33 years. The 17-OH steroids were determined before treatment, after 16 to 21 weeks of therapy, and, in three cases, 6 to 8 weeks after stopping the medication. In the 23-year-old unmarried female a fifth determination was made after resumption of the treatment. The results show that under the influence of norethynodrel the 17-OII level increased up to 3 to 4 times above normal. On the other hand, total urinary 17-OH steroid levels tend to fall as the plasma levels rise. There was no substantial lowering of the free 17-OH level, so that it was possibly the conjugated 17-OH levels that decreased most under the influence of norethynodrel. An increase in the plasma 17-OH levels of up to three to four times the normal has been reported during normal pregnancy (15–17) following the administration of oestrogens (18–20) and in women at their menopause (18). As norethynodrel is producing two different effects, one progestational and other oestrogenic, the increase in the plasma 17-OH levels is not unexpected. The exact mechanism of the favourable influence of pregnancy on rheumatoid arthritis is not known. Nevertheless, pseudo-pregnancy induced by norethynodrel reproduces not only the clinical picture of pregnancy; it produces also a pseudo-decidua similar to pregnancy in addition to an elevation of the level of the 17-hydroxycorticosteroids of the plasma.

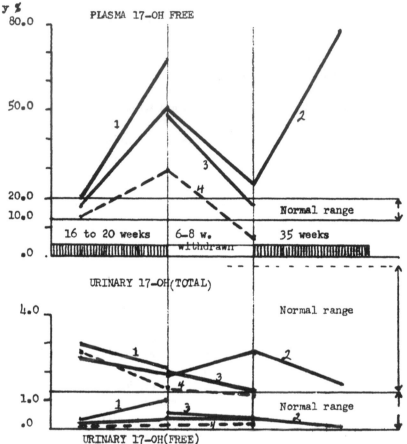

FIG. 1. A graphic representation of the level of the free plasma
17-OH and total and free urinary 17-OH in four women, before,
during, and after treatment with norethynodrel. There is a corresponding decrease in the urinary 17-OH (total) when the plasma-free
17-OH is increased. Curve 1, age 33; 2, age 23, new peak when
treatment resumed; 3, age 72, menopausal, no pre-treatment control;
4 (broken line), age 33, endometriosis without arthritis (control).

SUMMARY AND CONCLUSION

Under the influence of norethylnodrel administration the latex fixation
tests seem to have no correlation with the clinical improvement; E.S.R. is
not significantly improved. In anaemic patients the haemoglobin concentration
can be increased by 1 or 2 grams if there is better appetite and nutrition.
Liver function tests are altered in a great proportion of the patients and a

cholestatic type of jaundice can develop. The 17-hydroxycorticosteroids of the plasma are increased up to three to four times the normal level as during normal pregnancy.

Should the alteration of liver function tests be considered a more serious objection to the use of norethynodrel than in the case of gold salts, which can cause nephritis, or cortisone, which can cause many serious side actions? In our opinion the drug can be used in rheumatoid arthritis provided that two liver function tests are made routinely all along the treatment period, mainly B.S.P. and transaminases SGO and SGP.

ACKNOWLEDGMENT

We are grateful to Doctor Roland Dussault and to Doctor K. R. Mackenzie for their assistance and criticism in the preparation of this report and to Doctor Jacques Genest for his co-operation in carrying out 17-hydroxysteroid determinations.

REFERENCES

1. DRILL, V. A., and SAUNDERS, F. J. Biological activity of norethynodrel. Proceedings of a Symposium on 19-nor Progestational Steroids, Searle Research Laboratories, Chicago, Ill. (January 1957).
2. GARCIA, C. R., and PINCUS, G. Ovulation inhibition by progestin-oestrogen combination. Internat. J. Fertil. 9: 95–105 (1964).
3. GOLDZIEHER, J. W. Newer drugs in oral contraception. Med. Clin. North Am. 48: 529–45 (1964).
4. AARON, M. L., and FARROW, I. J. The liver in rheumatoid arthritis. Ann. Rheumat. Dis. 14: 162–9 (1955).
5. ROY, L. M. H., WIGZELL, F. W., DEMERS, R., SINCLAIR, P. J. G., DUTHIE, J. J. R., ATHERDEN, S. M., and MARRIAN, G. F. Liver function in relation to possible abnormalities of steroid metabolism in rheumatoid arthritis. Ann. Rheumat. Dis. 14: 183–90 (1955).
6. NETTELBLADT, E. Rheumatoid arthritis and hepatocellular injury. Acta rheumat. Scand. 6: 256–66 (1960).
7. MOVITT, E. R., and DAVIS, A. E. Liver biopsy in rheumatoid arthritis. Am. J. M. Sci. 226: 516–20 (1953).
8. KORY, R. C., BRADLEY, M. H., WATSON, R. N., CALLAHAN, R., and PETERS, B. J. A six-month evaluation of an anabolic drug, Norethandrolone, in underweight persons. II. Bromsulphalein (BSP) retention and liver function. Am. J. Med. 26: 243–8 (1959).
9. SCHAFFNER, F., POPPER, H., and CHESROW, E. Cholestasis produced by the administration of Norethrandolone. Am. J. Med. 26: 249–54 (1959).
10. WILDER, E. M. Death due to liver failure following the use of Methandrostenolone. Canad. M. A. J. 87: 768–9 (1962).
11. PEREZ-MERA, R. A., and SHIELDS, C. E. Jaundice asociated with Norethindrone acetate therapy. New England J. Med. 267: 1137–8 (1962).
12. MARQUARDT, G. H., FISHER, C. I., LEVY, P., and DOWBEN, R .M. Effects of anabolic steroids on liver function tests and creatinine excretion. J.A.M.A. 175: 851 (1961).
13. HOGARTH, W. J. Jaundice associated with Methandrostenolone (Danabol) administration. Canad. M. A. J. 88: 368–71 (1963).
14. ZIMMERMAN, H. J. Clinical and laboratory manifestations of hepatotoxicity. Ann. New York Acad. Sci. 104: 954–87 (1963).

15. GEMZELL, C. A. Blood levels of 17-hydroxycorticosteroids in pregnancy. J. Clin. Endocrinol. *13*: 898–902 (1953).
16. BAYLISS, R. I. S., BROWNE, J. C., ROUND, B. P., and STEINBECK, A. W. Plasma 17-hydroxycorticosteroids in pregnancy. Lancet, *1*: 62–64 (1955).
17. MIGEON, C. J., BERTRAND, J., and WALL, P. E. Physiological disposition of 4-C^{14}-cortisol during late pregnancy. J. Clin. Invest. *36*: 1350 (1957).
18. WALLANCE, E. Z., SILVERBERG, H. I., and CARTER, A. C. Effect of ethinyl estradiol on plasma 17-hydroxycorticosteroids, ACTH responsiveness and hydrocortisone clearance in man. Proc. Soc. Exper. Biol. & Med. *95*: 805–8 (1957).
19. TALIAFERRO, I., COBEY, F., and LEONE, L. Effect of diethylstilbestrol on plasma 17-hydroxycorticosteroids levels in humans. Proc. Soc. Exper. Biol. & Med. *95*: 742 (1956).
20. MILLS, I. H., SCHEDL, P. H., CHEN, P. S., and BARTTER, F. C. The effect of estrogen administration on the metabolism and protein binding of hydrocortisone. J. Clin. Endocrinol. *20*: 515–28 (1960).

The Treatment of
Persistent Knee Effusions with
Intra-Articular Radioactive Gold

BARBARA M. ANSELL,* ANNE CROOK,†
J. R. MALLARD,† E. G. L. BYWATERS,* and J. R. TOPP‡

A PRELIMINARY REPORT on this subject was published by Ansell, Crook, Mallard, and Bywaters in 1963. This is a brief communication to present a short follow-up on that report.

In the original paper it was explained that the rationale behind this therapy was to produce a radiation synovectomy. This was thought to be possible because AU^{198} has a half-life of 2.7 days and emits both beta and gamma rays. The average range of beta rays in tissue is 1 mm. and therefore destruction of the superficial cells of the synovial membrane should occur if a sufficiently large radiation dose could be delivered.

Pilot studies established that tracer doses of radioactive gold injected into the knee joint diffused evenly throughout the synovial cavity, and after 24 hours there was no radioactivity detectable in the blood or regional lymph nodes, and only 1 per cent of the injected radioactivity was present in the synovial fluid.

Autoradiographs have been done on several needle biopsies taken a day or two after the injection, and these show radioactive particles uniformly dispersed in the superficial layers of the synovium.

It was decided that a dose of between 600 and 1000 rads should be delivered to the surface of the synovium. A formula to calculate the number of millicuries necessary to produce this amount of radioactivity was worked out on the assumption that the effusion of the knee was spherical. The size of the effusion was assessed on the basis of an aspiration done sometime prior to the injection. It happened that most patients were given between one and two millicuries.

Only patients who had persistent large effusions for many months and

*Taplow, England.
†London, England.
‡Toronto, Ontario.

in many cases several years were selected for this treatment. All had received conventional therapy including intra-articular steroid.

Following the injection the patients were seen frequently for the first few weeks and then about every three months. If an uncomfortable effusion was present, the knee was aspirated to dryness but steroid was not injected. In many cases a needle biopsy was performed a day or two after the injection and then at three months, six months, and one year. Most of the biopsies were done with the Parker–Pearson needle.

The results were classed in four grades (Table I):

1. Good, i.e. there was no clinically detectable effusion, good range of movement, and absence of pain and soft-tissue swelling.

2. Improved, i.e. the parameters had all improved but the knee was not symptom free.

3. No change.

4. Worse.

TABLE I

RESULTS OF INJECTING Au[198] INTO THE KNEE JOINT

	Good	Improved	No change	Worse
3 weeks	0	4	19	7
3 months	8	15	7	0
1 year	16	7	7	0
1 year*	16	2	2	0
Total follow-up at year	32	9	9	0

*An additional 20 patients excluding patients whose knees had a grossly thickened synovial membrane.

The last 20 patients are listed separately because by this time it seemed apparent that effusions without grossly thickened synovium were doing best.

In 14 patients there were bilateral knee effusions. One knee was treated and the other used as a control. The follow-up after one year for these patients is shown in Table II.

TABLE II

STATE OF BILATERAL KNEE EFFUSIONS ONE YEAR AFTER INJECTION OF Au[198]

Knee	No effusion	Smaller effusion	No change
Treated	10	1	3
Control	4	2	8

Most of the patients in this series had classical rheumatoid arthritis, but there were other cases of varying aetiology. The results in the rheumatoid arthritis patients were not as favourable as in the other cases, but when cases with grossly thickened synovial membrane were avoided, this difference was less marked.

The biopsies of the treated cases did not show consistent findings, but by three months many showed the following changes:

1. The surface layer of the synovial cells, which at first becomes irregular, finally no longer shows hyperplasia.

2. Sclerosis around vessels with occasional obliteration of lumen.

3. Some fibrosis.

4. Decrease in inflammatory cells.

These changes are consistent with reactions occurring elsewhere following radiation.

It is concluded from this study that the intra-articular injection of colloidal radioactive gold may be useful in the treatment of some cases of persistent knee effusions. Those with large effusions and not too greatly thickened synovium appear to have done best.

REFERENCE

ANSELL, B. M., CROOK, A., MALLARD, J. R., and BYWATERS, E. G. L. Evaluation of intra-articular colloidal gold Au 198 in the treatment of persistent knee effusions. Ann. Rheum. Dis. 22: 435 (1963).

Effect of Short-Term
Glucocorticoid Administration on
Pituitary—Adrenal Function*

E. J. PINTER, A. B. HOOD,
B. E. P. MURPHY, and C. J. PATTEE

WHILE INTENSIVE SHORT-TERM GLUCOCORTICOID THERAPY is frequently administered, little is known about the functional aspects of the pituitary and the adrenals within the period immediately following such regimens. It is also of practical importance to determine the extent and duration of pituitary and adrenal suppression. The first part of this study consists of measurements of the functional capacity of the pituitary and adrenal glands in patients before and after intensive glucocorticoid treatment for periods ranging from 11 to 28 days. Patients receiving oral glucocorticoid (dexamethasone) therapy for various articular and respiratory conditions were studied in the following manner: (1) blood corticoid levels before, during, and up to 7 days after steroid therapy were determined at 2–4-day intervals; (2) pituitary responsiveness was estimated by intravenous SU 4885 tests before and 7 days following therapy; (3) intravenous ACTH test before, 48 hours after, and 7 days after the steroid administration for the measurement of functional capacity of the adrenal glands. Of these, half showed a reduced pituitary reserve whereas all had normal responses to ACTH when these tests were done within one week of stopping therapy.

The second part of the study was based on our observations that the responsiveness to exogenous ACTH was found to be impaired during dexamethasone therapy as early as one week after initiating dexamethasone therapy. As far as we are aware, this observation has not been reported previously in the human. To investigate this effect further, 12 patients with normal pituitary–adrenal function were given small doses of dexamethasone for periods of a few hours to several days. A pretreatment intravenous ACTH test was compared with an ACTH test at various times after initiating steroid administration. An inhibition of adrenal response could be demonstrated within 24 hours of administration. Since this period is short to attribute this effect to pituitary suppression, it was felt that dexamethasone may exert a direct inhibitory action on the adrenal gland.

*From the Clinical Investigation Unit, Queen Mary Veterans Hospital, Montreal.

New Concepts in
Bracing and Splinting*

C. M. GODFREY, B.A., M.D., CERT. PHYS. MED.

THIS is a report on clinical research trials that are going on at the University of Toronto, Rheumatic Diseases Unit, the Wellesley Hospital (Sunnybrook Division). It deals primarily with four problems encountered by the physiatrist in the rehabilitation of patients with rheumatoid disease.

A common problem seen in the treatment of patients with acute rheumatoid disease is that of immobilization and splinting for relief of pain. It is a problem, inasmuch as using the standard plaster splints for immobilization usually causes pain after application of more than an hour or two. It has been remarked by the nursing staff that at twelve o'clock midnight at Sunnybrook Hospital the sound of the velcro being removed is deafening.

To surmount this difficulty it must be realized that to hold any joint in an immobile position for more than a few hours is painful, whether the joint be diseased or not. Furthermore, it is not imperative that the joint be held in an optimum position, for example an anatomical or functional position, in order to relieve pain. Thus a wrist may be immobilized at any one of five positions and still result in relief of pain for the patient. Consequently, it has been considered advantageous to build into the resting plaster a simple hinge joint which permits various degrees of flexion or extension. The splint is applied in the usual fashion, but after two hours the degree of flexion or extension is altered by 10°, which prevents the painful immobilization pattern, while still immobilizing the wrist. The hinges are made so that they are altered by a lug which is large enough to be manipulated even by the patient himself, though he may be severely deformed with arthritis.

A similar alteration may be made to the posterior leg splint, with the hinge being placed posterior to the knee, permitting "active immobilization." It is suggested, however, that a kneecap leather be incorporated into the splint in order to keep the knee from popping anteriorly when the infra- and suprapatellar straps are applied.

*From the University of Toronto, Rheumatic Diseases Unit, the Wellesley Hospital (Sunnybrook Division).

A second problem arises when a painful knee is required to bear weight. In order to get around the problem of weight bearing during walking a simple modification has been made of the Thomas long-leg walking caliper. This incorporates the principle of an ischial weight-bearing thigh corset, a functional knee joint, and transference of the weight to the floor by a yoke attached to the shoe. By these means the weight can be short-circuited by the ischial tuberosity through the side irons to the floor. The amount of weight borne on the leg itself can be varied from none to partial depending on the level at which the thigh corset is set. The joint of the knee is placed posterior so that it is stable when the patient is in the weight-bearing phase, but at toe off the knee bends and the leg is then swung through as in a normal gait.

This ischial weight-bearing functional long-leg brace has been tried on 28 patients with a variety of diseases of the knee, and in some cases of the hip, and they have been able to walk relatively pain free. It is a highly functional apparatus, and the patient can go back to work wearing it without any difficulty. One patient, an elevator repairman who has returned to work, can climb in and around elevators with the brace on his leg.

Another problem we have is fitting shoes to our female arthritic patients. Traditionally this has been done well in males, where a boot type shoe can be applied, but the females have always caused a good deal of trouble, largely because of the weight of the boot-type shoe, and because of their refusal to accept the boot because of its appearance. We have fitted a number of patients with a general shoe which has an application to most rheumatoid patients. We have fitted 80 patients during the past two years with satisfactory acceptance in 75 per cent on the basis of a follow-up done four months later and eight months later. One of the criteria of satisfactory acceptance was the question of whether the patients would be prepared to pay for the shoes. The shoe is light weight, of oxford construction, with wooden heels, a rigid arch of metal, a metatarsal bar, and bull noses with a sponge rubber insole. It must be pointed out that it is necessary to check shoes constantly on the rheumatoid, to make sure that a "boat form" is not being developed in the sole of the shoe with resulting compression of the second, third, and fourth metatarsals.

Another problem is the management of patients with canes. Usually people use canes in order to short-circuit some of the weight to the ground, as well as to give them stability with their weak lower extremities. However, a cane causes a great deal of stretching, particularly on the ulnar side of the hand, during manipulation, and often patients cannot take sufficient weight through their affected hands in order to relieve their complaint of pain due to weight bearing. If the patient uses crutches, he more effectively short-circuits the weight to the ground; however, these are unwieldy. Modifications of the crutch, such as the triceps crutch or the elbow crutch, are clumsy and the patient frequently does not have sufficient skill to manipulate the appliances correctly.

A simple modification can be made to a cane so that the patient can bear some of his weight with his forearm, and still have the advantage of a single stick cane. It consists of a board with a hole through which the shaft of the cane passes. This 8-inch board is shaped to fit the distal portion of the forearm so that when the patient holds the cane in his hand naturally, his forearm rests along the board. Thus the patient can walk bearing weight on the forearm as well as on the hand. The hand is also in a functionally good position, in contrast to that of the usual cane walker, who develops a good deal of deformity at the wrist, either radial or ulnar depending on where he puts his hand on the cane.

The above describes four simple modifications that can be made to normal appliances for use by the rheumatoid patient.

The Treatment of Rheumatoid Arthritis in
a Rehabilitation Hospital:
Results of a Staged Programme*

L. H. TRUELOVE, M.A., M.R.C.P., D.PHYS.MED.

IN WINNIPEG we have been interested in the problems of organizing a programme of physical treatment for patients with rheumatoid arthritis. Our object has been to treat people as far as possible in groups so that they could benefit from the competitive and social atmosphere and to some extent learn about the disease from one another. A further advantage, of course, is that maximum use can be made of therapists' time. The scientific object has been to define the various stages of treatment so that we would be able to assess progress in terms of the various levels of physical activity and disease activity.

The programme which has evolved is based on the hypothesis that disease activity can be controlled by adequate rest in the initial stages of treatment in hospital and that subsequent physical activity should depend on the activity of the disease.

The arthritic unit consists of 54 beds in a comprehensive rehabilitation hospital of 160 beds; there are several physicians within the unit, each with his own group of patients. We wanted, therefore, to design a programme which would have the advantages of a uniform regimen in a unit, and yet be sufficiently flexible to allow for individual variation.

The first idea was to treat these patients on the same basis as other individuals in the rehabilitation hospital, i.e. to have them attend the same classes as patients with other disabilities. This has been advocated by various authorities, but we had no success with it, mainly because the classes were too strenuous for the arthritic group and also because the classes did not take into account the systemic nature of the disease. We quickly realized the need for a separate programme for the patients with rheumatoid arthritis. The programme was divided into six stages as will be detailed later. The stages are intended as a framework to allow for individual prescriptions within the stages. Division between the stages is on the basis of the total amount of physical

*From the Manitoba Rehabilitation Hospital, Winnipeg.

activity undertaken at each stage. When a patient is ready to move into a given stage the prescription consists simply of the number of the stage and details of any necessary modifications or individual requirements.

The principles of our staged programme have been criticized on the grounds that the results cannot be as good as a more individual approach and that we are sacrificing individual results in favour of a scientific and administrative advantage. For this reason the results have been compared with other published series, and an attempt has also been made to assess the patients' reactions to the programme.

METHODS

The first two stages involve mainly rest in bed. In the first stage meals are given in bed and patients are conveyed to the bathroom in a wheelchair. Rest splints are made from Plaster of Paris and provided for hands and legs. Serial plasters are applied to correct flexion deformity where necessary. Physiotherapy is given in the form of a short period of general exercises once a day. The occupational therapist sees the patient, assesses the functional difficulties before admission, and outlines some of the functional goals of treatment.

Stage 2 includes a second period of exercises in bed each day, a period of general exercises in a group in the hydrotherapy pool twice a week, and, if indicated, light occupational therapy in the ward.

In stage 3 patients have exercises in bed twice a day as before. Light general exercises in the hydrotherapy pool are given three times a week, and patients attend the occupational therapy department for about an hour three times a week to partake in social activities in groups. Walking is usually discouraged and maximum use made of wheelchairs. In addition, patients perform light craft work on the ward to encourage function in normal patterns.

In stage 4 patients attend the physiotherapy department on the days they do not have treatment in the pool, and limited walking is allowed in the departments, although they are still taken there in wheelchairs. Lower limb activities without weight bearing and graded upper limb activities are undertaken in the occupational therapy department. Work saving methods are demonstrated in the home unit, and necessary aids and gadgets are provided. During this stage patients are seen by therapists from the Canadian Arthritis and Rheumatism Society. These therapists assess difficulties in the home and do the follow-up visits.

The fifth stage is one of maximum physiotherapy. Patients stop using wheelchairs if they can. They have daily exercises in the physiotherapy department, both individually and in groups. They wear their own clothes, make their own beds, and do their own laundry.

The sixth stage is intended as a final preparation to return home or to work. All physiotherapy is stopped except for specific individual exercises in a few patients. Treatment in the occupational therapy department is designed to be the equivalent of a full day's work. A work assessment is made where applicable. The patients are encouraged to go out on shopping trips, look after their own needs in hospital, and cook at least one luncheon for their companions.

This programme has had to be modified on several occasions but the basic division of the stages has remained the same. Two main modifications have been necessary. First, the amount of physical activity, particularly in the early stages, was too heavy in the earliest programmes so that patients were exhausted by the end of the day or were unable to keep up with the programme and became discouraged. Secondly, it became necessary to distinguish in the later stages between those patients who could achieve a high level of independence and those who, in spite of treatment, would remain severely disabled. Stages 4 and 5 were therefore subdivided into A and B programmes. B programmes involved less physical activity and had a greater emphasis on activities in wheelchairs and self-care. In spite of necessary modifications it has proved possible to maintain the principle of treatment in groups and thus conduct a progressive programme for arthritics along parallel lines with those organized for other patients in the rehabilitation setting.

Other treatment was conservative. All patients were given maximum tolerable doses of acetylsalicylic acid. A number of patients, 55 in all, were receiving steroid drugs at the time of admission; some reduction in dosage was achieved in 22 of these.

Patients were admitted because of disability or activity of the disease or frequently both. They were assessed in four grades of functional capacity, the most important division being between grades II and III. Patients in grades I and II are socially and economically independent, whereas those in grades III and IV are essentially dependent. Assessments were done on admission, on discharge, and on a follow-up examination 6 to 24 months after discharge, the average being 15 months. Ninety-eight per cent of the patients were accounted for at this time.

RESULTS

The characteristics of the group are shown in Table I. The group is very similar to those reported on in other surveys. The average duration of 11 years

TABLE I

CHARACTERISTICS OF THE
RHEUMATOID ARTHRITICS (200 CASES)

Sex	44 men, 156 women
Age	Average 55 years
Duration	Average 11 years
Length of stay	Average $10\frac{1}{2}$ weeks
Rheumatoid factor	Positive 74%

is somewhat greater. By the time the follow-up study was done 11 of the original 200 patients had died and 4 could not be traced. The progress of the 185 patients who were followed up is shown in Fig. 1. This demonstrates the

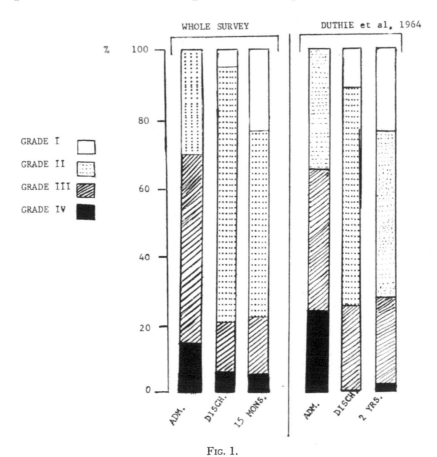

FIG. 1.

progressive improvement in the group as a whole and shows continued improvement from the time of discharge until follow-up examination. For comparison I have included in this figure the early results obtained from a series of 300 patients treated in Edinburgh and reported by Duthie *et al.* (1) earlier this year. The methods of assessment were the same in the two series. The basic principles of conservative treatment were the same. The main differences were in the staging of the programme and the treatment in groups. The Edinburgh series had a rather lower average age and a shorter duration of disease. There is a marked similarity between the two sets of results although on the basis of duration of disease on admission one would expect the results

in the Edinburgh series to be superior. In our series 35 patients were admitted
within the first 18 months from the onset of the disease and the progress of this
group, compared with the whole series, is shown in Fig. 2. The progress in
this group is obviously better than that in the survey as a whole and confirms
a tendency that has been reported in other series. The striking feature once
more is the continued improvement following discharge, particularly in the

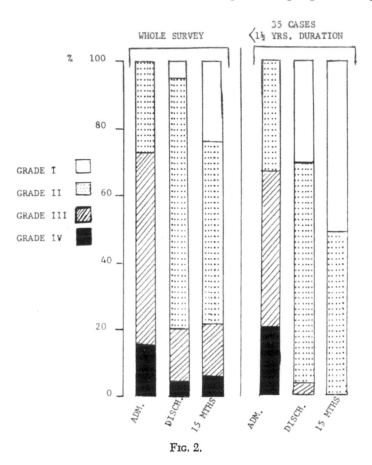

FIG. 2.

increased proportion in grade I on follow-up examination. It seemed likely that
this group, which contains 35 patients, would influence the results in the whole
series and perhaps account for the improvements observed. This was so only
to a minor extent, however, as is shown on Fig. 3, which shows the results
excluding the short-duration group compared with the results already seen.
There are 150 patients in this group and the trends are very much the same as
in the survey as a whole. An attempt was made to find out the patients' reactions to the programme by circulating a questionnaire among the patients who

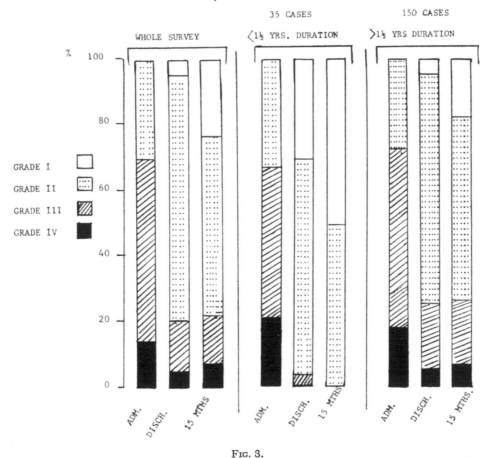

FIG. 3.

are at present in hospital. This was filled in anonymously and indicated that with few exceptions patients of all age groups and various stages of disability find the programme satisfactory.

CONCLUSIONS

This series shows that substantial gains are possible by this kind of organized treatment in a group of patients with rheumatoid arthritis of this duration and age, and that improvement is maintained and to some extent continued during the follow-up of 15 months. The staged programme that has been outlined is practicable, acceptable to patients, and the results compare well with other reported series. By using this method the requirements of a rheumatic unit can be met in a general rehabilitation hospital in such a way that the various programmes fit in well with each other.

REFERENCE

1. DUTHIE, J. J. R., BROWN, P. E., TRUELOVE, L. H., BARAGAR, F. D., and LAWRIE, A. J.
   Ann. Rheum. Dis. 23: 193 (1964).

Index of Authors

Lightning Source UK Ltd.
Milton Keynes UK
UKHW030611210722
406167UK00006B/714